Clinical Management of Children's Voice Disorders

Clinical Management of Children's Voice Disorders

Christopher J. Hartnick and Mark E. Boseley

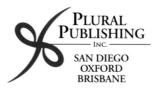

PLURAL
PUBLISHING
INC.

SAN DIEGO
OXFORD
BRISBANE

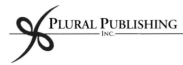
PLURAL PUBLISHING
INC.

5521 Ruffin Road
San Diego, CA 92123

e-mail: info@pluralpublishing.com
Web site: http://www.pluralpublishing.com

49 Bath Street
Abingdon, Oxfordshire OX14 1EA
United Kingdom

Typeset in 10½/13 Garamond book by Flanagan's Publishing Services, Inc.
Printed in Malaysia by Four Colour Print Group

Library of Congress Cataloging-in-Publication Data:
Clinical management of children's voice disorders / [edited by] Christopher J. Hartnick
and Mark E. Boseley.
     p. ; cm.
 Includes bibliographical references and index.
 ISBN-13: 978-1-59756-354-3 (alk. paper)
 ISBN-10: 1-59756-354-4 (alk. paper)
 1. Voice disorders in children. I. Hartnick, Christopher J. II. Boseley, Mark E.
 [DNLM: 1. Voice Disorders. 2. Child. 3. Voice–physiology. WV 500 C6405 2010]
 RF511.C45C55 2010
 616.89'855–dc22
                          2009044501

Contents

Preface

This book is the second book by our group whose focus is on pediatric voice disorders. Although this book is still the product of a group of pediatric otolaryngologists, pulmonologists, gastroenterologists, psychologists, psychiatrists, and speech-language pathologists with an interest in caring for children with a wide variety of voice disorders, the target audience for this book is speech-language pathologists who care for children with vocal disorders. To that end, we have removed certain chapters from the previous book, *Pediatric Voice Disorders*, which focuses on the techniques of surgical care, and reshaped others to highlight issues of office-based diagnosis and intervention. We have added several new chapters, including a fascinating and comprehensive chapter by Kittie Verdolini et al. which reviews the literature regarding voice therapy in children as well as an additional chapter on the work-up and treatment of children with velopharyngeal insufficiency. What we hope is novel, exciting, and educational about this book is the cross-fertilization of thoughts and ideas that comes from putting together a seemingly diverse group of specialists and having them focus on specific pediatric disease-based and pediatric voice pathology-based topics. Within this book, members of each specialty attend to these questions and comment on how the specialties can best work together towards obtaining diagnoses and rendering unified and comprehensive treatment. We hope you enjoy!

Contributors

Jean E. Ashland, Ph.D., CCC-SLP
Speech-Language Pathologist
Massachusetts General Hospital
Boston, Massachusetts
Chapter 16

Mark E. Boseley, M.D., M.S.
Assistant Professor of Surgery,
Uniformed Services University of the
    Health Sciences
Chief Pediatric Otolaryngology,
Madigan Army Medical Center
Children's Hospital and Regional Medical
    Center
Seattle, Washington
Chapters 1, 2, 4

Matthew T. Brigger, M.D.
Pediatric Otolaryngology Fellow
Massachusetts Eye and Ear Infirmary
Harvard Medical School
Chapters 12, 13, 16

Venu Divi, M.D.
Assistant Professor, Department of
    Otolaryngology-HNS
Drexel University College of Medicine
Philadelphia, Pennsylvania
Chapter 17

Abigail L. Donovan, M.D.
Assistant Psychiatrist
Massachusetts General Hospital
Clinical Instructor of Psychiatry
Harvard Medical School
Boston, Massachusetts
Chapter 18

Robert Edwin
Robert Edwin Studio
Associate Editor, NATS *Journal of Singing*
National Association of Teachers of
    Singing (NATS)
American Academy of Teachers of Singing
    (AATS)
Cinnaminson, New Jersey
Chapter 10

Shirley Gherson, M.A., CCC-SLP
Speech-Language Pathologist
Voice Specialist
Voice and Speech Lab at Massachusetts
    Eye and Ear Infirmary
Boston, Massachusetts
and Voicewize
Dedham, Massachusetts
Chapter 3

Stephen C. Hardy, M.D.
Pediatric Gastroenterology and Nutrition
Massachusetts General Hospital for Children
Assistant Professor of Pediatrics
Harvard Medical School
Boston, Massachusetts
Chapter 5

Christopher J. Hartnick, M.D., M.Epi.
Associate Professor
Department of Otolaryngology
Massachusetts Eye and Ear Infirmary
Harvard Medical School
Chapter 1, 2, 4, 8, 12, 13, 16

Kenan E. Haver, M.D.
Assistant Professor of Pediatrics, Harvard
    Medical School

Associate Pediatrician, Massachusetts
General Hospital
Director, Pediatric Pulmonary Fellowship
Program, Massachusetts General Hospital
Co-Founder and Co-Director, Pediatric
Airway, Voice and Swallowing Center,
Massachusetts Eye and Ear Infirmary
Boston, Massachusetts
Chapter 6

Mary J. Hawkshaw, RN, BSN, CORLN
Research Associate Professor
Department of Otolaryngology-Head and
Neck Surgery
Drexel University College of Medicine
Philadelphia, Pennsylvania
Chapter 17

Rita Hersan, M.S., CCC-SLP
Speech-Language Pathologist
Voice Clinician
University of Pittsburgh Medical Center,
Voice Center
Pittsburgh, Pennsylvania
Chapter 9

Al Hillel, M.D.
Professor, Otolaryngology-Head and Neck
Surgery
University of Washington Medical Center
Seattle, Washington
Chapter 7

Leslie S. Kessler, M.A., CCC-SLP
Director, The Voice Experience and
The Language Experience
Lecturer, University of Maryland's Graduate
Course in Motor Speech Disorders
Rockville, Maryland
Chapter 9

Nicole Yee-Key Li, Ph.D.
Research Scientist
Department of Communication Science
and Disorders

University of Pittsburgh
Pittsburg, Pennsylvania
Chapter 9

Bruce J. Masek, Ph.D., ABPP
Clinical Director of Outpatient Child and
Adolescent Psychiatry
Massachusetts General Hospital
Associate Professor of Psychology
(Psychiatry)
Harvard Medical School
Boston, Massachusetts
Chapter 18

J. Scott McMurray, M.D., FAAP, FACS
Associate Professor
Department of Surgery, Division of
Otolaryngology-Head and Neck Surgery,
and
Department of Pediatrics
University of Wisconsin Medical School
Madison, Wisconsin
Chapter 11

Nelson Roy, Ph.D., CCC-SLP
Associate Professor
Department of Communication Sciences
and Disorders
University of Utah
Salt Lake City, Utah
Chapter 15

Robert T. Sataloff, M.D., D.M.A.
Professor and Chairman, Department of
Otolaryngology-HNS
Senior Associate Dean for Clinical
Academic Specialties
Drexel University College of Medicine
Philadelphia, Pennsylvania
Chapter 17

Cara Sauder, M.A., CCC-SLP
Clinical Director
University of Utah Voice Disorders Center
Salt Lake City, Utah
Chapter 15

Andrew R. Scott
Chapter 8

Marshall E. Smith, M.D., FACS, FAAP
Associate Professor, Division of
    Otolaryngology/Head and Neck Surgery
Primary Children's Medical Center
University of Utah School of Medicine
Salt Lake City, Utah
Chapter 15

**Katherine Verdolini Abbott, Ph.D.,
CCC-SLP**
Professor
Department of Communication Science
    and Disorders,
Department of Otolaryngology
Member, McGowan Institute for
    Regenerative Medicine
Member, Center for the Neural Basis of
    Cognition

University of Pittsburgh
Pittsburgh, Pennsylvania
Chapter 9

**Barbara Wilson-Arboleda, MS,
CCC-SLP**
Beth Israel Deaconess Medical Center
Boston, Massachusetts
and Voicewize
Dedham, Massachusetts
Chapter 3

Karen B. Zur, M.D.
Assistant Professor, Otolaryngology-Head
    and Neck Surgery
University of Pennsylvania School of
    Medicine
Director, Pediatric Voice Program
Children's Hospital of Philadelphia
Philadelphia, Pennsylvania
Chapter 14

1

Developmental, Gross, and Histologic Anatomy of the Larynx

Mark E. Boseley
Christopher J. Hartnick

INTRODUCTION

Understanding the embryologic development of the larynx is important when trying to comprehend the pathophysiology and treatment options we face as pediatric voice specialists. This chapter first focuses on the maturation of the anatomic structures. We then discuss the gross and histologic development of the true vocal folds ex utero. Our specific aims are to provide an anatomic review, as well as to add additional facts that might prove helpful in a clinical context.

EMBRYOLOGIC ANATOMY OF THE LARYNX

The larynx and pharynx are derived from the branchial arches in utero. Each branchial arch consists of mesenchyme, and is covered externally by ectoderm and internally by endoderm. Neural crest cells migrate into the branchial arches and eventually surround the central core of mesenchyme. It is important to note here that each branchial arch has an associated nerve, muscle, and skeletal structure.[1] These relationships are shown in Table 1–1.

The laryngeal framework, consisting of the epiglottis, hyoid bone, and the laryngeal and cricoid cartilages, begins to develop during the fourth week of gestation. These structures form from the mesenchyme of the second through fifth branchial arches. The cartilage of the epiglottis actually forms from the mesenchyme in the hypobranchial eminence (third and fourth brancial arches). The hyoid bone is also derived from two branchial arches (the second and third). The second arch contributes to the lesser cornu and superior part of the body. The

Table 1–1. Structures Derived from the Branchial Arches

Arch	Nerve	Muscles	Skeletal Structures
First	Trigeminal (V)	Muscles of mastication, mylohyoid and anterior belly of the diagastric, tensor tympani, and tensor veli palatini	Malleus and incus
Second	Facial (VII)	Muscles of facial expression, stapedius, stylohyoid, and posterior belly of diagastric	Stapes, styloid process, lesser cornu and upper part of body of hyoid
Third	Glossopharyngeal (IX)	Stylopharyngeus	Greater cornu and lower part of hyoid
Fourth, fifth and sixth	Superior laryngeal and recurrent laryngeal branches of vagus (X)	Cricthyroid, levator veli palatini, constrictors of the pharynx, intrinsic muscles of the larynx, and striated muscles of the esophagus	Thyroid cartilage, cricoid cartilage, arytenoid cartilage, corniculate cartilage, and cuneiform cartilage

third arch becomes the greater cornu and inferior portion of the body of the hyoid. Finally, the fourth and six arch mesenchyme fuse to form both the laryngeal and cricoid cartilages.[1]

The internal structures of the larynx also begin to develop during the fourth week of gestation. The endoderm lining the laryngotracheal groove begins to invaginate, forming a laryngotracheal diverticulum. Longitudinal folds then fuse to become the tracheoesophageal septum. Proliferating mesenchyme at the cranial end of the laryngotracheal apparatus diiferentiates into what will become the arytenoid, corniculate, and cuneiform cartilages. This process changes the narrow slitlike glottic aperture into a T-shaped opening. Also of note is that the laryngeal epithelium is rapidly proliferating during this time and actually obliterates the lumen of the larynx before later recanalizing by the 10th week of gestation. This recanalization is instrumental in the maturation of the false and true vocal folds, as well as the laryngeal ventricles. Failure of this to occur leads to congenital cartilaginous subglottic stenosis. When present, the cricoid cartilage is usually abnormally shaped with prominent lateral shelves obstructing the subglottic lumen. A further consequence of failure of recanalization is the presence of a supraglottic or glottic web. Glottic webs are the more common of the two and often extend into the subglottis. They are subdivided into types I to IV, with a type I representing a thin anterior web involving up to 50% of the glottis, progressing to a type IV which is a thick web involving 75 to 90% of the glottis and often extending into the subglottis.[2]

GROSS ANATOMY OF THE LARYNX

Muscles of the Larynx

The laryngeal muscles are derived from the fourth and sixth branchial arches and are innervated by the nerves that supply each (see Table 1–1).[1] The muscles of the larynx can be divided into extrinsic and intrinsic. The extrinsic muscles move the larynx as a whole. These include the depressors of larynx which are the omohyoid, sternohyoid, and sternothyroid. The elevators of the larynx are the stylohyoid, diagastric, and mylohyoid. There are also muscles that modify the pharyngeal inlet. The stylopharyngeus and palatopharyngeus elevate the pharynx,

whereas the middle and inferior pharyngeal constrictors participate in changing the shape of the air passage.[3]

The intrinsic muscles of the larynx are the cricothyroid, posterior and lateral cricoarytenoids, interarytenoid, thyroarytenoid, and vocalis (Figs 1–1 and 1–2). The posterior cricoarytenoid muscle slides the arytenoids laterally and is the only abductor of the true vocal folds. The cricothyroid muscle tilts the cricoid lamina in a backward direction and thus lengthens, tenses, and adducts the true vocal folds. The lateral cricoarytenoid muscle pulls the vocalis process of the vocal fold forward and laterally and therefore adducts the folds. The interarytenoid muscle approximates the arytenoid cartilages and subsequently is also an adductor of the vocal folds. The thyroarytenoid muscle

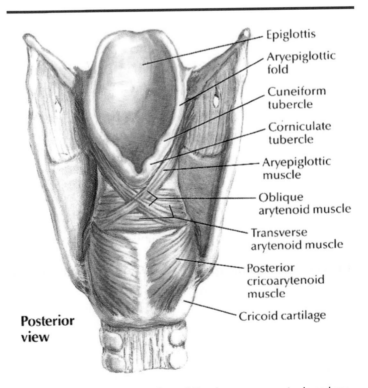

Epiglottis

Aryepiglottic fold

Cuneiform tubercle

Corniculate tubercle

Aryepiglottic muscle

Oblique arytenoid muscle

Transverse arytenoid muscle

Posterior cricoarytenoid muscle

Cricoid cartilage

Posterior view

Fig 1–1. Intrinsic muscles of the larynx—posterior view.

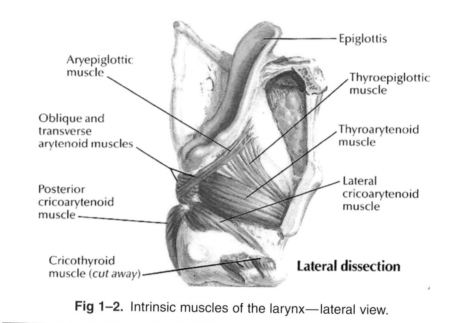

Aryepiglottic muscle

Epiglottis

Thyroepiglottic muscle

Oblique and transverse arytenoid muscles

Thyroarytenoid muscle

Lateral cricoarytenoid muscle

Posterior cricoarytenoid muscle

Cricothyroid muscle (*cut away*)

Lateral dissection

Fig 1–2. Intrinsic muscles of the larynx—lateral view.

draws the arytenoids forward and medially and adducts the true and false folds. The last of the intrinsic laryngeal muscles is the vocalis. This muscle is difficult to discern anatomically from the thyroarytenoid, but is instrumental in adducting and tensing the true vocal folds.[3]

Blood Supply of the Larynx

The larynx's blood supply is supplied from the superior and inferior laryngeal arteries. The superior laryngeal artery arises from the superior thyroid artery and runs horizontally across the thyrohyoid membrane. The artery then penetrates the membrane and lies in the submucosa of the lateral wall and floor of the piriform sinus; supplying the mucosa and musculature of the larynx. The inferior laryngeal artery is a branch of

the inferior thyroid artery (itself a branch of the thyrocervical trunk) and enters the larynx below the inferior constrictor muscle. This artery anastomoses with the superior laryngeal artery to also supply the laryngeal mucosa and muscles.[3]

Nerves of the Larynx

The innervation to the larynx is via the superior and inferior laryngeal nerves (Fig 1–3). Both of these nerves are branches of the vagus nerve. The superior laryngeal nerve passes down the vagal trunk and lies medial to the internal and external carotid arteries. This nerve has an external and internal branch. The external branch travels down the lateral surface of the inferior constrictor and ends at the cricothyroid muscle. The internal branch takes a similar course to

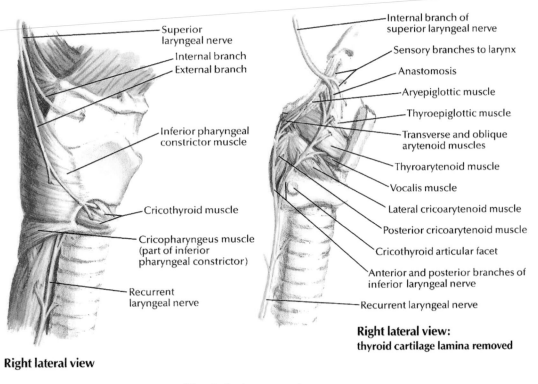

Right lateral view

Right lateral view:
thyroid cartilage lamina removed

Fig 1–3. Laryngeal nerves.

the superior laryngeal artery, penetrating the thyrohyoid membrane. Sensory fibers from the internal branch supply the posterior aspect of the tongue, valleculae, epiglottis, piriform recesses, vestibular folds, ventricles, and the posterior laryngeal and anterior pharyngeal walls at the level of the cricoid cartilage.[3]

The inferior laryngeal nerve is an extension of the recurrent laryngeal nerve. It enters the larynx with the inferior thyroid artery just posterior to the cricothyroid articulation. There are usually at least two branches from this nerve which may occur before or after it enters the larynx. The anterior branch, or adductor of the larynx, supplies the lateral cricoarytenoid, thyroarytenoid, and vocalis muscles. The posterior

branch, or abductor of the larynx, supplies the posterior cricoarytenoid and the interarytenoid musculature.[3]

Framework of the Larynx

External changes in position and structure of the larynx itself can be seen as a child matures. The larynx descends in the neck in relationship to the cervical vertebrae from infancy (where the inferior aspect of the cricoid approximates the fourth cervical vertebra) to the mature position (C6-C7) by mid-adolescence (see Fig 1–2).[4] Kahane[5] discovered that the laryngeal and cricoid cartilages also undergo significant changes as a child grows. He compared specimens before and after puberty and noted changes that included increase in length, height, width, and weight of both cartilages. As one might expect, these changes were greater in male than in female specimens.

Internal laryngeal changes are equally important as the child grows. There have been two studies published utilizing MRI scans to examine changes in laryngeal anatomy over time.[6,7] One of these was a report from the anesthesia literature which looked at 99 children between the ages of 2 months to 13 years. They determined that the anterior-posterior and transverse measurements at the levels of the true vocal folds, subglottis, and cricoid all increased linearly with age. The narrowest region was the transverse dimension at the true vocal fold level.[6] A second study compared serial MRI scans in two pediatric patients over the first 4 years of life. Their most significant finding was that laryngeal and tongue descent appeared to be the most influential in vocal fold lengthening over time.[7]

The actual growth of the true vocal folds has also been studied. Male vocal folds undergo over twice the growth of female true vocal folds.[5] Hirano[8] measured the length of the developing vocal fold and its anatomic components, namely, the membranous and cartilaginous portions. The measurements comparing newborn with adult male and female vocal folds are presented in Table 1–2. Important to note is the vocal fold at birth has nearly equal contribution of the membranous and cartilaginous portions. The membranous portion of the vocal fold is dominant by 3 years of age (Fig 1–4).[8]

HISTOLOGIC ANATOMY OF THE LARYNX

The "modern" description of the micro-anatomy of the human vocal folds has been properly attributed to Dr. Hirano with his seminal work in 1975 entitled "Phono-surgery: Basic and Clinical Investigations."[9] It was here that Hirano defined the trilaminar structure of the human vocal fold. He labeled these the superficial, intermediate and deep layers of the lamina propria. The layers were defined by examining the elastin and collagen concentrations within each layer in adult autopsy specimens (Fig 1–5).[9-11]

Lamina Propria Development

The lamina propria is instrumental in modulating voice. This is often explained with the cover-body theory of phonation. Defin-

Table 1–2. True Vocal Fold Lengths

Age	Overall Vocal Fold Length	Membranous Vocal Fold Length	Cartilaginous Vocal Fold Length
Newborn	2.5–3.0 mm	1.3–2.0 mm	1.0–1.4 mm
Adult Males	17–21 mm	14.5–18 mm	2.5–3.5 mm
Adult Females	11–15 mm	8.5–12 mm	2.0–3.0 mm

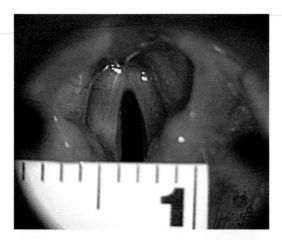

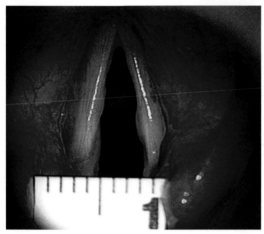

Fig 1–4. Suspension laryngoscopy of an infant (*top*) and adolescent (*bottom*) larynx. Note that ratio of the length of the arytenoid cartilage to membranous vocal fold changes significantly with age as the membranous vocal fold lengthens.

itions of what layers of the vocal fold make up the cover and body vary. Perhaps the most common definition is that the cover consists of the epithelium and superficial portion of the intermediate layers of the lamina propria. This relatively pliant layer moves over the stiffer vocal ligament (composed of the middle and deep layers of the lamina propria), rests upon the vocalis muscle, and allows the vocal fold to vibrate with consistency and control.[8]

As the lamina propria has such an important role in voice production, it is important that we attempt to understand both how and when it develops into its final three-layered form. We know that the lamina is not fully developed in the newborn. Studies have shown that it appears to be a uniform, one-layered structure at birth.[12-15]

There are areas of more abundant cells in the anterior and posterior portions of the fold that are adjacent to the thyroid cartilage and vocalis process. These areas are labeled the anterior and posterior macula flavae, respectively. Cells within the macula flavae appear to be important in the growth and maturation of lamina propria.[12-14]

Macula Flavae and Lamina Propria Cells

Immature fibroblasts are the primary cells found within the infant macula flavae. They appear to be more abundant than the mature form seen in the adult. The mechanism of how these cells differentiate into mature cells has yet to be elucidated. One theory is that the trauma produced as a child begins to develop speech might stimulate differentiation of the cells within the lamina propria. These fibroblasts produce collagen, elastin, and reticular fibers, as well as glycoprotein (fibronectin) or ground substance; substances that are vital for maintenance of strength and elasticity of the vocal fold.[12-13]

The cells within the lamina propria layers are also believed to be important in the differentiation of the three-layered vocal fold. Fibroblasts are again the most prominent cell type.[12,13] Macrophages and myofibroblasts (differentiated fibroblasts believed to be

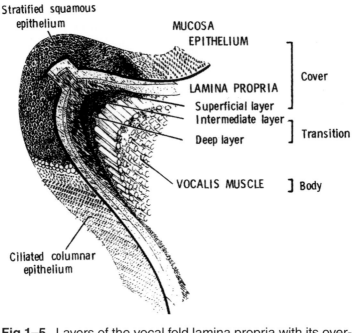

Fig 1–5. Layers of the vocal fold lamina propria with its overlying epithelium. Also labeled are the layers that are typically thought to make up the cover and body of the vocal fold.

important in the reorganization of tissues) are also found within the lamina. The discovery that the cytoplasm of these cells contain proteoglycans indicates that they, along with fibroblasts, are involved with the development and maintenance of the vocal fold.[16]

Catten[17] expanded on this work by looking at the concentration of fibroblasts, myofibroblasts, and macrophages in each layer of the lamina propria. He found that fibroblasts were most abundant in the deepest layer of the lamina propria and myofibroblasts were found in more superficial regions. Macrophages were only seen in 36% of his specimens and, when present, were also found in the superficial layer.[17] The cell signaling mechanisms that are

instrumental in cell differentiation have yet to be determined.

The early work by Catten looking at differences in cellular concentration in the three layers of the lamina propria was important as before that time the layers were defined only by elastin and collagen concentrations. Hartnick[15] was the first to look cellular differences as the vocal fold develops from infancy until adolescence He found that the newborn vocal fold contained only a monolayer of cells, which agreed with what had been previously described by Sato and Hirano.[12,13] This became two layers of cells by 5 months and three layers by 7 years (Fig 1–6). The results of the study helped support the notion that the three-layered vocal fold might develop earlier than what had previously been

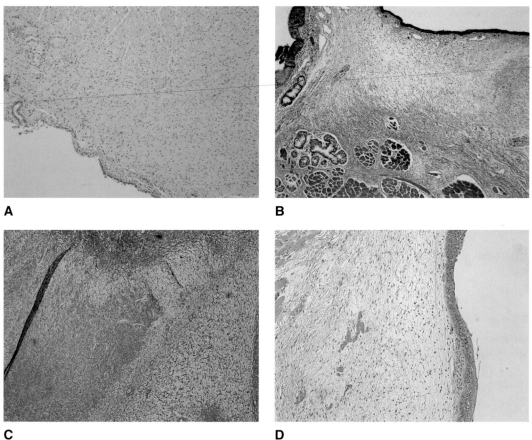

Fig 1–6. Four micrometer sections of 2-day-old (*A*), 2-year-old (*B*), 7-year-old (*C*), and 13-year-old (*D*) true vocal folds. **A.** Hematoxylin-eosin stain at 10x magnification showing single hypocellular layer of the lamina propria. **B.** Alcian blue stain at 40× magnification showing two distinct cellular populations within the lamina propria. **C.** Trichrome stain at 100x magnification showing the beginning of middle layer of the lamina propria. There are superficial and deep areas of hypocellularity with a middle layer that is more cellular. **D.** Hematoxylin-eosin stain at 40x magnification showing the fully developed three-layered lamina propria.

described by using elastin and collagen content.[15]

Boseley and Hartnick[18] later duplicated Catten's study, looking specifically at the concentrations of macrophages and myofibroblasts in the lamina propria. These cells were first seen by the age of 11 months.

This work provided additional evidence that both are predominately found in the superficial layers of the lamina.

Measurements of the depth of the entire lamina propria and the superficial lamina propria were also reported. The superficial layer appeared to become thinner with age, encompassing approximately 20% of the entire lamina propria in the 7-year-old specimen. In addition, the total depth of the lamina propria reached 1,300 μm in the specimen of a 10-year-old child (Fig 1–7). These two measurements approximate what is seen in the adult. Therefore, one could conclude that the vocal fold may be fully developed at some point within this age range. The small sample size in the study, however, prevents making definitive conclusions.[18]

Lamina Propria Proteins

Elastin

Elastin plays a significant role in the biomechanics of the lamina propria. These fibers are primarily found in the intermediate layer of the lamina propria in the fully developed vocal fold and are intimately associated with a glycosaminoglycan (hyaluronic

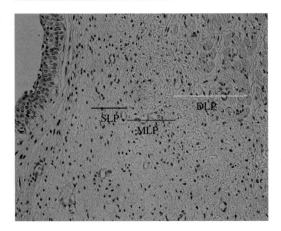

Fig 1–7. Histologic photomicrograph of a 10-year-old child's TVF. Lines are drawn to demonstrate how the individual layers of the lamina were measured using an optical analysis computer software program. The total depth of the three layers was 1300 μm.

acid) and a proteoglycan (fibromodulin). Here elastin can stretch up to two times its resting length.[19]

Elastin is found in low concentrations in the newborn, but its fibers aren't fully developed (thin, coiled fibers). The concentration increases with age, with the highest concentrations found in geriatric male and female specimens. This fact doesn't necessarily mean that vocal fold elasticity is increased with age. One theory is that cross-linking may cause decreased elasticity despite the higher concentrations. It should also be noted here that there does not appear to be gender-related differences in elastin concentrations.[19]

Collagen

Collagen is another important protein found in the lamina propria. Unlike elastin, collagen is typically found immediately under the surface epithelium and also in the deep layer of the lamina propria. The deep layer and the underlying vocalis muscle make up part of the vocal ligament (in addition to the deep portion of the intermediate layer). This accounts for the relatively stable body, over which the cover of the vocal fold can move.[20]

Collagen concentration within the basement membrane of the epithelium is actually greater in infant specimens than what is found in adult and geriatric specimens. However, the collagen within the deep layer of the lamina propria increases significantly until adulthood and then appears to level off. Furthermore, there seems to be a significantly higher concentration of collagen in males compared to females. The reason for this is not completely understood. This is particularly puzzling if one suspects that collagen production is in response to tension exerted on the fold which should be the same in both sexes. Other gender specific environmental (voice use) and physiologic (hormones, etc) factors may also play a role, although this has not been definitively proven.[20]

CONCLUSION

Although much knowledge has been gained regarding the development of the human vocal fold, there are still many questions to be answered. Thus far, definitive conclusions have been difficult to reach due, in part, to the small sample size restraints in most published studies. To this end, new technologies are being developed that may allow us to examine the histologic make-up of the vocal fold in vivo. In addition to continuing to examine the anatomic development of the vocal fold, we also need to examine the mechanisms of cellular differentiation and the biomechanical properties of the various layers of the vocal fold. The hope is that this information will be helpful in treating various pathologies that are seen in the pediatric population.

REFERENCES

1. Moore KL. *The Developing Human.* Philadelphia, Pa: Saunders; 1988:170–210.
2. Cotton RT, Myer CM. *Practical Pediatric Otolaryngology.* Philadelphia, Pa: Lippincott-Raven; 1999:497–513.
3. Hollinshead WH. *Anatomy for Surgeons The Head and Neck.* Philadelphia,Pa: Lippincott, Williams & Wilkins; 1982:418–432.
4. Cummings CW, Fredrickson JM, Harker LA, Krause CJ, Richardson MA, Schuller DE. *Otolaryngology-Head and Neck Surgery.* St. Louis, Mo: Mosby; 1998.
5. Kahane JC. Histologic structure and properties of the human vocal folds. *Ear Nose Throat J.* 1988;67:322–330.
6. Litman RS, Weissend EE, Shibata D, Westesson P. Developmental changes of laryngeal dimensions in unparalyzed, sedated children. *Anesthesiology.* 2003;98:41–45.
7. Vorperian HK, Kent RD, Gentry LR, Yandell BS. Magnetic resonance imaging procedures to study the concurrent anatomic development of vocal tract structures: preliminary results. *Int J Pediatr Otorhinolaryngol.* 1999;49:197–206.
8. Hirano M. Growth, development, and aging of human vocal folds. In: Abbs J. *Vocal Fold Physiology.* San Diego,Calif: College-Hill Press; 1983:23–43.
9. Hirano M. Phonosurgery. Basic and clinical Investigations. *Otologia (Fukuoka).* 1975; 21(suppl 1):239–260.
10. Hirano M. Structure and vibratory behavior of the vocal folds. In: Sawashima M, Franklin S, eds. *Dynamic Aspects of Speech Production.* Tokyo, Japan: University of Tokyo Press; 1977:13–30.
11. Hirano M. Structure of the vocal fold in normal and disease states: anatomical and physical studies. *ASHA Reports.* 1981;11:11–30.
12. Sato K, Hirano M. Histologic investigation of the maculae flavae of the human vocal fold. *Ann Otol Rhinol Laryngol.* 1995;104: 556–562
13. Sato K, Hirano M, Nakashima T. Fine structure of the human newborn and infant vocal fold mucosae. *Ann Otol Rhinol Laryngol.* 2001;110:417–424.
14. Ishii K, Akita M, Yamashita K, Hirose H. Age-related development of the arrangement of connective tissue fibers in the lamina propria of the human vocal fold. *Ann Otol Rhinol Laryngol.* 2000;109:1055–1064.
15. Hartnick CJ, Rehbar R, Prasad V. Development and maturation of the pediatric human vocal fold lamina propria. *Laryngoscope.* 2005;115:4–15.
16. Pawlak A, Hammond TH, Hammond E, Gray SD. Immunocytochemical study of proteoglycans in vocal folds. *Ann Otol Rhinol Laryngol.* 1996;105:6–11.
17. Catten M, Gray SD, Hammond TH, Zhou R, Hammond E. Analysis of cellular location

and concentration in vocal fold lamina propria. *Otolaryngol Head Neck Surg.* 1998; 118:663–667.

18. Boseley ME, Hartnick CJ. Development of the human vocal fold: depth of cell layers and quantifying cell types within the lamina propria. *Ann Otol Rhinol Laryngol.* 2006; 115:784–788.

19. Hammond TH, Gray SD, Butler J, Zhou R, Hammond E. Age- and gender-related elastin distribution changes in human vocal folds. *Otolaryngol Head Neck Surg.* 1998;119:314–322.

20. Hammond TH, Gray SD, Butler JE. Age- and gender-related collagen distribution in human vocal folds. *Ann Otol Rhinol Laryngol.* 2000;109:913–920.

PART I

Evaluation of a Child With a Voice Disorder

2

Pediatric Laryngology: The Office and Operating Room Setup

Mark E. Boseley
Christopher J. Hartnick

INTRODUCTION

The field of pediatric laryngology has grown as the equipment and technology available to us has expanded. Where we were once limited by pediatric flexible fiberoptic laryngoscopes with poor optics, we now have distal-chip camera scopes with digital quality images displayed on a video monitor. Videostroboscopy is now possible using these scopes, a diagnostic tool that was often not used previously as it required the use of rigid telescopes that were not tolerated by pediatric patients. We are also now able to archive images and videos from both the office and operating room, making pre- and post-treatment evaluations more accurate than in the past. Furthermore, we are utilizing the services of our pulmonary and gastroenterology colleagues more and more in the care of these often complex patients with multiple medical problems. This has taken the form of pediatric aerodigestive clinics in several of our academic centers around the country. As this occurs, we have to be able to acquire digital images of both flexible bronchoscopies and esophagoscopies and archive them in some unified fashion to complement our rigid tracheobronchoscopies.

This chapter discusses both the office and operating room personnel and equipment important in the practice of pediatric laryngology. This is not intended to be an exhaustive list, but should provide a useful foundation if one is beginning a practice (or expanding one) to care for pediatric voice patients.

OFFICE-BASED PRACTICE

Personnel

Developing a pediatric laryngology clinic involves having at your disposal the appropriate personnel and equipment needed to diagnose and treat these patients. The personnel usually includes an otolaryngologist (usually pediatric otolaryngologist) who has an interest in caring for children with voice disorders. Another vital member of the team is the speech-language pathologist (SLP) who has a specific interest and training in treating pediatric patients. A clinic nurse is also invaluable for patient/parent teaching and helping with the care of the complex equipment that is utilized in the clinic.

Children with voice complaints often present with numerous aerodigestive symptoms. Medical histories can uncover such symptoms as chronic cough, wheezing, exercise intolerance, and feeding difficulties, in addition to the voice concern that brought them to your office. Prior experience suggests that these children were sent to other specialists, required multiple visits, and often involved poor communication between specialties. This problem can be alleviated by establishing a close working relationship with our pediatric pulmonary and gastroenterology colleagues. This may take the form of a formal aerodigestive workup or might simply involve an informal design where there is an open line of communication between the clinicians.

A visit to the aerodigestive clinic involves essentially three complete evaluations of the child. This is followed by a conference among the specialists involved and typically generates a detailed treatment plan before the patient leaves the office. Occasionally this plan involves an endoscopic evaluation in the operating room, where flexible bronchoscopy and flexible esophagoscopy can yield valuable information.

Equipment

We have included pictures and videos of the equipment outlined in this chapter in a CD compendium that accompanies the text. This chapter and subsequent chapters that have either photographs or videos that enhance the didactic portion the text have a second section where the images are explained in detail. This second section includes detailed information about list costs and catalog numbers if you are interested in purchasing any item discussed. We hope this will be a valuable tool for better understanding the equipment and techniques that are currently being utilized in the field of pediatric laryngology.

The diagnostic equipment available in the office has changed considerably over the past several years. The Kay Pentax Stroboscope Model 9100B is the latest in the line of videostroboscopic equipment allowing for digital quality imaging of the larynx, utilizing either a flexible rhinolaryngoscope or a 70-degree rigid peroral telescope. A 3.4-mm (Olympus) or 3.7-mm (Kay Pentax) flexible distal-tip-chip camera strobsocope can allow for full screen high-resolution images and stroboscopic observation of younger children's vocal folds (Fig 2–1). Alternatively, 2.7-mm and 3.0-mm angled rigid stroboscopes are available from Karl Storz (Fig 2–2).

Stroboscopy is not always possible in young children. This is not always due to their chronologic age, but may be more a function of their age-independent maturity. The skill and experience of the endoscopist is also important in this regard. Also, young

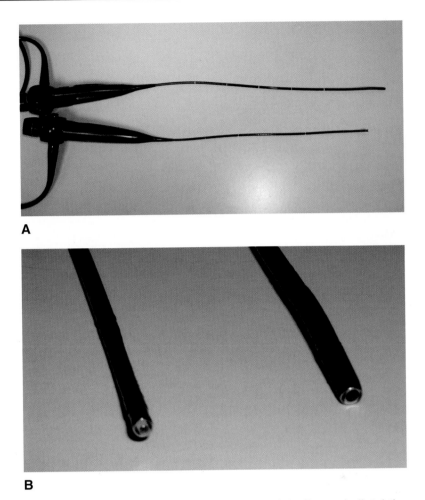

Fig 2–1. 3.4-mm (Olympus) and 3.7-mm (KayPentax) distal-tip-chip camera flexible rhinolaryngoscopes.

children are not always able to produce the asynchronous prolonged mucosal wave vibration needed to obtain stroboscopic images. Despite these potential hindrances, distal-chip camera technology allows for a more detailed evaluation of the vocal fold anatomy and of glottal aperture abnormalities even without the use of stroboscopy.

This new equipment can provide valuable information. One example of this is a flexible transnasal videostroboscopic examination on a 6-year-old child. The resolution of the digital video is much better than traditional flexible laryngoscopes and much easier accomplished than rigid peroral stroboscopy. Examination for glottal insufficiency, as well as examination of the mucosal wave to identify overall pliability of the mucosa and points of stiffness, is now feasible. Mucosal wave abnormalities may also be useful in differentiating vocal fold pathologies. Additionally, acoustic measurements can be recorded and saved for future comparison.

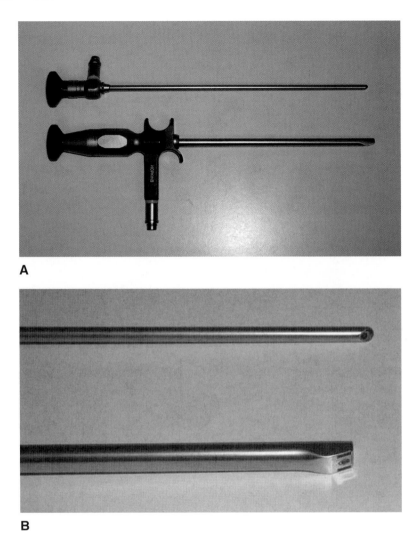

Fig 2–2. 70-degree pediatric rigid Hopkins rod strobscopes (Karl Storz Inc.).

Another office examination made both more practical, and perhaps more accessible by the new technology described above, is pediatric functional endoscopic evaluation of swallowing (FEES). FEES can be useful in the workup of children with swallowing difficulties or in those children whom you suspect may be aspirating. This is demonstrated by a 14-year-old girl who presents after skull base resection of a clival chordoma with signs of aspiration.

Archiving of digital images and videos in the office is very important for determining treatment outcomes. There are several programs that can be used for this purpose. We have experience with products from Karl Storz and NStream. Both were easy to use and we do not necessarily endorse one over the other. There are undoubtedly other programs that either are currently or soon will be on the market. The important message here is that archiving in both the operating room and the clinic setting is vital to assessing treatment outcomes in our voice patient population.

OPERATING ROOM-BASED PRACTICE

Equipment

The operating room equipment that should be available to the pediatric laryngologist can be thought of in several distinct categories. These include tools for visualization, airway access instruments, microsurgical instruments, and video/picture capabilities with an archiving system. Each of these categories is described in detail.

Tools for Visualization

Most pediatric cases can be managed with the infant, adolescent, or adult Lindholm laryngoscopes (Fig 2–3) which can be sus-

pended from either a Mayo or Mustard stand using the Benjamin suspension apparatus (Fig 2–4). Another laryngoscope that can be useful in the difficult-to-expose patient is the pediatric universal glottis-

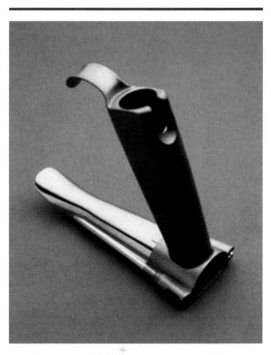

Fig 2–3. Lindholm laryngoscopes.

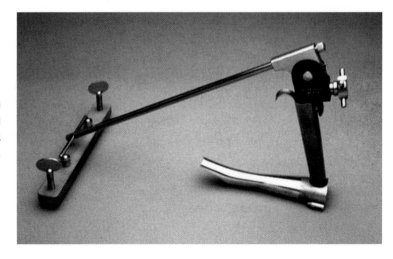

Fig 2–4. Benjamin suspension device which can rest on either a Mustard or Mayo stand.

cope with the gallows suspension device (Fig 2–5). This device takes advantage of torsion-fulcrum principles to achieve better exposure of the vocal folds.

All the aforementioned laryngoscopes may be used to visualize the larynx with a small endotracheal tube in place, or (as our preference) utilizing a tubeless spontaneous ventilation/apneic anesthetic technique. Magnification can be achieved with either a 4.0-mm Hopkins rod telescope with a camera attachment or with an operating microscope with a 400-mm lens. (We prefer the Leica M520S3 microscope although there are other microscopes that would suffice.) The latter is particularly useful when performing phonosurgical procedures that require bimanual manipulation. With these instruments and microscopes, close inspection of pediatric vocal folds is

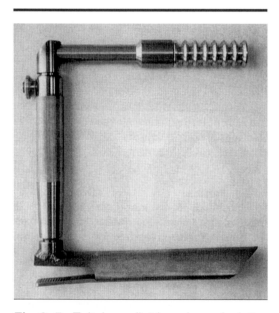

Fig 2–5. Zeitels pediatric universal glottoscope with gallows suspension. This instrument can be utilized when the Lindholm laryngoscopes are unable to give adequate visualization of the glottis.

possible. This often allows us to discriminate between lesions such as vocal nodules and cysts and allows for proper treatment and therapy plans to be developed (Fig 2–6). It is tantamount to realize that not all children will allow office visualization of their vocal folds, and that there is a time when operative endoscopy will be essential.

Tools for Airway Access

Although not always required, it is important that a variety of ventilating bronchoscopes are available and assembled to handle the difficult airway. A size 2.5 rigid bronchoscope with an inner diameter of 3.5 mm and an outer diameter of 4.2 mm with a 18-cm 1.9-mm Hopkins rod telescope is a scope that we have available for most of our infant airway cases. This is the smallest bronchoscope on the airway cart and should be able to be passed through most stenotic lesions that are encountered. If a tight distal airway stenosis is suspected, a modified endotracheal tube can be fashioned to get access to the distal airway (Fig 2–7). The point that must be emphasized is that a child with a suspected difficult airway **does not get muscle relaxants** until the airway is stabilized.

Microsurgical Instruments

The surgeon is only as good as the instruments that he or she has available. There is no place where this dictum is more true than when attempting to perform phonosurgical procedures. Developing microsurgical flaps between the vocal fold epithelium and superficial layer of the lamina propria requires great skill, but also necessitates the avail-

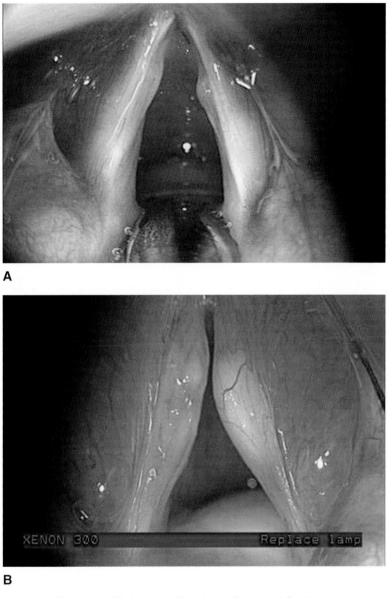

A

B

Fig 2–6. High magnification of a vocal fold cyst

ability of the proper instruments. These instruments should be analyzed routinely to be sure that they are sharp and of good working order. A typical microlaryngeal instrument set is pictured in Figure 2–8. The minimum requirements should be microscopic scissors (right, left, straight, and upbiting), atraumatic graspers such as the Sataloff forceps (right and left), a sickle knife, a microsurgical dissector, and set of laryngeal suctions. One-quarter-inch neurologic cotton pledgets soaked in oxymetazoline on a sponge carrier are often helpful to achieve hemostasis.

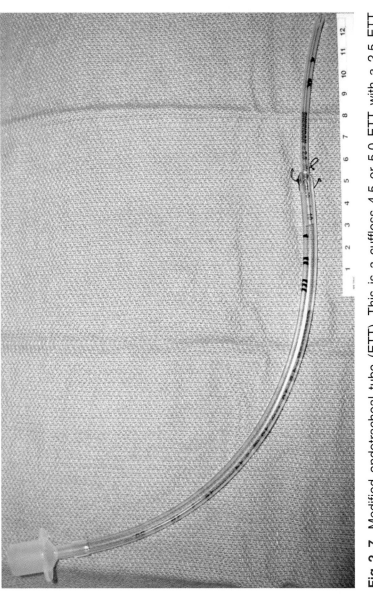

Fig 2–7. Modified endotracheal tube (ETT). This is a cuffless 4.5 or 5.0 ETT with a 2.5 ETT secured to the end with 4.0 silk sutures. The outer diameter of the 2.5 ETT is 3.6 mm which is smaller than the diameter of the 2.5 bronchoscope. This can be used to bypass a distal tracheal stenosis.

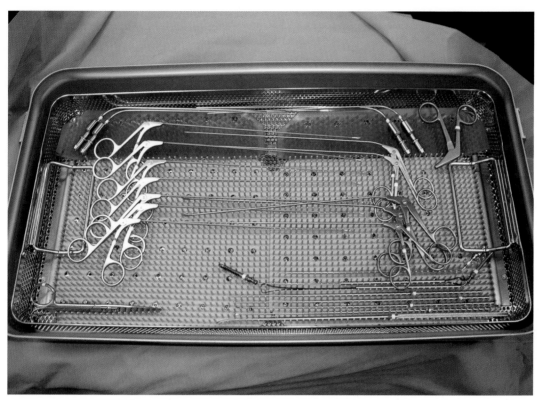

A

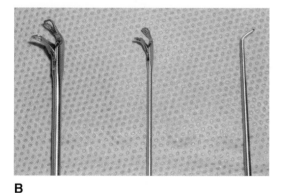

B

Fig 2–8. Example of a complete pediatric voice set for the operating room.

Archiving

Archiving images from the operating room are equally as important as in the office. This is extremely valuable for patients who make frequent trips to the operating room (ie, children following airway reconstruction and children with the diagnosis of juvenile onset recurrent respiratory papillomatosis). Photographs are also useful when discussing treatment plans with parents.

CONCLUSION

This chapter has described how to set up a pediatric voice clinic. It focused on those personnel and equipment that we find invaluable in the office and operating room.

We have attempted to consolidate the list of equipment to make ordering these items much easier than searching through numerous catalogues (Appendix 2). We hope this information will be helpful to those of you considering starting or expanding a pediatric voice practice.

APPENDIX 2

Pediatric Vocal Fold Instrument Set*

Description	Company	Model #	# Required	List Price
Straight cup forceps (*straight*)	Karl Storz	8591A	1	$695.00
Curved cup forceps (*right*)	Karl Storz	8591C	1	$695.00
Curved cup forceps (*left*)	Karl Storz	8591D	1	$695.00
Alligator forceps (*right*)	Instrumentarium	L.70.925	1	$572.90
Alligator forceps (*left*)	Instrumentarium	L.70.926	1	$572.90
Small Sataloff forceps (*right*)	Instrumentarium	L.70.991	1	$776.40
Large Sataloff forceps (*right*)	Instrumentarium	L.70.191	1	$516.45
Large Sataloff forceps (*left*)	Instrumentarium	L.70.190	1	$516.45
Scissors (*angled up*)	Karl Storz	8594BM	1	$875.00
Scissors (*straight*)	Karl Storz	8594AM	1	$875.00
Scissors (*right*)	Karl Storz	8594DM	1	$875.00
Scissors (*left*)	Karl Storz	8594CM	1	$875.00
Universal knife handle	Pilling	506888	1	$391.06
Jako sponge carrier (26-cm)	Pilling	506751	2	$265.20 ea
Holinger laryngeal dissector	Pilling	506882	1	$153.00
Phono curved sickle knife	Pilling	506882	1	$229.50
Phono blunt probe elevator (60-degree)	Pilling	506832	1	$142.80
Zeitels vocal fold infusion needle	Endocraft	ZIN-100A	Box of 5	$500.00

*2007 list prices

VIDEO TOWER

Description	Company	Model #	# Required	List Price
Computer w/ DV/SDI	Karl Storz	22200011U102	1	$16,270.00
Flat panel monitor	Karl Storz	9319NR-A24	1	$8,920.00
3-chip camera	Karl Storz	22220130-3	1	$15,230.00
Sony printer	Karl Storz	9512C	1	$10,140.00
175-watt xenon light source	Karl Storz	201315-20	1	$3,075.00
Light cable	Karl Storz	495ND	1	$570.00
Cart	Karl Storz	9801T	1	$1,255.00

TELESCOPES

Description	Company	Model #	# Required	List Price
Hopkins II 0-degree (4-mm × 18-cm)	Karl Storz	7230AA	1	$3,980.00
Hopkins II 0-degree (2.7-mm × 18-cm)	Karl Storz	7219AA	1	$4,425.00
Hopkins II 0-degree (1.9-mm × 18-cm)	Karl Storz	10017AA	1	$4,660.00
Hopkins II 70-degree (4-mm × 18-cm)	Karl Storz	7230CWA	1	$4,110.00
Hopkins II 70-degree (4-mm × 15-cm)	Karl Storz	7228CA	1	$3,795.00
Hopkins II 70-degree (3-mm × 14-cm)	Karl Storz	7220CA	1	$3,570.00
Hopkins II 70-degree (2.7-mm × 18-cm)	Karl Storz	7219CA	1	$4,425.00
Hopkins II 120-degree (4-mm × 18-cm)	Karl Storz	7230EA	1	$3,980.00

LARYNGOSCOPES

Description	Company	Model #	# Required	List Price
Infant Lindholm	Karl Storz	8587 P	1	$1,645.00
Light carrier	Karl Storz	8587 PF	1	$515.00
Child Lindholm	Karl Storz	8587 N	1	$1,645.00
Adult Linholm	Karl Storz	8587 A	1	$1,645.00
Light carrier	Karl Storz	8587 GF	1	$515.00
Pediatric universal glottiscope	Endocraft	UMG-100A	1	$3,900.00
Light cable for universal glottiscope	Endocraft	UMG-100 LC	1	$450.00
Gallows suspension	Endocraft	ZVG-100A	1	$3900.00
Benjamin suspension & chest support	Karl Storz	8574 KW	1	$1,470.00

BRONCHOSCOPES AND ACCESSORIES

Description	Company	I.D.	O.D.	Model #	# Required	List Price
2.5 × 20 cm	Karl Storz	3.5 mm	4.2 mm	10339F	1	$875.00
3.0 × 20 cm	Karl Storz	4.3 mm	5.0 mm	10339D	1	$875.00
3.5 × 20 cm	Karl Storz	5.0 mm	5.7 mm	10339CD	1	$875.00
3.5 × 30 cm	Karl Storz	5.0 mm	5.7 mm	10339DD	1	$875.00
4.0 × 30 cm	Karl Storz	6.0 mm	6.7 mm	10339C	1	$875.00
4.5 × 30 cm	Karl Storz	6.6 mm	7.3 mm	10339BB	1	$875.00
5.0 × 30 cm	Karl Storz	7.2 mm	7.7 mm	10339B	1	$875.00
6.0 × 30 cm	Karl Storz	7.5 mm	8.2 mm	10339A	1	$875.00

Description	Company	Model #	# Required	List Price
Prism light defelector	Karl Storz	10101FA	1	$445.00
Glass plug window	Karl Storz	10338M	1	$80.00
Rubber telescope guide	Karl Storz	10338N	1	$65.00
Adapter for respirator	Karl Storz	10924D	1	$15.00

OFFICE EQUIPMENT

Fiberoptic Scopes (flexible and rigid)

Description	Company	Model #	# Required	List Price
ENF-V2 flexible video rhinolaryngoscope with video system (3.4-mm diameter)	Olympus	K230000229	1	$26,350.00
ENF-XP flexible fiberoptic rhinolaryngoscope (2.2-mm diameter)	Olympus	1111900	1	$8,820.00
ENF-GP flexible fiberoptic rhinolaryngoscope (3.6-mm diameter)	Olympus	1113308	1	$6,325.00
Rigid endoscope (70-degrees, 10-mm diameter)	Kay Pentax	9106	1	$4,195.00

Videostroboscopic Equipment

Description	Company	Model #	# Required	List Price
Rhinolaryngeal stroboscope	Kay Pentax	9100B	1	$15,995.00
Camera, 3-CCD	Kay Pentax	9106	1	$4,195.00
22-37-mm zoom lens coupler	Kay Pentax	9118	1	$1,375.00
Digital video capture module	Kay Pentax	9200C	1	$16,995.00
Color printer	Kay Pentax	9264C	1	$325.00
Electroglottograph	Kay Pentax	6103	1	$1,995.00
Cart	Kay Pentax	9271	1	$1,995.00
Setup/training	Kay Pentax	9198	1	$995.00

Evaluation of the Child With a Vocal Disorder

Shirley Gherson
Barbara M. Wilson Arboleda

INTRODUCTION

Voice disorders in the pediatric population are as varied as those in the adult population, but present special considerations for the voice evaluation team. Chronic hoarseness in children can stem from functional, structural, or neurologic bases. Reflux, asthma, allergies, and medication side effects may be complicating factors even among very young children. Recent advances in neonatal intensive care, although life-saving, often present a series of traumas to the airway and voicing mechanism.[1,2] A child's voice disorder may be congenital, acquired after a period of normal voicing or may present from the earliest stages of communication. Congenital problems include: laryngeal papillomas, glottic web, paralysis, vocal fold sulcus, laryngomalacia, and subglottic stenosis.[3,4] Acquired voice problems include use-related injuries, trauma, and those secondary to intubation.

The diversity of etiology, presentation, and perception of voice disorders among children is a complicating factor in discerning the presence of a voice disorder and in making management decisions. Vast variability in prevalence rate has been reported. Most often quoted is 6 to 9%, but some authors report prevalence as high as 38%.[5-7] One study revealed vocal fold nodules in almost 17% of a large cohort of children, regardless of voicing or functional status.[8] Comparison across studies is complicated by the differing criteria applied to each study. For example, parent and physician questionnaires tend to report a lower incidence than clinic or speech-language pathologist evaluation.[9] Overlooking the presence of a pediatric voice disorder may lead to undertreatment. In one study by Powell,[10] 82 children out of 203 identified with a voice disorder continued to demonstrate symptoms in a 4-year follow-up. By nature, children with congenital abnormalities of the larynx and those who have had surgical intervention to the airway will have a higher incidence of voice disorders. In one study by Zalzal, cited by Baker,[2] 15 of 16 children status postlaryngotracheal reconstruction were considered to be dysphonic by the voice clinician.

Differences in prevalence based on gender are different between the adult and the pediatric voice populations. In the school-aged population, more males present with use-related voice disorders.[5,7,8] This is reversed for adults, where over two-thirds of patients diagnosed with vocal fold nodules are female.[8,11]

Parents are not always certain what represents typical variation versus disordered voicing. In particular, parents may not be tuned in to their child's voice if hoarseness has been present since birth. One study in which a voice screening was administered to over 7,000 children revealed a disparity between clinician reporting of atypical voice versus parents' reporting of atypical voice.[5] Young children are not able to express functional limitations and parents may not understand the implications a voice disorder will have on their children as they grow. For this reason, parents will be heavily reliant on the judgment of the voice evaluation team to understand prognosis and propose treatment solutions.

The voice evaluation may also be a portion of a larger review of the child's speech, language, and developmental skills. One study found that over half of children with voice disorders had a concomitant articulation disorder and language disorders were found in over 40% of the children in the study.[12] Children who have gone through periods of intubation or tracheostomies are at high risk for language and speech delays due to prolonged periods of aphonia.[1]

All the above considerations make the voice evaluation team pivotal in the care of a child with a voice disorder. Undiagnosed voice disorders can result in difficulties in school and later in life. The team, in consultation with parents and teachers, will be required to present an argument for treatment based at times on current functional limitations, but also at times based on presumed functional limitations that will present if the disorder is allowed to continue to run its course. These recommendations must be clinically correlated and prioritized appropriately among other, sometimes complex, medical conditions. A thorough voice evaluation will not only tell us about the quality and function of the voice, but can also provide us with a guide for how we might remediate the problem with therapy.

The purpose of this chapter is to provide a guideline for understanding the unique factors at play in the evaluation of a child with a voice disorder and to provide a framework for structuring the evaluation and eliciting the vocal behaviors needed for decision making.

CHILDREN VERSUS ADULTS— A COMPARISON

Guidelines and protocols for use in the pediatric realm are extremely limited. Most of the protocols for voice diagnostics have been written for adults. Most of the textbooks are also based on the adult model. In this section, we present several broad areas of consideration when approaching evaluation of a child with a voice disorder.

Anatomy and Physiology

A complete description of the anatomic and physiologic differences between children and adults can be found elsewhere in this book. Therefore, we offer only a brief summary here.

The infant larynx sits high in the neck with the lower border of the cricoid cartilage reportedly resting around the level of C2-C4.[13,14] The shape of the pediatric larynx is also different from that of adults, with the thyroid cartilage taking on a more semicircular shape[13,15] and the epiglottis more likely to be omega-shaped.[15] A greater percentage of the glottis is cartilaginous in children than in adults, with the ratio of the membranous to the cartilaginous portion progressing from 1.5 in the newborn to 5.5 in the adult male.[13] There is no differentiation of the vocal ligament until nearly 4 years of age[13-15] and the low calcification of laryngeal cartilages leaves the entire larynx more flexible than that of an adult.[15] An examination of the thyrohyoid space reveals that the hyoid bone overlaps the edge of the thyroid cartilage of the larynx, reducing the thyrohyoid space to a narrow seam.[15,16] Of particular importance in the management of airway issues is the size of the larynx in relation to the tracheobronchial tree, which is comparatively larger in infants than adults.[16]

One organizing factor in considering the differences between the child larynx and the adult larynx is the prioritization of food and the airway over other functions in early life. The position and shape of the mechanism at birth supports rapid alternation between swallowing and breathing.

Voice Norms

Given the vast anatomic and physical changes that take place in the vocal mechanism between birth and adulthood, it stands to reason that acoustic, aerodynamic, and perceptual parameters will be different between the two groups. Nonetheless, no reliable set of norms has been specifically developed for the pediatric population. Small sample sizes and differences in voice elicitation techniques make current studies difficult to interpret.

Acoustic measures will be impacted by children's high fundamental and formant frequencies due to their vocal tract being shorter and smaller in diameter than an adults'.[17] Tables 3–1 and 3–2 present normative acoustic and maximum phonation time measures for children. Separate normative values for jitter and shimmer have not been presented, but Leeper[7] did find increased jitter among children with vocal fold nodules when compared to matched peers without vocal fold lesions. Campisi and colleagues[18] determined that the acoustic profiles of prepubescent boys and girls were similar and that children with vocal fold nodules did have consistently increased perturbation measures. Of note, however, Boltezar[19] discovered increased instability overall in vowel production among children, in particular in boys. Therefore, perturbation measures must be interpreted with caution in the pediatric population. Repeated measures and female settings for vowel production tasks will minimize the impact of this instability and compensate for the fact that acoustic analysis programs are more likely to make mistakes in interpreting signals with a high fundamental frequency.[17] Nonetheless, Boltezar[19] cautions that no one voice analysis parameter used in his study was capable of discerning normal variation from pathology.

Increased fundamental and formant frequency values in children can make spectrograms difficult to interpret as high fundamental frequency creates less defined formants. This may be aided by setting a wider filter in order to read the formants more accurately.[17]

Table 3–1. Acoustic Normative Measures of Children

Average Fundamental Frequency: Speech			
Age/Sex	Norm	SD/Range	Source
7y/F	294	—	Fairbanks, Wiley, & Lassman (1949)[45]
7y/M	281	—	
8y/F	297	—	
8y/M	288	—	
8y2m/F	235	221–258	Bennet (1983)[46]
8y2m/M	234	204–270	
9y2m/F	228	215–239	
9y2m/M	226	198–263	
10y2m/F	228	215–239	
10y2m/M	224	208–259	
11y2m/F	221	200–244	
11y2m/M	216	195–259	
10 to 12y/F	237.5	198–271	Horii (1983)[47]
10 to 12y/M	226.5	192–269	
Average Fundamental Frequency: Sustained Vowels			
Age/Sex	Norm	SD/Range	Source
3y	298	30.8	Eguchi & Hirsh (1969)[48]
4y	286	20.9	
5y	289	46.3	
6y	271.2	27.9	
7y	262.5	38.5	
8y	261	31.1	
9y	262.5	35.9	
10y	261.9	32.9	
11y/F	252.5	42.5	
11y/M	244.2	24.4	
12y/F	248.6	19.2	
12y/M	243.2	26.8	
13y/F	239.8	19.6	
13y/M	221.1	66.4	

continues

Table 3–1. *continued*

Perturbation Measures: Sustained /a/			
Acoustic Measure	**Norm**	**SD**	**Source**
Jitter %	1.24	0.07	Campisi et al (2002)[18]
RAP	0.75	0.04	
Shimmer %	3.35	0.12	
NHR	0.11	0.002	

Intensity Measures (dB SPL) with SD: Sustained /a/				
Age/Sex	**Soft**	**Medium**	**Loud**	**Source**
4y/F	73.79 (2.30)	80.82 (3.44)	91.04 (5.54)	Stathopolous & Sapienza (1993)[21]
4y/M	73.12 (3.88)	82.49 (3.68)	89.91 (4.80)	
8y/F	74.58 (3.68)	81.14 (4.66)	90.01 (9.05)	
8y/M	73.66 (2.62)	80.8 (3.41)	91.34 (8.09)	

Speech: Fairbanks, Wiley, & Lassman, 1949.[45] Normal children reading a 52-word passage embedded in a longer reading passage.

Bennet, 1983.[46] 15 boys and 10 girls measured over the period of 3 years, reading "There is a sheet of paper in my coat pocket."

Horii, 1983.[47] 36 10- to 12-year-old children reading the Rainbow Passage and the Zoo Passage.

Sustained Vowels: Eguchi & Hirsh, 1969.[48] Average fundamental frequency of 6 vowels produced 5 times. Five subjects in each age group.

Perturbation Measures: Campisi et al, 2002.[18] 100 children (50 girls and 50 boys) sustaining 'ah' three times at a comfortable pitch. Multi-Dimensional Voice Program (MDVP) in conjunction with Computerized Speech Lab (CSL) was used for acoustic analysis.

Intensity Measures: Stathopolous & Sapienza, 1993.[21] Twenty 4-year-olds and 20 8-year-olds produced three trials of syllable trains on /pa/ at soft, comfortable, and loud vocal intensity levels.

When looking at volume dynamics, Stothopoulus[20] noted that children increase pitch more dramatically when asked to get louder as compared to adults because their vocal folds are smaller and more easily influenced by increases in subglottic pressure.

Aerodynamic measurements will be impacted by respiratory differences between children and adults. Table 3–3 presents normative subglottic measures for children. Stathopoulos and Sapienza[21] found children generate lung pressures 50 to 100% greater than adults. In association with this, rib cage excursion can be twice that of adults due to their smaller capacity and the need to move their rib cages more to achieve the same lung volume displacement. Compared to adults, children work harder to use their voices. They use a higher subglottic pressure and have shorter maximum phonation time.[13] Children use a high percentage of rib cage contribution to breathing, versus abdominal contribution when compared to adults.[20] Baker[2] cautions us that true vocal fold vibration is necessary for the accurate measurement of a number of aerodynamic parameters, including measurement of open quotient, speech quotient, and maximum flow declination rate. He proposes that average airflow rate in children who have undergone laryngeal-tracheal reconstruction, although more variable overall, is more accurate when assessing a child with true vocal fold vibration.

Given the complications and artifacts involved in the acoustic and aerodynamic assessment of children, the perceptual rating of voice remains a key component in determination of the severity of the functional voice limitation. For children, we may rate voice using a traditional GRBAS[22] scale or the CAPE-V.[23] The necessity of children to take more frequent breaths and use greater rib cage movement during speech must be taken into account during the perceptual evaluation.

Table 3–2. Normative Ranges in MPT Measures in Children

Age/Sex	Norm (range)	Source
3–5y	6–10 seconds	Finnegan (1984)[49]
6–9y	14–17 seconds	
10–12y	15–22 seconds	

Finnegan, 1984.[49] 286 normal children, ages 3 to 17, were instructed to sustain the vowel /a/ for as long as possible for 14 trials.

Table 3–3. Average Subglottal Pressure at Varying Intensity and Pitches

Average Subglottal Pressure (H_2O) at Varying Intensity (with SD)				
	Soft	**Medium**	**Loud**	**Source**
4y/F	5.37 (1.62)	8.46 (2.05)	14.55 (3.22)	Stathopolous & Sapienza (1993)[21]
4y/M	5.6 (2.49)	8.75 (4.15)	13.83 (4.44)	
8y/F	6.21 (1.57)	8.24 (2.11)	11.98 (3.11)	
8y/M	5.97 (2.23)	7.95 (2.03)	11.75 (3.47)	
Average Subglottal Pressure (H_2O) at Varying Pitches (with SD)				
	Low	**Comfortable**	**High**	**Source**
6y–10y11m	8.72 (2.91)	9.29 (2.97)	9.86 (3.16)	Weinrich et al (2005)[50]

Stathopolous & Sapienza, 1993.[21] Twenty 4-year-olds and 20 8-year-olds produced three trials of syllable trains on /pa/ at soft, comfortable, and loud vocal intensity levels.

Weinrich, Salz, & Hughes, 2005.[50] 75 children between the ages of 6 and 10 years 11 months were asked to produce a sustained /a/ at low, comfortable, and high pitches.

Cognition and General Speech and Language Development

Special consideration must be given to the child's level of cognitive development during the evaluation process. Age alone should not be the sole determinant of cognitive expectations. Rather, the child's functional cognitive level will guide the clinician in terms of the vocabulary he or she uses and the manner in which he or she elicits evaluation tasks.

Very young children may be shy around new people. Therefore, directing your initial introduction to the parent rather than the child may be helpful in allowing the child to get comfortable in the evaluation environment.

Children also tend to be concretely oriented. Cues that rest firmly in the five senses, such as seeing, feeling, and hearing will be more successful than abstract cues in eliciting the behaviors you are looking for. Young children, in particular, may be approached with games or play to elicit vocal behaviors.

Evaluation of the voice should also account for the possibility of concurrent speech, language and developmental delays.[12] There is some evidence to show that sensory motor or other oral motor deficits may coincide with voice disorders in children.[12]

Behaviors

Andrews[24] listed "high risk factors" with regard to interpersonal behaviors, such as talking too much, ignoring feedback, ignoring differences between people and situations, ignoring the needs and interests of others and aggressive behavior. Akif Kilic[8] suggested that boys who get vocal fold nodules are those who are active and who scream. Green[25] compared a group of children with vocal fold nodules to matched normal peers in terms of their parents' responses to the Walker Problem Behavior Identification Checklist. Those with vocal fold nodules rated significantly higher, in particular on the Acting Out scale and as a group were found to be distractible and immature with less stable peer relations.

Special Diagnoses

Advances in neonatal care have resulted in an increase in the number of children who have undergone sometimes numerous, invasive medical procedures at a very young age. It is currently estimated that approximately 12% of babies are born at less than 37 weeks gestation.[8] Although vocal fold nodules are the most common diagnosis for school-age children, very young children presenting with disorders of the laryngeal mechanism are more likely to have subglottic stenosis, laryngomalacia, or vocal fold paralysis.[26]

Knowledge of the specific anatomic and physiologic changes caused by these disorders is crucial in evaluating these medically fragile children. Detailed discussions can be found elsewhere in this text.

Considerations for Functional Impairment

Numerous children who are known to have dysphonia do not receive treatment for the disorder. This is often the result of a misunderstanding of or lack of knowledge regarding the long-term consequences of nontreatment. Conversely, parents of children who have struggled with life-threatening airway issues may consider dysphonic voicing to be a minor nuisance in comparison.[2]

Nonetheless, a voice disorder can have a significant impact on a child's ability to participate in daily activities. Ruddy[27] suggests that children with voice disorders may display decreased classroom participation that will negatively impact learning by decreasing their opportunity to benefit from instructor feedback and practice time. Among activities that are potentially negatively impacted by the presence of a voice disorder are peer interaction, teacher evaluation of the student, extracurricular activities (such as music or cheerleading), interviewing, and internship opportunities.[2,27]

Some parents and pediatricians believe that children will grow out of their voice disorder. Instead, a chronic voice disorder may prompt the child to develop maladaptive compensations that become habituated and more difficult to modify as the child grows to adulthood.[27] This is particularly important considering the large number of professions that require high-level spoken communication skills.

THE SPEECH-LANGUAGE PATHOLOGIST'S ROLE IN PEDIATRIC VOICE EVALUATION

Voice evaluations may be done in conjunction with the otolaryngologist, at a specialized clinic, in a hospital, or school setting. Referrals sources include parents, doctors, teachers, and school-based speech-language pathologists. Speech-language pathologists are often called on to address the nonmedical aspects of dysfunctional voice. With a strong background in the anatomy and physiology of the larynx, feeding and swallowing, cognition, and speech, speech-language pathologists are well equipped to assess behavioral issues that may be contributing to the voice disorder and subsequently establish an effective treatment program targeting these behaviors. The speech-language pathologist's holistic understanding of the communication process and the anatomic

and physiologic underpinnings allows him or her to treat the whole child in an integrated manner.

Medically complex children often have a history of emergency surgical intervention to preserve the airway, which by its nature does not consider the functional limitations imposed on the child once healing has taken place. In some cases, the speech-language pathologist may provide education to medical personnel regarding the benefits of speech therapy intervention in establishing a functional voice in the absence of a structurally normal voicing mechanism.

THE EVALUATION PROCESS

Multidisciplinary Teams

The evaluation of a child with a voice disorder is best accomplished in a multidisciplinary team that includes an otolaryngologist, a speech-language pathologist, the child's pediatrician, the child's parents, the school nurse, and perhaps specialists (eg, pulmonologist, gastroenterologist, neurologist, allergist). The speech-language pathologist often serves as the liaison between the parents, the school, and the medical team. Throughout the evaluation process the speech-language pathologist will gather and clinically correlate information from the various medical specialties and communicate this plainly to the parents and school. Important new information gleaned from the interview process may in turn be relayed to the doctor.

From Recognition to Diagnosis

Recognition of a voice disorder and the need for evaluation may originate from a variety of sources, including the child's parent, pediatrician, teacher or school-based speech-language pathologist. Once the need for evaluation has been identified, the child's first stop is usually to their pediatrician, who will refer the child to a pediatric otolaryngologist. The otolaryngologist will then refer appropriate children to the speech-language pathologist for evaluation. At this point in the process, evaluations from other specialists, such as allergists or gastroenterologists will be obtained as necessary.

The Pediatric Voice History

Basic History

Many components of a basic history for pediatric voice disorders are similar to those of the adult case history. These will include details regarding the onset of the dysphonia, the progression of symptoms, variability of voice, typical daily voice activities, psychosocial milieu (who lives at home, sibling structure), medications, allergies, surgical history, medical conditions, and vocal hygiene factors (hydration, vocal misuse, environmental exposure to inhaled irritants such as secondhand smoke, and reflux). Even when the child has had extensive medical intervention, a review of the medical history with the parent is important as it may reveal updated information or information that was previously forgotten by the parent. Table 3–4 presents a detailed review of history elements. Appendix 3 is a sample pediatric case history form.

Table 3-4. Pediatric Voice History

Onset	Congenital may include surgery after birth for airway obstruction or a malformation of the anatomy (eg, sulci, web)
	Acquired may include trauma (eg, external injury or intubation), use-related injury (eg, nodules, polyps)
	Was onset sudden or gradual?
	Has the child always been hoarse (eg, even when crying) or did the dysphonia begin with a certain event (medical or circumstantial) or under certain conditions?
Progression of Symptoms	Is the dysphonia progressing from intermittent to constant?
	Is the dysphonia improving overall or becoming worse over time?
Variability of Voice	Are there certain conditions under which the dysphonia worsens (eg, after school, with certain friends, during certain seasons, time of day, after eating certain foods)
Developmental History	Was the child born premature (at how many weeks)? Were there other complications in the birthing process?
	Is the child seeing any other therapists (eg, physical therapist, occupational therapist, psychotherapist)?
Speech-Language History	Are there other speech-language delays (articulation disorder, receptive/expressive language, learning disabilities, global delays)? Is the child dysfluent?

continues

Table 3-4. *continued*

Typical Daily Voice Activities	This question will help the speech-language pathologist to determine not only what behaviors may be maintaining the dysphonia, but what the child's functional needs are in his/her community.
	How often does the child use loud voice, scream, make character voices?
	What are the child's extracurricular activities (eg, sports, acting, singing)?
	Has the child had to stop any activities because of her voice problems?
Psychosocial Milieu	Who lives at home with the child? What communication style is used within the family (eg, constantly talking over each other versus quiet group activities)?
	Is anyone at home hard of hearing?
	How is the child's relationship with their siblings (Is there animosity or competition? Do they fight?)
	Is this child very talkative or does the child have an aggressive personality?
	Does the child have many friends? Is the child left out of group activities with other children due to his/her poor intelligibility or "funny sounding" voice?
Medications	Consider whether or not the child's medications may be impacting the dysphonia (eg, drying medications, medications that affect the child's energy level or affect).
	Special consideration should be given to asthma medications, which may contribute to hoarseness or laryngeal candidiasis.
Allergies	Have the child's allergies been properly diagnosed and treated?
	Is the child a chronic mouth-breather due to allergic congestion?
	Are allergies long-standing or recent?
	Are food allergies present? To what extent are these controlled?
Surgical History	Consider the impact of surgeries such as tracheal or laryngeal reconstruction, cardiac surgery, oromaxillary facial reconstruction.
Other Medical Conditions	These may include developmental disorders, chromosomal disorders, cerebral palsy, apraxia, seizures. These conditions may impact the child's cognitive level and ability to participate in therapy as well as suggest certain modifications that may be necessary to the therapy program.
Vocal Hygiene Factors	How much water does the child drink?
	Does the child have reflux (eg, mini throw-ups, repeat taste after dinner, soreness in the back of their throat)

Cultural considerations regarding family communication and the role of the child in the family and social structure may affect the manner in which evaluation tasks are conducted. Gaining an understanding of these factors prior to or during the initial interview with the child's parent or caregiver will aid you in acquiring the most accurate evaluation information possible. Some examples of this may include children who are raised to respond to but not initiate communication with adults, or a child in the social service system who lacks trust in the integrity of the intentions of adults.

Unique considerations for the pediatric population include: the details of the child's birth history, general development across domains (physical, cognitive, social/pragmatic, and communication—including articulation, vocabulary development, receptive language, and fluency).

Medically Complex Children

A history of airway complications and congenital conditions or acquired injuries will be particularly important for medically complex children. Examples of medically complex diagnoses include: laryngeal stenosis, papillomatosis, laryngomalacia, laryngeal web, craniofacial syndromes, infantile intubation injuries, vocal fold paralysis, and tracheostomy. A thorough understanding of these pediatric voice etiologies will be important in guiding the direction of your evaluation.

Specific Evaluation Tasks

Children have a shorter attention span than adults and tend to be more distractible. Directing the child in such a way as to collect the voice measures needed can be challenging. In this section, we outline specific voice evaluation tasks that may comprise a typical voice evaluation for a dysphonic child and provide ideas for how to obtain each measure as accurately and quickly as possible.

General Tips

Tips to improve child participation:

1. Do not present yourself too aggressively to younger children. Begin by speaking casually with the parent, addressing the child directly when the child has had the opportunity to adjust to the new environment.
2. As in early intervention, a young child may be more apt to carry out a task when accompanied by a favorite toy. Involve the parents by asking them to bring a favorite toy or book for discussion.
3. Take your time, allow the child to process what is going on.
4. For younger children, provide concrete instructions.
5. Never jump into the task without explaining first.
6. Make use of play in demonstrating the task using a child's favorite toy or puppet first. This may open them to performing the task themselves or engaging in imaginative play, taking on the persona of a puppet. This is often less threatening and more fun.
7. When recording the child, Visi-Pitch can offer a pleasing visual aid in guiding the child through maximum phonation time, pitch glides, and connected speech tasks.
8. Always repeat tasks several times (if possible) as performance may vary greatly.

Oral-Motor Assessment

The oral-motor assessment evaluates the strength, speed, coordination, and range of motion of the oral-facial mechanism as well as inspects for structural deviations that could be interacting with or exacerbating the child's vocal symptoms. A screening of the cranial nerves, as far as the child can comply with this, is useful in determining whether the child's voice disorder is related to a more broad reaching neurologic condition.[28] A thorough oral-motor assessment will help to rule out a motor speech disorder such as developmental apraxia of speech or dysarthria. There are three areas of particular interest to this assessment: oral structure, oral movement skills (lips, tongue, jaw), and motor speech function (articulation in single words, connected speech, and diadochokinesis).[29]

It is not uncommon to find that fluency and articulation disorders coincide with a voice disorder.[30] Articulation skills should be screened with regard to age-related articulatory processes and delayed phonological patterns. If one suspects a lingering articulation disorder that is not currently being treated, a quick screening test may be in order, for example, the Fluharty preschool speech and language screening test.[31]

Speech Sample and Perceptual Assessment

In this task, we are interested in several domains. These include the child's vocal characteristics, learning style, temperament, motivation, and social interaction with their caregiver.[32] The speech-language pathologist may use a simple GRBAS[22] scale (Grade, Roughness, Breathiness, Asthenia, Strain) or the CAPE-V[23] (Consensus Auditory Perceptual Evaluation of Voice) to rate aspects of the child's voice quality such as roughness, breathiness, strain, phonation breaks, and the presence of hard glottal attacks. Also, during this conversational task, one may observe the child's alertness, attention, muscle tone, and overall emotional stability.[32] Difficulty attending, poor emotional stability, and erratic social interaction may be symptomatic of more in-depth behavioral problems that may be driving or adding to the severity of the voice disorder.[25]

One easy way to elicit this task is to observe parent-child interaction during free play. If the child attends the evaluation with a sibling, the speech-language pathologist can document whether sibling relationship factors stimulate more stressful vocal patterns. If the child is reluctant to participate in free play in an unfamiliar environment, a structured activity such as book reading may engage the child in discussion of the characters and story line. Monologue can be encouraged by asking the child to retell the story you have just read. Use of picture description or open-ended questions (best for older children) such as "Tell me what you like to do in the summer time?" may also elicit longer utterances.

Rate of speech may be calculated from the speech sample as a simple count of syllables per minute.

Tension and Breath Patterns

As mentioned previously, children naturally take more frequent breaths with larger ribcage excursion. Nonetheless, truly uncoordinated breathing patterns may still be observed. In particular, one must attend to clavicular breathing, shallow or inadequate breath replenishment, and extraneous muscular effort in the strap muscles of the neck upon inhalation. Respiratory incoordination will impact speech patterns as well, including choppy/short sentences or running out of air at the ends of phrases.

Some of the information you need may be gleaned from parents, who may be important informants in reporting how much the child "works" to phonate at the end of the day and if they push through increasing hoarseness. To directly observe the child's respiratory patterns, you may try having the child count or say the alphabet and measure syllables per breath. Does the child have to push their breath to reach the end of the phrase? Does the child's breath pattern change as the child progresses through the numbers or letters?

Pitch and Volume Range

Pitch and volume measures are important in mapping out the parameters of vocal flexibility. Many times children with voice problems may exhibit increased instability at the extremes of their range where vocal quality is more easily disrupted by changes in biodynamic quality of vocal folds. As pitch and volume are the major building blocks of spoken inflection, vocal inflexibility can negatively impact intelligibility and speech naturalness. Volume irregularities also may also be indicative of the state of the vocal folds. For example, some children with voice problems have difficulty producing soft voicing and use increased volume in compensation for poor glottal valving.[14]

As young children do not have an abstract understanding of pitch and volume control, cues to obtain these measures should be concrete and related to sounds with which they are familiar. Modeling and frequent praise for attempts is important in this realm.[33]

Pitch Flexibility. High and low pitch may be obtained with visual aids such as the Visi-Pitch with which the child can use his or her voice to draw a hill on the screen. If you have no access to this type of equip-

ment, simpler means may include having the child trace his or her finger up and down a hill on a piece of paper while vocalizing. Moya Andrews[34] uses an image of stairs on which the child can move his or her voice up to the "attic" of a house and then down to the "basement." In addition, she describes using an animal in order to "climb" to the top and bottom of the stairs for maximal high and maximal low pitches.[34]

Volume Flexibility. Volume, like pitch, may be approached through the use of metaphors such as animals. Large animals elicit a louder voice; small animals elicit a softer voice.[35] One may also utilize prompts that elicit naturalistic behavior, such as "A voice you would use in the library" or "the voice you would use on the playground." Cognitive cues[36] like "shhh don't wake the baby" or "hey there!" are another route to naturalistic volume variation.

Inflection. Observation of volume and pitch use during conversation may be revealing as well. Inflection may be assessed during collection of the speech sample.

Maximum Phonation Time

This measure will provide the speech-language pathologist with important information regarding the efficiency of coordination between the respiratory and phonatory systems. Maximum phonation time may be difficult to attain depending on the cognitive level of the child.

A stuffed animal may be used to demonstrate the task, with the child repeating.[34] Tracing the path of an object from start to finish, such as a "walking" stuffed animal or a toy truck or car driving across the floor makes the task request more concrete. Use of an object getting to its destination, tracing the path of an object from start to finish, or stretching a slinky across a table or floor all suggest prolongation. As maximum phonation time is an unfamiliar task for most children, multiple trials will lead to more accurate results.

Recording Acoustic and Aerodynamic Measures

When recording acoustic measures, it is ideal to have a headgear-mounted microphone to avoid the effect of body shifting and maintain consistency of mouth to microphone distance. For very young children, use of a table microphone or a lapel microphone allows for gross method of recording the child's voice (but is not sensitive enough for research purposes).

Aerodynamic measures must be collected using a Rothenberg mask. Use of this equipment requires proper sizing. In addition, some children may experience anxiety associated with the placement of the mask and the need to create a seal around the nose and mouth.[37]

Stimulability Tasks

The child's response to stimulability tasks will provide the therapist with information regarding the child's ability to participate in direct therapy methods and which task types elicit the best voicing. Stimulability techniques may focus on decreasing muscular tension, improving airflow or improving vocal quality. These may include decreasing or increasing rate, increasing attention to resonance, exaggerating articulation, negative practice, or imitation of therapist.[14]

Quality of Life Survey

A quality of life (QOL) questionnaire reveals information about the way in which a voice disorder is affecting a patient's life. It is typ-

ically used as a supplementary tool in the context of a complete evaluation. Although several questionnaires have been developed and widely used to measure QOL in adults (Voice Handicap Index,[38] Voice Outcome Survey,[39] Voice-Related Quality of Life[40]), questionnaires for children, in regard to voice, remain somewhat underdeveloped.[41] Each of the adult questionnaires has been modified to address pediatric voice concerns. These include the Pediatric Voice Outcomes Survey (PVOS),[42] the Pediatric Voice-Related Quality of Life questionnaire (PV-RQOL),[43] and the Pediatric Voice Handicap Index (pVHI).[44]

The PVOS is a 4-item parent-proxy questionnaire that rates the overall severity of the child's speaking voice, level of strain, and limitations faced by the child in social and noisy environments. The PVOS is simple to administer and to complete and sensitive to changes in voice-related quality of life; however, it is thought to be somewhat limited in scope. The PV-RQOL is a 10-item parent-proxy questionnaire that was designed to measure both social-emotional and physical functioning aspects of voice problems. More recently, the pVHI is a 23-item parent proxy questionnaire developed by Zur et al.[44] This tool focuses on the functional, physical, and emotional impacts of a voice disorder on a child's daily activities. Both the PV-RQOL and the pVHI are broader in scope than the PVOS and therefore thought to be more sensitive to subtle changes in voice QOL over time.

Stroboscopic Examination

Most children being evaluated for a voice disorder will experience some anxiety surrounding the stroboscopic examination. Children with complex medical conditions, in particular, may have a history of invasive and painful procedures. For this reason, the environment in which the stroboscopic examination will be conducted should be calming and the examiner should not appear to be rushed.

The examiner may wish to conduct a brief "show and tell" session with an anxious child, allowing the child to touch the instrument or put it to their tongue in order to acclimate to the feeling and increase the child's feeling of control over the environment. Some children may be motivated by the promise of seeing the photographs after the examination is complete. Younger children may be more comfortable supported on their parent's lap. Regardless of the manner in which the child is prepared for stroboscopy, the examination should be completed as quickly as possible.[14]

Discussion with Parent

Discussion with the parent begins with the initial interview and continues through the review of the findings and generation of the treatment plan.

During the initial interview, the therapist should praise the parent for things they have already done to improve their child's voice, even if those attempts were small or ultimately unhelpful. This establishes an internal locus of control within the family network and encourages the family taking future steps to help the child through the intervention process.

At the completion of the evaluation, the therapist should discuss the plan of intervention and answer any questions. The parent should understand what is happening and why and have the opportunity to participate in the formulation of the treatment plan. Interventions should be discussed in terms of the family's daily life schedule. The therapist may need to help the family problem solve for creation of practice time.

The conclusion of the evaluation may be a good time to introduce simple guidelines for vocal hygiene or to present a "voice tracker" sheet on which they can keep track of potentially harmful vocal behaviors.

CASE STUDIES

Case #1: A Child with Vocal Abuse

Comprehensive History

Emily was a 7-year-old second grader and well adjusted socially and academically. Her mother noted that Emily's voice had been "hoarse and husky" since she was able to talk, but found that in the past 6 to 7 months her voice quality had become much more "gravelly" and hoarse. Symptoms included persistent hoarseness, difficulty getting loud, frequent pitch breaks, frequent voice loss (especially after increased or aggressive voice use or at the end of the day), and vocal fatigue with strain. Additional medical history was significant for Hashimoto's disease (hypothyroidism) and juvenile arthritis.

The otolaryngologic report indicated Emily had a right vocal fold cyst with a left vocal fold reactive nodule. In addition, there were indications of laryngopharyngeal reflux (edema and erythema surrounding the arytenoids). Closure patterns revealed an hourglass shape. Emily had not been sick or suffering from allergies when her voice worsened.

Emily's mother described her as a very loud and verbal child who talked constantly at home and in school. She was the "leader of the pack" often raising her voice to be heard above others and gaining attention through grunting or squealing. Her mother reported that Emily would often yell in anger when fighting with her older sister, yell in excitement when playing with her friends, and engage in a guttural grunting sound when playing or refusing to do something. She noted that by the end of the day, Emily talked in a whisper, or pushed her voice to a much louder volume; "There's no middle ground." Her vocal symptoms were mild to moderately disruptive and lowered her overall intelligibility. When asked, Emily noted that her voice was not a problem; however, her mother found Emily's frequent voice loss to be worrying as people were having more difficulty understanding her. Emily drank 2 to 3 glasses of water per day and had 1 glass of chocolate milk per day.

Speech Sample and Perceptual Measures

During the interview and in spontaneous conversation, Emily was noted to talk relatively fast with a markedly monotone intonation pattern. Her voice was consistently too low for her and nearly all of her phrases ended in vocal fry. Emily's voice quality was noted to be consistently severely hoarse and breathy with frequent voice breaks and delayed voiced onset. Resonance was severely reduced, although during maximum phonation, voice quality was markedly better at the beginning of her production and deteriorated by the end of the tone.

Tension and Breathing Patterns

During conversation and in more structured tasks, Emily appeared to be straining most visibly in her strap muscles and also in her shoulders and jaw. Respiratory behaviors during conversation and reading included shallow, audible, and seemingly effortful inhalation initiated with her chest and shoulders raised. Once having taken a breath,

Emily often spoke too long on one breath, pushing past her resting expiratory level in attempts to force out the rest of the phrase.

Pitch and Volume Range

Emily's pitch was consistently too low for her age and sex. In addition, pitch flexibility or intonation was also noticeably reduced, lending to a monotone pattern which often dropped off into vocal fry. She had difficulty controlling her volume during loud and soft tasks. In loud tasks, voicing was effortful, and often felt uncomfortable to her. In softer tasks, voicing was moderately inconsistent and she had difficulty sustaining easy, soft voicing and frequently vacillated between aphonic intervals and louder abrupt onset phonation.

Acoustic Measures

1. Pitch Range = 238 to 440 Hz (A#3–A4 = 11 ST)
2. Loudness Range = 64 to 119 dB SPL
3. Average Fundamental Frequency (taken on sustained "ah") = 277 Hz
4. Loudness (during reading of Rainbow Passage) = 67 dB SPL
5. Perturbation Measures (taken on sustained "ah"): jitter (1.6%) and shimmer (4.9%)
6. MPT = 4.0

Aerodynamic Measures

Emily exhibited increased subglottal air pressure in both comfortable and loud phonation (taken with the pneumotachometer using inverse filtering on "pae-pae-pae" repetitions).

Quality of Life Survey

Both Emily and her mother filled out a QOL survey, which revealed a difference in perceived difficulty in the efficiency of voice use. Emily's mother's rating was much higher, indicating more functional limitations; whereas Emily's ratings were low. When this was discussed during the evaluation, both Emily and her mother came to an agreement that her vocal quality was beginning to get in the way of playing with friends and speaking up in class.

Impressions

When taking acoustic measures, an analysis of a sustained 'ah' in her speaking pitch revealed increased pitch and volume perturbation (jitter and shimmer %). Her fundamental frequency was too low for her age and sex. Her volume during reading (Rainbow Passage) was slightly above normal dB SPL. Further vocal testing revealed a markedly limited maximum phonation time and pitch range. When asked to sustain the quietest voice possible, Emily had difficulty getting below 64 dB SPL, a volume considered to be more akin to conversational voice.

Emily presents with a typical profile of a patient with a diagnosis of vocal fold masses. Her videoendoscopic evaluation findings of poor vocal fold closure coincides with perceptual measures of increased breathiness and acoustic findings of reduced maximum phonation time. In addition, a large vocal fold cyst, in Emily's case, may explain reduced vocal loudness and pitch dynamics, lowered pitch (due to increased vocal fold mass), and increased hoarseness (which coincides with high perturbation measures of jitter and shimmer).

Trial Therapy

When Emily was asked to breathe easily before each trial of sustained phonation on "ah," her vocal quality became clearer and more resonant, although breathiness was still present. She was then introduced to the concepts of "easy" versus "strained" voicing. Easy voice was characterized as smooth and relaxed with somewhat increased airflow; strained voicing was described at gravelly and tense. Initially, Emily relied on frequent models from the therapist. She quickly identified when the therapist used strained versus easy voicing and benefited from negative practice. This helped her to gain a better understanding of the effects of deliberately increased tension on her own voice quality. Easy voicing was then carried into humming with continued focus on smooth quality and relaxed sense of production. This was initiated with vowels and then slowly carried into m-initial words and phrases. Emily was attentive to tasks and noticed the difference in levels of effort when using an easy voice versus strained. Emily's "smooth" voice revealed reduced vocal strain and increased breathiness.

Therapy Plan

Emily was referred for voice therapy in order to decrease vocal strain and improve vocal function. While surgical excision would be an appropriate option for an adult presenting with Emily's profile, a child of this age cannot be expected to maintain absolute voice rest throughout the postsurgical period. Due to the danger of scarring associated with noncompliance with postsurgical voice rest, this option will have to be postponed until Emily reaches a more mature age.

Case #2: A Child with a History of Intubation

Comprehensive History

Jeff was a 3½-year-old boy with a history of premature birth followed by several weeks of intubation. He had a history of pulmonary compromise as well as laryngomalacia. He had global delays in expressive and receptive language and fine and gross motor skills. Jeff had received early intervention and at that time was noted to have a pronounced raspy voice quality to his cry which became more noticeable when he began talking.

Jeff was seen by a pediatric otolaryngologist who performed a brochoscopy with examination of his vocal folds. This examination revealed marked bilateral vocal fold sulci. Closure and mucosal wave could not be evaluated due to the nature of bronchoscopy (Jeff was under general anesthesia).

His mother complained that friends and family found his speech to be extremely difficult to understand and complained of a low-pitched, gravelly, "froggy" voice quality when Jeff became excited or during play. She reported that when Jeff was more relaxed, or when singing, his voice was much higher and softer. This contrast was also noted by his preschool teachers.

Speech Sample and Perceptual Evaluation

Jeff's vocal quality was severely hoarse, breathy, and strained with frequent periods of an abnormally low-pitched, monotone, rough voice quality. Notably, there were moments of voicing that revealed increased breathiness, reduced volume, and a higher pitch more appropriate to a boy his age and size. This was also apparent when he sang a song with his mother.

Tension and Breath Patterns

Visible strain was noted in his upper torso and in the strap muscles of his neck during all voicing tasks. This was much more prominent during loud voicing or when Jeff became excited. Breathing patterns included shallow breathing. Utterances were relatively short during the evaluation; therefore, true documentation of breathing during longer phrases was not available. By parent report, his breathing was more labored when excited.

Pitch and Volume Range

During conversational speech, volume was either extremely loud or too soft. Observation of pitch control revealed a somewhat high, soft quality of voice during relaxed moments of speech and abnormally low speech when excited. During the course of a conversation with his mother, pitch and volume were highly variable depending on context and subject matter.

Acoustic Measures

1. Pitch Range = unattainable due to poor participation
2. Loudness Range = unattainable due to poor participation
3. Average Fundamental Frequency (taken on sustained "ah") = 168 Hz
4. Perturbation Measures (taken on sustained "ah"): jitter (0.73%) and shimmer (7.74%)
5. MPT = 5.3
6. s/z ratio = 0.78

Aerodynamic Measures

Aerodynamics taken with the Rothenberg mask were unachievable due to Jeff's increased activity levels and cognitive level.

Quality of Life Survey

A parent-proxy QOL questionnaire revealed considerable limitations at home and during preschool. Jeff's preschool teacher found it difficult to understand him and interaction with other children was also limited given his low intelligibility. In addition, Jeff was becoming aware of his voice limitations. He was starting to display behavioral indicators of frustration at his inability to be understood by other children, teachers, and family members. His mother became visibly upset when describing the fact that other children often avoided playing with him due to his voice quality and the way in which he became frustrated during communicative exchanges to the point where he simply abandoned the attempt.

Impressions

Pitch and volume control was poor, which contributed to low intelligibility. Articulation delays added to this. Acoustic measures revealed extremely high measures of shimmer and jitter percent, and abnormally low fundamental frequency. Perceptual assessment revealed severely limited frequency and intensity range. Acoustic measures coincided well with perceptual measures and further defined the severity of Jeff's dysphonia.

Jeff's use of false vocal fold vibration as a vocal quality when excited is not uncommon in children who have significant difficulty achieving vocal fold closure prior to language development. It is a strong compensatory strategy used to effectively access increased volume. True vocal fold vibration, in this case, would only yield a soft, breathy vocal quality. In Jeff's case, the use of false vocal fold vibration correlates with perceptual measures of abnormally low, hoarse, monotone, and strained vocal quality. Moments of higher pitch and breathy, weak vocal quality is likely the result of true vocal fold vibration, but may have been too weak for his functional environment. The poor closure pattern created by the bilateral vocal fold sulci would encourage the use of false vocal fold phonation to solve this problem.

Trial Therapy

Trial therapy revealed a higher more stable sound quality with inhalation phonation and increased involvement in therapy activities using musical instruments. For example, when Jeff sang songs with slower rhythms while beating on a drum, his voice quality became more stable.

Treatment Plan

Young children under the age of 5 are best involved in therapy using child-directed techniques as well as implementing small changes in daily routines and places. It was clear that in trial therapy, Jeff had a propensity for playing musical instruments and singing. This was used as the basis for further exploration and treatment at home. Jeff was already receiving speech therapy services for delayed articulation. A phone conference with the voice specialist and the current therapist was planned for integrating several voice activities (musical in nature) into his regular therapy sessions. The goals were to begin increasing Jeff's vocal repertoire and comfort with adapting to different vocal pitches using the easier, but slightly softer voice. With continued focus on building coordination between respiration, phonation, and resonance, overall vocal strength should continue to grow.

Case #3: The Medically Complex Child

Comprehensive History

Molly was a 10-year-old girl with a medically complex background. She was born 3 months premature. Seven chest tubes were placed at birth and she underwent numerous surgical procedures for airway compromise (including laryngomalacia and subglottic stenosis). Laryngeal surgeries included an initial tracheotomy (in infancy) and laryngeal reconstruction using a right floating rib at 5 years of age, which resulted in necrotic tissue formation. She underwent a revision laryngeal reconstruction with tracheotomy and an arytenoid trim several month as a result of these complications. One year later, she underwent t tube placement (airway stent) to maintain airway patency.

Molly had been diagnosed with reflux and was put on a trial of Protonix in the past which did not appear to be helpful (as per Molly's mom). Additional medical history includes adenoidectomy and tonsillectomy. Molly had significant global delays including fine and gross motor development and language and articulation (verbal apraxia). She was receiving speech/language services at school 4 times per week in addition to occupational and physical therapy. A recent stroboscopic examination revealed bilateral vocal fold scarring, limited motion of the left arytenoid cartilage and severe supraglottal constriction during phonation, which limited visualization of vocal fold vibratory characteristics.

Perceptual Assessment and Speech Sample

Voicing during conversation was noted to be severely hoarse, harsh, gravelly, and raspy in quality. Frequent aphonic breaks, low volume, and frequent use of inhalation false vocal fold phonation also noted. Voice quality during inhalation phonation was predominantly low-pitched and somewhat louder, causing erratic shifts in volume and pitch. In turn, this disrupted articulation and

intelligibility. Articulation revealed backed consonants and stopping of sibilants. Overall speech intelligibility was extremely poor.

Tension and Breath Patterns

Respiration was uncoordinated, extremely effortful, audible, and shallow. Visibly low tone was noted in Molly's torso. Respiration patterns during conversation revealed poor breath replenishment with use of inhalation phonation with engagement of the false vocal folds during conversation. Phrase length was particularly long, because Molly used a strategy of inhalation phonation to continue voicing after her breath was depleted. Visible tension sites were noted in the jaw, neck, shoulders, and chest.

Pitch and Volume Range

During spontaneous speech and structured speech tasks, pitch was noted to be consistently too low for Molly's age and size. Pitch variation during speech was also noted to be severely restricted leading to a monotone quality. Volume range was reduced. Although she could attain softer and louder voicing, keeping volume stable for longer than several seconds was difficult.

Acoustic Measures

1. Pitch Range = 149 to 246 Hz (D3–B3 = 9 ST)
2. Loudness Range = 48 to 97 dB SPL
3. Average Fundamental Frequency (taken on sustained "ah") = 182 Hz
4. Loudness (during reading of Rainbow Passage) = 51 dB SPL
5. Perturbation Measures (taken on sustained "ah"): jitter (20%) and shimmer (21%)
6. MPT = 5.0

Aerodynamic Measures

Molly demonstrated extremely high airflow and subglottal pressure at both conversational and loud phonation.

Quality of Life Survey

A QOL questionnaire revealed difficulty academically and socially. In school, teachers had difficulty understanding her and she was often reluctant to participate in class. She was required to use an amplifier in the classroom to be heard. In addition, she had limited interaction with her peers during play and in the classroom due poor intelligibility. Molly was showing signs of embarrassment and social stigma due to the sound of her voice.

Impressions

Respiratory and phonatory coordination was disrupted in several ways; vocal fold closure was inadequate, and expiratory pressure was not sufficient to meet the needs of vocal fold vibration. The use of inhalation phonation in children who are status post-laryngotracheal reconstruction has been documented several times in literature.[1,2] Molly's weak inspiration was insufficient to generate enough force on exhalation to meet the needs of phonation, particularly in the context of having such a stiff vocal mechanism. Therefore, she used her false vocal folds in the context of inhalation phonation to generate greater volume during conversation.

Trial Therapy

In Molly's case, inhalation phonation engaged false vocal fold phonation instead of true vocal fold phonation. This resulted in an extremely low, hoarse voice quality that did not match Molly's age and gender. Intelligibility was significantly negatively impacted by intermittent inhalation phonation, which also appeared to effect articulation. Molly demonstrated little ability to generate the oral pressure needed for plosives and many of her forward consonants were backed.

Abdominal effort released false vocal fold tension, but resulted in weak voice production due to Molly's low muscle tone. A combination of louder volume and increased abdominal support was slightly easier for Molly to manage and resulted in a consistent voice. Negative practice was employed to help Molly distinguish between inhalation phonation and exhalation phonation.

Case #4: The Child with Laryngeal Candidiasis

Comprehensive History

Gary is a 10-year-old boy who complained of chronic hoarseness, lowered pitch, decreased volume, decreased stamina, frequent coughing, and throat clearing. Gary had a long-standing chronic cough. He was diagnosed with asthma the year before and placed on Advair. His mother noted that Gary's voice symptoms began 4 to 5 months previous to his voice evaluation and 2 weeks after starting Singulair. Medical history was otherwise unremarkable.

A stroboscopic examination revealed bilateral nodules on the mid-third of the vocal folds, bilateral medial surface scarring, bilateral medial and superior surface varices, bilateral erythema, laryngopharyngeal reflux, periarytenoid and posterior cricoid edema, and vocal hyperfunction. Results were consistent with a probable fungal infection. During the evaluation, Gary reported that his voice was slowly improving since starting to take Fluconozol, Zantac, and initiating behavioral and dietary precautions for reflux.

Gary and his parents denied any vocally abusive activities (screaming/yelling, incessant talking, creating guttural sounds). Due to his dysphonia, Gary stopped singing in the school choir and at home on the recommendation of his choir teacher. He felt it strained his voice to sing for even short periods of time.

Perceptual Assessment and Speech Sample

Gary was consistently severely hoarse and strained; consistently moderately breathy; with intermittent throat clearing, pitch, and phonation breaks. Vocal pitch was adequate; however, vocal loudness was intermittently too soft. He also exhibited consistently severely decreased oral resonance.

Tension and Breath Patterns

Gary demonstrated shallow breath replenishment with increased visible tension noted in the shoulders, chest, neck, and jaw. Respiratory coordination was noted to be poor with occasional audible inspiration.

Pitch and Volume Range

These measures were within normal limits with the exception of quiet voicing. This would be expected, given the edema and erythema noted on examination.

Acoustic Measurements

1. Pitch Range = 171 to 617 Hz (F3–D#5 = 22 ST)
2. Loudness Range = 65 to 94 dB SPL
3. Average Fundamental Frequency (taken on sustained "ah") = 243 Hz
4. Loudness (during reading of rainbow passage) = 67 dB SPL
5. Perturbation Measures (taken on sustained "ah"): jitter (1.8%) and shimmer (6.3%)
6. MPT = 12.0

Aerodynamic Measurements

Increased airflow and increased subglottal pressure for both conversational and loud voicing.

Quality of Life Survey

Gary was unable to sing with ease; he felt extremely frustrated by his vocal quality and restricted volume range (especially when playing sports or with his friends).

Impressions

Gary was a typically developing child with no history of voice problems prior to this most recent incident. A fungal infection brings about increased edema and erythema of the vocal fold tissue. This leaves the phonatory system much more susceptible to vocal fold injury with use. Gary became increasingly dysphonic as his laryngeal infection progressed. As a result of the vocal fold changes caused by the infection, there was greater pressure required to initiate phonation, which resulted in a change in his voicing patterns for both speech and singing.

Trial Therapy

Increased attention to oral resonance through sustained hums with decreased tension during production resulted in improved voice quality. Carryover into words and phrases revealed decreased breathiness and hoarseness, and diminished laryngeal strain (as evidenced by decreased visible tension).

Gary was quick to learn therapy techniques and found his resonant voice to be much easier to use.

Treatment Plan

Continue using resonance based therapy techniques in order to reduce compensatory behaviors and restore vocal function.

CONCLUSION

Evaluation of pediatric voice disorders is complicated by the vast physical and cognitive differences between children and adults. The majority of research on voice disorders to date has been conducted on adults and is not necessarily applicable to the pediatric population. Special considerations regarding the high survival rate of premature babies and the multiple airway issues that can present also require specialized knowledge. A thorough pediatric voice evaluation may involve input from multiple medical specialties, the child's parents, and school personnel. Evaluation tasks will be similar to those presented in an adult evaluation; however, they may need to be adapted to the needs of various age groups. At times, some measures may be unattainable. The therapy plan is a natural progression from the observations made during the evaluation and will be tailored to each child's specific needs.

REFERENCES

1. Smith ME, Marsh JH, Cotton RT, Myer CM 3rd. Voice problems after pediatric laryngotracheal reconstruction: videolaryngostroboscopic, acoustic, and perceptual assessment. *Int J Pediatr Otorhinolaryngol.* 1993; 25(1-3):173-181.

2. Baker S, Kelchner L, Weinrich B, et al. Pediatric laryngotracheal stenosis and airway reconstruction: a review of voice outcomes, assessment, and treatment issues. *J Voice.* 2006;20(4):631-641.

3. Harvey GL. Treatment of voice disorders in medically complex children. *Lang Speech Hear Serv Schools.* 1994;27:282-291.

4. Gray SD, Smith ME, Schneider H. Voice disorders in children. *Ped Clin North Am.* 1996;43(6):1357-1384.

5. Carding PN, Roulstone S, Northstone K, Team AS. The prevalence of childhood dysphonia: a cross-sectional study. *J Voice.* 2006;20(4):623-630.

6. Lee L, Stemple JC, Glaze L, Kelchner LN. Quick screen for voice and supplementary documents for identifying pediatric voice disorders. *Lang Speech Hear Serv Schools.* 2004;35:308-319.

7. Leeper L. Diagnostic examination of children with voice disorders: a low-cost solution. *Lang Speech Hear Serv Schools.* 1992;23:353-360.

8. Akif Kilic M, Okur E, Yildirim I, Guzelsoy S. The prevalence of vocal fold nodules in school age children. *Int J Pediatr Otorhinolaryngol.* 2004;68(4):409-412.

9. McKinnon DHM, McLeod S, Reilly S. The prevalence of stuttering, voice, and speech-sound disorders in primary school students in Australia. *Lang Speech Hear Serv Schools.* 2007;38:5-15.

10. Powell M, Filter MD, Williams B. A longitudinal study of the prevalence of voice disorders in children from a rural school division. *J Comm Dis.* 1989;22(5):375-382.

11. Roy N, Bless DM. Personality traits and psychological factors in voice pathology: a foundation for future research. *J Speech Lang Hear Res.* 2000;43(3):737-748.

12. St. Louis KO, Hansen GR, Buch JL, Oliver TL. Voice deviations in coexisting communication disorders. *Lang Speech Hear Serv Schools.* 1992;23:82-87.

13. Smith ME, Gray SD. Developmental laryngeal and phonatory anatomy and physiology. *Perspect Voice Voice Dis.* 2002;12.

14. Hersan R, Behlau M. Behavioral management of pediatric dysphonia. *Otolaryngol Clin North Am.* 2000;33(5):1097–1110.

15. Sapienza CM, Ruddy BH, Baker S. Laryngeal structure and function in the pediatric larynx: clinical applications. *Lang Speech Hear Serv Schools.* 2004;35:299–307.

16. Elluru RG. Reconstruction techniques for the treatment of anatomical upper respiratory tract anomalies in children. *Perspect Voice Voice Dis.* 2006;15(3):3–10.

17. Shrivastav R. Acoustic analysis of children's voices. *Perspect Voice Voice Dis.* 2002;12.

18. Campisi P, Tewfik TL, Manoukian JJ, Schloss MD, Pelland-Blais E, Sadeghi N. Computer-assisted voice analysis: establishing a pediatric database. *Arch Otolaryngol Head Neck Surg.* 2002;128(2):156–160.

19. Boltezar IH, Burger ZR, Zargi M. Instability of voice in adolescence: pathologic condition or normal developmental variation? *J Pediatr.* 1997;130(2):185–190.

20. Stathopoulos ET. Consideration of children's voices: understanding age-related processes. *Perspect Voice Voice Dis.* 2002;12(1):8–10.

21. Stathopoulos ET, Sapienza C. Respiratory and laryngeal measures of children during vocal intensity variation. *J Acoust Soc Am.* 1993;94(5):2531–2543.

22. Hirano M. *Clinical Examination of Voice.* New York, NY: Springer-Verlag Wein; 1981.

23. Association TAS-L-H. Consensus auditory-perceptual evaluation of voice. Retrieved May 14, 2007 from: http://www.asha.org/NR/rdonlyres/79EE699E-DAEE-4E2C-A69E-C11BDE6B1D67/_0/CAPEVform.pdf

24. Andrews M. *Voice Therapy for Children.* San Diego, Calif: Singular Publishing Group, Inc; 1986.

25. Green G. Psycho-behavioral characteristics of children with vocal nodules: WPBIC ratings. *J Speech Hear Dis.* 1989;54(3):306–312.

26. Saniga RD, Carlin MF. Vocal abuse behaviors in young children. *Lang Speech Hear Serv Schools.* 1993;24:79–83.

27. Ruddy BH, Sapienza, CM. Treating voice disorders in the school-based setting: working within the framework of idea. *Lang Speech Hear Serv Schools.* 2004;35:327–332.

28. Witzel MA, Riski J. *The Oral Mechanism Examination for Children and Young Adults: Craniofacial and Oral Evaluation.* Rockland, Md: American Speech-Language Hearing Association; 2003.

29. McCauley R, Strand E. *Assessment of children's oral and speech motor skills: A review.* Retrieved March 4, 2007 from: http://www.asha.org/NR/rdonlyres/48052BC4-6AC7-4BD6-82AF-0899858D4F90/_0/985Handout.ppt

30. McAllister A. Voice disorders in children with oral motor dysfunction: perceptual evaluation pre and post oral motor therapy. *Logoped Phoniatr Vocol.* 2003;28(3):117–125.

31. Fluharty NB. *Fluharty-2 Preschool Speech and Language Screening Test.* Austin, Tex: Pro-Ed; 2001.

32. Batshaw ML. *Children with Disabilities.* 5th ed. Baltimore, Md: Paul H. Brookes Publishing Company; 1997.

33. Verdolini K. *Pediatric LMRVT.* Paper presented at: Pittsburgh Voice Conference, 2006; Pittsburgh, Pa.

34. Andrews M. *Voice Treatment for Children and Adolescents.* 2nd ed. San Diego, Calif: Singular Thompson Learning; 2002.

35. Champley EH, Adrews ML. The elicitation of vocal responses from preschool children. *Lang Speech Hear Serv Schools.* 1993;24:146–150.

36. Bohnenkamp TA, Andrews M, Shrivastav R, Summers A. Changes in children's voices: the effect of cognitive cues. *J Voice.* 2002;16(4):530–543.

37. Shrivastav R. Acoustic analysis of children's voices. *Perspect Voice Voice Dis.* 2002;12(1):11–12.

38. Jacobson BH, Johnson A, Grywalski C, et al. The Voice Handicap Index (VHI): development and validation. *Am J Speech-Lang Path.* 1997;6:66–70.

39. Gliklich RE, Glovsky RM, Montgomery WW. Validation of a voice outcome survey for unilateral vocal cord paralysis. *Otolaryn-*

gol-Head Neck Surg. 1999;120(2):153–158.

40. Hogikyan ND, Sethuraman G. Validation of an instrument to measure voice-related quality of life (V-RQOL). *J Voice*. 1999;13(4): 557–569.

41. Zur KB, Cotton S, Kelchner L, Baker S, Weinrich B, Lee L. Pediatric Voice Handicap Index (pVHI): a new tool for evaluating pediatric dysphonia. *Int J Pediatr Otorhinolaryngol*. 2007;71(1):77–82.

42. Hartnick CJ. Validation of a pediatric voice quality-of-life instrument: the pediatric voice outcome survey. *Arch Otolaryngol-Head Neck Surg*. 2002;128(8):919–922.

43. Boseley ME, Cunningham MJ, Volk MS, Hartnick CJ. Validation of the pediatric voice-related quality-of-life survey. *Arch Otolaryngol Head Neck Surg*. 2006;132(7):717–720.

44. Zur KB, Cotton S, Kelchner L, Baker S, Weinrich B, Lee L. Pediatric voice handicap index (pvhi): a new tool for evaluating pediatric dysphonia. *Int J Pediatr Otorhinolaryngol*. 2007;71(1):77–82.

45. Fairbanks G, Wiley JH, Lassman FM. An acoustical study of vocal pitch in seven- and eight-year-old boys. *Child Devel*. 1949; 20(2):63–69.

46. Bennet S. A 3-year longitudinal study of school-aged children's fundamental frequencies. *J Speech Hear Res*. 1983;26:137–142.

47. Horii Y. Automatic analysis of voice fundamental frequency and intensity using a Visi-Pitch. *J Speech Hear Res*. 1983;25:467–471.

48. Eguchi S, Hirsh IJ. Development of speech sounds in children. *Acta Oto Laryngologica Supplement*. 1969;257:1–51.

49. Finnegan DE. Maximum phonation time for children with normal voices. *Folia Phoniatrica*. 1985;37:209–215.

50. Weinrich B, Salz B, Hughes M. Aerodynamic measurements: normative data for children ages 6:0 to 10:11 years. *J Voice*. 2006;19(3): 326–329.

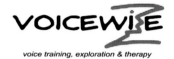

PEDIATRIC CASE HISTORY FORM

Date:_____   Person filling out this form (include relation): _____

Patient Name:_____Date of Birth: _____   Sex: M F
          First   M. I.   Last

Address:

Contact #: Home (   )_____   Work (   )_____
          Email: _____
School and Grade:_____

Background Information

1. Briefly describe your child's voice problem and what you believe is its cause:

2. When was the voice problem first noticed? Was it sudden or gradual?

3. Describe any events or conditions which you associate with the onset of the problem (e.g., cold, increased voice use, yelling, injury)?

4. Over time, has the problem changed (e.g., better, worse, stayed the same)?

5. Has your child had voice problems in the past?

6. Does someone else in your family have a similar problem? If so, who?

7. Is your child's voice worse during certain seasons? Or at a certain time of day (e.g., upon awakening, after school)

8. Are there any situations in which your child's voice is better or seems to improve?

9. Vocal Symptoms (check all that apply)
____**NONE**
____hoarse voice quality   ____effortful/strained speaking
____raspy/scratchy voice quality   ____voice tires easily
____weak/breathy voice quality   ____nasal voice quality
____voice too low   ____stuffed nose quality
____voice too high   ____ trouble speaking loud or soft
____ other: _____

PO Box 126, Dedham, MA 02027   (781) 329 – 2262

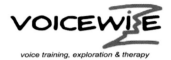

VOICEWISE

voice training, exploration & therapy

10. Voice Use: Does your child engage in these behaviors?

Screaming/yelling (in anger):	Rarely	Sometimes	Constantly
Yelling/Cheering (sports, games, play):	Rarely	Sometimes	Constantly
Talking loudly:	Rarely	Sometimes	Constantly
Talking over noise:	Rarely	Sometimes	Constantly
Aggressive Crying/Tantrums:	Rarely	Sometimes	Constantly
Coughing:	Rarely	Sometimes	Constantly
Throat Clearing:	Rarely	Sometimes	Constantly
Singing:	Rarely	Sometimes	Constantly
Talking on the phone or cell:	Rarely	Sometimes	Constantly
Making Noises during Play (animals, cars):	Rarely	Sometimes	Constantly

11. Has your child ever received voice therapy? If so, please list when, where, and for how long.

Other Symptoms/Circumstances
12. Check the following symptoms or circumstances that apply to your child:
____**NONE**

____frequent sore throats   ____hoarseness first thing in the morning
____chronic cough/throat clearing   ____ night coughing that interrupts sleep
____bad breath / "smelly" burps   ____ regurgitation or "mini throw-ups"
____antacid use   ____anxiety/depression
____other (specify:_____)

13. Does your child frequently eat or drink:
- Sweets/Candy
- Orange Juice/Lemonade
- Very spicy foods
- Heavily fried foods
- Large meals
- Late at night
- On the run

14. Estimate the combined daily servings of; water _____ soda _____ chocolate _____ coffee/tea ___

Medical History
15. Please check any medical conditions:
____**NONE**

____Gastroesophageal reflux   ____Ear infections
____Bronchitis/pneumonia   ____Diabetes
____Asthma   ____Seizures
____Sinus problems   ____Cancer
____Cleft palate   ____Tracheostoma (when: _____)
____ADD and/or Hyperactivity   ____Injury to head/neck/chest
____Medically diagnosed depression/anxiety

PO Box 126, Dedham, MA 02027   (781) 329 – 2262

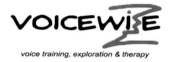
voice training, exploration & therapy

16. Please list any surgical or medical procedures your child has had (include date and place performed)

17. Please list all medications (prescription and over-the-counter) that your child has taken or is currently taking:

18. List all allergies (e.g., dust, animals, foods, medications) and include treatments:

19. Does your child have any diagnosed speech-language learning difficulties?

20. Does your child receive therapeutic/education services? If so list type of therapy and frequency:

PO Box 126, Dedham, MA 02027   (781) 329 – 2262

Voice Quality of Life Instruments

Mark E. Boseley
Christopher J. Hartnick

CORE INFORMATION

1. Validity—face, criterion, and discriminant validity are defined.
2. Reliability—test-retest reliability and internal consistency are defined.
3. The Voice Outcomes Survey (VOS) and Pediatric Voice Outcomes Survey (PVOS) are described.
4. The Voice-Related Quality of Life (V-RQOL) and the Pediatric Voice-Related Quality of Life (PV-RQOL) are described.
5. The Voice Handicap Index (VHI) and Pediatric Voice Handicap Index (pVHI) are described.
6. Conclusion—voice quality of life instruments are important in voice outcomes research and the PV-RQOL seems to offer the most information for the least amount of required time.

INTRODUCTION

One of the difficulties that we have faced in treating children with voice disorders is that we have lacked quantitative data to assess the results of our treatments. Normative acoustic measurements have been published utilizing computer assisted voice analysis software. However, until recently, there was no tool available to determine how this would affect a child's quality of life. The need for such instruments has spurred interest in clinicometrics and psychometrics, which provide the methods to construct and evaluate quality of life surveys. This chapter briefly describes the steps in validating these tools. We also discuss the validated pediatric voice surveys that currently exist and their adult counterparts.

VALIDITY

Before an instrument can be used in a clinical setting, it must first be proven to be valid and reliable. Validity is typically described in terms of face validity, criterion validity, and discriminant validity. The first of these can be explained simply as whether the survey is deemed valid by a group of experts in the field. Criterion validity is then tested by comparing the scores from the instrument with other well-established means of testing. Validating a voice survey in this fashion would involve comparing test scores to results obtained from acoustic measurements and other valid voice instruments that were obtained from the same group of subjects. Discriminant validity describes the ability of a survey to discriminate between two groups of individuals. In the case of patients with voice disorders, the instrument should be able to discriminate patients with voice concerns from those who have no voice concerns.

Reliability must also be tested before a quality of life instrument can be utilized in the office. The two most common means employed to test reliability are test-retest reliability and internal consistency. Test-retest reliability usually involves having a patient complete the instrument twice in a 2-week interval. There is no treatment given during that period of time. Ideally, the answers would be the same on both surveys, thus a change in score could only be explained by the treatment rendered. Internal consistency is tested by sequentially eliminating questions on the survey to determine if the remaining questions are more reliable without the deleted item. This is typically reported as a Cronbach's alpha value with a score >0.55 deemed acceptable.[1]

Until recently, there were no validated voice-specific quality of life surveys for the pediatric population. Fortunately, our adult laryngology colleagues have created several voice instruments that have been used for adult patients. However, these instruments were not, until recently, validated for use in the pediatric population. The three most commonly utilized of these are the Voice Outcome Survey (VOS), the Voice-Related Quality of Life Survey (V-RQOL), and the Voice Handicap Index (VHI). The Pediatric Voice Outcome Survey (PVOS), the Pediatric Voice-Related Quality of Life Survey (PV-RQOL), and the Pediatric Voice Handicap Index (pVHI) are the parent-proxy instrument counterparts that may now be utilized in the general pediatric population. The Pediatric Voice Outcome Survey (PVOS) has also been validated for use in pediatric patients with velopharyngeal insufficiency.

VOS/PVOS

The Voice Outcomes Survey (VOS) was initially validated as a tool to assess voice outcomes following surgery for unilateral vocal fold paralysis. The VOS (Fig 4–1) is a 5-item instrument that was found to be valid, reliable, and responsive to change in a group of patients who had undergone an Isshiki thyroplasty. The brevity of the VOS has both advantages and disadvantages. Although it is easy to administer and to score, the VOS is unable to discern subcategories such as physical and emotional components that contribute to one's quality of life.[2]

The Pediatric Voice Outcome Survey (PVOS) was developed as a modification of the VOS to be given to a parent-proxy of a child. This was first validated by comparing two groups of pediatric patients. These groups consisted of children who previously had a tracheotomy that had subsequently

Voice Outcomes Survey (VOS)

1. In general, how would you say your speaking voice is:
   - ☐ Excellent
   - ☐ Good
   - ☐ Adequate
   - ☐ Poor or inadequate
   - ☐ I have no voice

The following items ask about activities that your child might do in a given day.

2. To what extent does your voice limit your ability to be understood in a noisy area?
   - ☐ Limited a lot
   - ☐ Limited a little
   - ☐ Not limited at all

3. During the past 2 weeks, to what extent has your voice interfered with your normal social activities or your work?
   - ☐ Not at all
   - ☐ Slightly
   - ☐ Moderately
   - ☐ Quite a bit
   - ☐ Extremely

4. How often do you have with your food or liquids going "down the wrong pipe" when you eat or find yourself coughing after eating or drinking?
   - ☐ All the time
   - ☐ Most of the time
   - ☐ Sometimes
   - ☐ Rarely
   - ☐ Never

5. Do you find yourself "straining" when you speak because of your voice problem?
   - ☐ Not at all
   - ☐ A little bit
   - ☐ Moderately
   - ☐ Quite a bit
   - ☐ Extremely

Fig 4–1. Voice Outcomes Survey (VOS)

been decannulated and a group of children who remained tracheotomy dependent.[1] The final version of the PVOS consisted of 4 questions (Fig 4-2), with one question being dropped after determining the inter-nal consistency was improved when it was excluded (question 4 on the VOS).

Normative data were later obtained for the PVOS by administering the survey to a group of 385 parents of children and ado-

---

Pediatric Voice Outcomes Survey (PVOS)

1. In general, how would you say your child's speaking voice is:
   - ☐ Excellent (25 pts)
   - ☐ Good (18.75 pts)
   - ☐ Adequate (12.5 pts)
   - ☐ Poor or inadequate (6.25 pts)
   - ☐ My child has no voice (0 pts)

The following items ask about activities that your child might do in a given day.

2. To what extent does your child's voice limit his or her ability to be understood in a noisy area?
   - ☐ Limited a lot (0 pts)
   - ☐ Limited a little (12.5 pts)
   - ☐ Not limited at all (25 pts)

3. During the past 2 weeks, to what extent has your child's voice interfered with his or her normal social activities or with his or her school?
   - ☐ Not at all (25 pts)
   - ☐ Slightly (18.75 pts)
   - ☐ Moderately (12.5 pts)
   - ☐ Quite a bit (6.25 pts)
   - ☐ Extremely (0 pts)

4. Do you find your child "straining" when he or she speaks because of his or her voice problem?
   - ☐ Not at all (25 pts)
   - ☐ A little bit (18.75 pts)
   - ☐ Moderately (12.5 pts)
   - ☐ Quite a bit (6.25 pts)
   - ☐ Extremely (0 pts)

Fig 4–2. Pediatric Voice Outcomes Survey (PVOS).

lescents; most of whom presented to the pediatric otolaryngologist for reasons other than their voice. The mean score obtained was 80.5 ± 19.9.[3] The PVOS was also validated for use in determining the functional impact of surgery to correct velopharyngeal insufficiency. The PVOS scores in that study were 38.3 ± 12 prior to surgery and 72.3 ± 22.7 after surgical intervention in a group of 12 patients which was a statistically significant change.[4]

Using the PVOS

Scores on the PVOS range from 0 to 100 points with higher scores indicating a relative better quality of life. The questions and point values are found in Figure 4–2.

V-RQOL/PV-RQOL

The Voice-Related Quality of Life Survey (V-RQOL) is a 10-item instrument that was validated in a group of 109 adult voice patients. There are also two subdomains within the V-RQOL which consist of scores for physical functioning and social-emotional components of quality of life. This survey was shown to be responsive to change in voice in patients who had treatment for their disorder. The V-RQOL has an advantage over the VOS in that it provides more information to the clinician at very little cost in terms of time required to complete and score.[5]

The Pediatric Voice-Related Quality of Life (PV-RQOL) instrument is the parent-proxy form that was validated in a group of 120 parents of children with a variety of otolaryngologic problems (Fig 4–3).[6] This instrument contained all of the 10 questions that are on the V-RQOL; simply reworded

for parent administration (ie, instead of "do you have . . . " the question was changed to "my child has . . . "). The PV-QROL was shown to have excellent internal consistency and had a high correlation to scores on the previously validated PVOS (criterion validity). The instrument was also able to discriminate between patients who had a voice change during treatment (adenoidectomy patients) and those who had procedures that should not have affected their voice (discriminant validity).[6]

Using the PV-RQOL

The PV-RQOL has 10 questions that each has scores from 0 to 10 points (10 points = no problem, 0 points = problem is "as bad as it can be"). Thus the raw scores can range from 0 to 100 points with higher scores indicating a better quality of life. There are also 2 subdomains within the PV-RQOL. The social-emotional score is determined by adding the scores from questions 4, 5, 8, and 10. The physical functioning score is calculated by adding the scores of questions 1, 2, 3, 6, 7, and 9. The questions and point values for responses are given in Figure 4–3.

VHI/PVHI

The Voice Handicap Index (VHI) is the other commonly cited adult vocal quality of life instrument. The VHI was validated in 1997 and consists of 30 questions, equally distributed in 3 subdomains (10 questions each in functional, physical, and emotional categories).[7] These additional questions were added to prior instruments in an attempt to better differentiate between the different areas in a person's life that a voice

Pediatric Voice-Related Quality of Life Survey (PV-RQOL)

Please answer these questions based upon what your child's voice (your own voice if you are the teenage respondent) has been like over the past 2 weeks. Considering both how severe the problem is when you get, and how frequently it happens, please rate each item below on how "bad" it is (that is, the amount of each problem that you have). Use the following rating scale:

    1 = None, not a problem (10 pts)
    2 = A small amount (7.5 pts)
    3 = A moderate amount (5 pts)
    4 = A lot (2.5 pts)
    5 = Problem is "as bad as it can be" (0 pts)
    6 = Not applicable

Because of my child's voice, how much of a problem is this?

1. My child has trouble speaking loudly or being heard in noisy situations.

   1   2   3   4   5   6

2. My child runs out of air and needs to take frequent breaths when talking.

   1   2   3   4   5   6

3. My child sometimes does not know what will come out when s/he begins speaking.

   1   2   3   4   5   6

4. My child is sometimes anxious or frustrated (because of his or her voice).

   1   2   3   4   5   6

5. My child sometimes gets depressed (because of his or her voice).

   1   2   3   4   5   6

6. My child has trouble using the telephone or speaking with friends in person.

   1   2   3   4   5   6

7. My child has trouble doing his or job schoolwork (because of his or her voice).

   1   2   3   4   5   6

8. My child avoids going out socially (because of his or her voice).

   1   2   3   4   5   6

9. My child has to repeat himself/herself to be understood.

   1   2   3   4   5   6

10. My child has become less outgoing (because of his or her voice).

   1   2   3   4   5   6

Fig 4–3. Pediatric Voice-Related Quality of Life Survey (PV-RQOL).

disorder can affect. The necessary tradeoff is the additional time burden required. Scores for each question range from 0 to 4 points (0 = never, 4 = always). The scores range from 0 to 120 points with higher scores representing worse perceived quality of life.[7]

Two variations of the VHI have recently been added to our armamentarium. The VHI-10 is a 10-item variation of the VHI that has been shown to correlate well with the scores obtained from the VHI. [8] The pediatric VHI (pVHI) is a 23-item parent-proxy version of the original VHI.[9] The pVHI was validated in a group of 45 nonvoice pediatric patients. Scores were compared to visual analogue scale and 10 open-ended questions regarding the impact of the child's voice quality on his or her overall communication, development, education, and social and family life. Normative scores were 1.47 for the functional, 0.20 for the physical, and 0.18 for the emotional components. The pVHI was then administered to children before and after laryngeal reconstruction. A correlation matrix comparing the overall pVHI scores with the subscores showed moderate correlation. Also, the visual analogue scores where compared to the pVHI scores and revealed moderate correlation. Furthermore, test-retest reliability was moderately high.[9]

Using the pVHI

The pVHI has 23 questions that each has scores from 0 to 4 points (0 points = no problem, 4 points = always a problem). Thus, the raw scores can range from 0 to 92 points with higher scores indicating a worse quality of life. There are also 3 subdomains within the pVHI. The functional score is determined by adding the scores from the first 7 questions and the physical score by adding the final 7 questions. The questions and point values for responses are given in Figure 4–4.

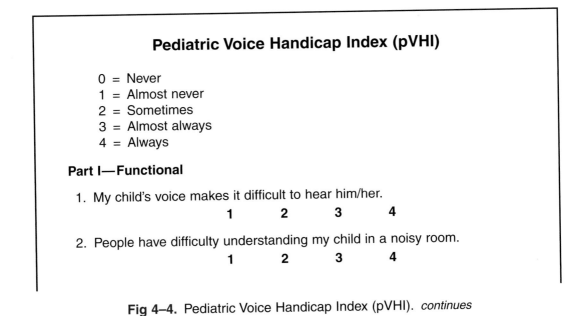

Pediatric Voice Handicap Index (pVHI)

0 = Never
1 = Almost never
2 = Sometimes
3 = Almost always
4 = Always

Part I—Functional

1. My child's voice makes it difficult to hear him/her.
   1   2   3   4

2. People have difficulty understanding my child in a noisy room.
   1   2   3   4

Fig 4–4. Pediatric Voice Handicap Index (pVHI). *continues*

3. At home, we have difficulty hearing my child when he/she calls through the house.

          1   2   3   4

4. My child tends to avoid communicating because of his/her voice.

          1   2   3   4

5. My child speaks with friends, neighbors, or relatives less often because of his/her voice.

          1   2   3   4

6. People ask my child to repeat him/herself when speaking face-to-face.

          1   2   3   4

7. My child's voice difficulties restrict personal, educational and social activities.

          1   2   3   4

Part II—Physical

8. My child runs out of air when talking.

          1   2   3   4

9. The sound of my child's voice changes throughout the day.

          1   2   3   4

10. People ask, "What's wrong with your child's voice?"

          1   2   3   4

11. My child's voice sounds dry, rasp, and/or hoarse.

          1   2   3   4

12. The quality of my child's voice is unpredictable.

          1   2   3   4

13. My child uses a great deal of effort to speak (eg, straining).

          1   2   3   4

14. My child's voice is worse in the evening.

          1   2   3   4

15. My child's voice "gives out" while speaking.

          1   2   3   4

16. My child has to yell in order for others to hear him/her.

          1   2   3   4

Fig 4–4. *continues*

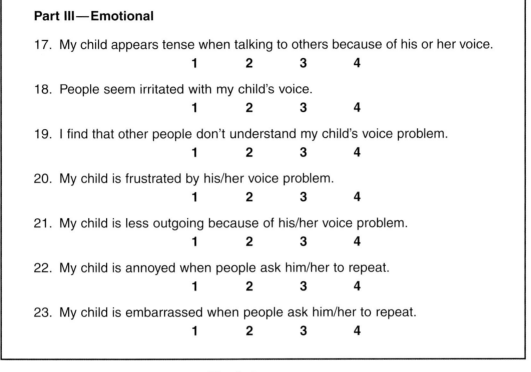

Part III—Emotional

17. My child appears tense when talking to others because of his or her voice.

    1   2   3   4

18. People seem irritated with my child's voice.

    1   2   3   4

19. I find that other people don't understand my child's voice problem.

    1   2   3   4

20. My child is frustrated by his/her voice problem.

    1   2   3   4

21. My child is less outgoing because of his/her voice problem.

    1   2   3   4

22. My child is annoyed when people ask him/her to repeat.

    1   2   3   4

23. My child is embarrassed when people ask him/her to repeat.

    1   2   3   4

Fig 4–4. *continued*

FUTURE DIRECTIONS

Quantitative analysis of voice outcomes following medical or surgical intervention is imperative if we are to advance the field of pediatric laryngology. Although we are gradually gathering normative data for both acoustic and quality of life instruments, widespread acceptance of their use has been slow to develop. Pediatric voice quality of life instruments are now available, but seem not to be utilized as often as they might be. There are now three such devices to choose from. It will be important, as we go forward, to adopt a standard instrument so that we can both track the voice results in our patients and compare results across institutions.

REFERENCES

1. Hartnick CJ. Validation of a pediatric voice quality-of-life instrument. *Arch Otolaryngol.* 2002;128:919–922.

2. Gliklich RE, Glovsky RM, Montgomery WW. Validation of a voice outcome survey for unilateral vocal cord paralysis. *Otolaryngol Head Neck Surg.* 1999;120:153–158.

3. Hartnick CJ, Volk M, Cunningham M. Establishing normative voice-related quality of life scores within the pediatric otolaryngology population. *Arch Otolaryngol Head Neck Surg.* 2003;129:1090–1093.

4. Boseley ME, Hartnick CJ. Assessing the outcome of surgery to correct velopharyngeal insufficiency with the pediatric voice outcomes survey. *Int J Pediatr Otorhinolaryngol.* 2004;68:1429–1433.

5. Hogikyan ND, Sethuraman G. Validation of an instrument to measure Voice-Related Quality of Life (V-RQOL). *J Voice.* 1999;13:557–567.

6. Boseley ME, Cunningham MJ, Volk MS, Hartnick CJ. Validation of the pediatric voice-related quality-of-life survey. *Arch Otolaryngol Head Neck Surg.* 2006;132:717–720.

7. Jacobson B, Johnson A, Grywalsky C. The Voice Handicap Index (VHI): development and validation. *Am J Speech Lang Path.* 1997;6:66–70.

8. Rosen CA, Lee AS, Osborne J, Zullo T, Murry T. Development and validation of the voice handicap index-10. *Laryngoscope.* 2004; 114:1549–1556.

9. Zur KB, Cotton S, Kelcher L, Baker S, Weinrich B, Lee L. Pediatric Voice Handicap Index (pVHI): a new tool for evaluating pediatric dysphonia. *Int J Pediatr Otorhinolaryngol.* 2007;71:77–82.

Laryngopharyngeal Reflux and the Voice

Stephen C. Hardy

INTRODUCTION

Gastroesophageal reflux disease (GERD) is a relatively common problem encountered by otolaryngologists. Symptoms in the adult population include throat clearing, chronic throat irritation, chronic hoarseness, and chronic cough.[1] Infants, on the other hand, often present initially with complaints of frequent "spitting up" during feeds. Others have a more worrisome history to include failure to thrive, hematemesis, anemia, or recurrent pneumonia.[2] It is these patients that often require a multidisciplinary approach to management. Pediatric otolaryngologists, working alongside our pediatric pulmonology and gastroenterology colleagues, play an important role in this regard. This chapter addresses the timing of evaluating children suspected to have GERD, the diagnostic tests currently available, and the treatment options that should be considered. This chapter aims to elucidate our role as otolaryngologists in treating GERD.

The true incidence of GERD in children is difficult to ascertain as many infants can spit up without any untoward complications. Premature infants, however, seem to have a higher likelihood of having reflux than other children. Marino found that in a group of 75 such patients, 63% were found to have GERD.[3] The good news is that the majority of these patients improve as they grow. It appears that 55% have resolution of their symptoms by 10 months of age and an additional 16% improve by 18 months.[4]

The reason for the apparent higher incidence of reflux in infants than in adults is likely multifactorial. There are several anatomic differences that have been noted. The angle between the esophagus and the axis of the stomach (angle of His) is more obtuse in the infant. Children with hiatal hernias are also more subject to GERD as the lower esophageal sphincter (LES) is exposed to negative intrathoracic pressure, rendering it less effective as a barrier to gastric acid. Although these anatomic factors play a role, currently it is believed that transient LES relaxation (TLESR) is the major factor causing clinically significant reflux in infants.[2]

In addition to these anatomic factors, physiologic considerations must also be considered. Infants are usually fed large fluid boluses in order to lengthen the duration of time between feeds. Children are also usually placed in a supine position following feeding. Food allergy can also masquerade as GERD. Some have proposed that allergy might be the cause in up to 42% of cases.[5] Increasing the frequency and decreasing the volume of feeds may be helpful in decreasing symptoms. Placing the infant in a prone, head-elevated position should decrease the incidence of reflux. Thickening feeds may also be beneficial. Finally, a trial of hypoallergenic protein hydrolysate infant formula can be considered before initiating a formal workup for GERD.[6]

Sutphen has advocated that children under the age of 12 months must have failure to thrive, weight loss, pulmonary disease, and/or an apparent life-threatening episode (ALTE) before a workup should be undertaken. Beyond the age of 12 months, persistent spitting up is adequate to pursue further testing.[6]

DIAGNOSTIC TESTS

Once the decision is made to evaluate for GERD, there are several tests that are in our armamentarium. These include an upper gastrointestinal series (upper GI series), pH-probe testing, impedance monitoring, and endoscopy. The upper GI series consists of having the child swallow barium during a fluoroscopic examination of the upper aerodigestive tract. We often involve our speech and swallowing therapist during this evaluation as they are often more adept

at commenting on the oropharyngeal component of swallowing. This study can be helpful in determining whether there is any evidence of laryngeal penetration. It is also useful to look for anatomic abnormalities such as a hiatal hernia, esophageal stricture, or tracheoesophageal fistula. However, when it comes to evaluating for GERD, some feel that this study is limited as the child is being tested under nonphysiologic conditions.

The 24-hour pH probe has become the procedure of choice for the diagnosis of GERD in infants and children. This probe has traditionally been placed through the nose and is attached to an external monitor. The recordings that have been commonly recorded are the number of reflux episodes (pH < 4), the percentage of time that the pH is less than 4 (reflux index), the number of reflux events of at least 5 minutes in duration, the average esophageal acid clearance time per reflux episode, the longest reflux episode, and the total time of pH less than 4.[6] It should be noted that there has not been a consensus on the values of these various variables as predictors to clinical disease.[6] However, one study in children with pulmonary disease showed a correlation between duration of reflux and evidence of esophagitis on esophageal biopsy specimens.[7] Another study looked specifically at reflux index and time with a pH less than 4 as predictors of esophagitis. The sensitivity for detecting GERD was 96% and 93%, respectively. However, the specificity was only 50% for the reflux index and 88% for time with a pH less than 4.[8]

The number of positions within the esophagus being tested has also varied over the years. One published report documented the sensitivity and specificity for detecting GERD at the levels of the lower esophageal sphincter and pharynx improved to nearly

100% when a double-probe was utilized.[9] Another study showed that 46% of children who had normal pH readings at the distal probe had abnormal pH values at the proximal probe, suggesting that the pharyngeal probe is necessary.[10] Finally, a report on the use of a four-probe device (pharynx, proximal, middle, and distal esophagus) showed a 87% sensitivity and 93% specificity in detecting GERD and LPR.[11]

Another option for esophageal pH monitoring is the Bravo pH-monitoring system. The Bravo involves a pH-capsule, about the size of a gel cap, that is temporarily attached to the wall of the esophagus, usually during an endoscopic exam (Figs 5–1 and 5–2). The Bravo pH capsule measures the pH of the surrounding esophagus and transmits the information continuously via radio telemetry to a receiver worn on the patient's belt, or kept nearby. As with a pH probe, the patient (or caregiver) records symptoms he or she experiences in a diary by pressing buttons on the receiver. The Bravo pH capsule collects pH measurements for up to 48 hours. After the study, data from the receiver is uploaded to a computer and diary information is entered for analysis to aid in the diagnosis and plan treatment. The capsule is released from the esophageal wall and passes through the alimentary tract until discarded with the patient's feces. The obvious advantage that this device has over standard pH monitoring is that there is no need for a probe to stay in the nose, and thus is better tolerated by children.

There are inherent problems with having so many different types of measurements and different types of probes when trying to define what makes up an abnormal study. Even if the results are consistent with GERD, this does not necessarily correlate with the child's symptoms. Finally, a pH

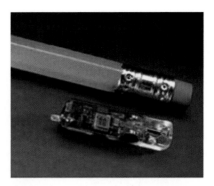

A

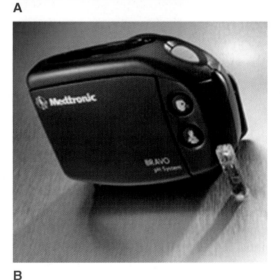

B

Fig 5–1. Bravo probe and receiver. **A.** The size is comparable to the size of a pencil eraser. **B.** The receiver is worn on the patient's belt.

probe study fails to address reflux of bile acids that have a pH greater than 5, but could still potentially be clinically significant.

One technique to better delineate a correlation of GERD with symptoms (particularly with pulmonary symptoms, such as apnea or ALTE) is to perform a Bernstein test. This test consists of placing a nasogastric tube into the esophagus and instilling alternating solutions of a low concentration of hydrochloric

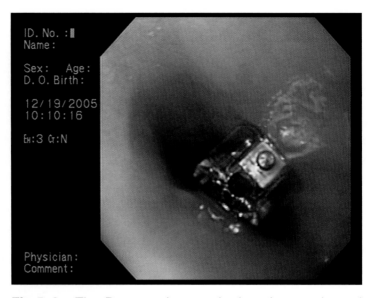

Fig 5–2. The Bravo probe attached to the esophageal mucosa.

acid and normal saline to see if the symptoms are reproduced. The second issue of nonacidic reflux is better addressed with multiple intraluminal impedance monitoring (MII). MII measures alterations in electrical impedance along multiple intraluminal electrodes during swallowing. This allows for detection of anterograde swallows and retrograde reflux, regardless of the acidity of the refluxate.[12] Perhaps the best evaluation for GERD would be a combination of a pH probe to measure acidity with MII to measure directional flow of fluid in the esophagus.

Endoscopy of the aerodigestive tract can be extremely useful when trying to make the diagnosis of GERD, particularly in those that have failed medical management. This group of children includes those with failure to thrive, chronic cough, and airway symptoms (including those with recurrent croup, pneumonias, and/or suspicion for aspiration). We have found it useful to include both our pediatric pulmonologist and gastroenterologist for this evaluation in the operating room.

The examination begins with a thorough inspection of the larynx with a 4.0-mm Hopkins rod telescope. Any signs of pharyngeal reflux are noted to include erythema and/or intra-arytenoid or true vocal fold edema. Also, care is taken to inspect for a laryngeal cleft as this could be the underlying cause for aspiration. A laryngeal mask airway is then placed to facilitate flexible bronchoscopy. A cobblestone appearance of the tracheal wall is a visual clue on endoscopy that the child may be aspirating (Fig 5–3). A bronchoalveolar lavage should be performed to confirm a suspicion of aspiration. Specifically, 100 macrophages are collected and stained with oil red O to test for lipid. Lipid-layden macrophages (LLM) become positive approximately 6 hours after a reflux episode and remain positive for up to 3 days.[13] The sensitivity for this test is believed to be near 85%.[14]

The child may be intubated prior to performing the esophagoscopy. A flexible grasping biopsy forceps is passed through the working port of the scope. Four sets of biopsies are taken from the duodenum, the stomach, and the distal and proximal esophagus. These specimens are examined for evidence of Barrett's esophagus or eosinophils which would suggest chronic reflux or allergic esophagitis. A endoscopic finding of "trachealization" or ringed appearance of the esophageal mucosal can be suggestive of esosinophilic esophagitis (Fig 5-4). Although uncommonly seen in the pediatric population, the clinician should also be aware of the distinct appearance of erosive esophagitis (Fig 5-5). This condition would obviously warrant more aggressive reflux therapy.

Once the diagnosis of GERD is made by clinical suspicion, pH probe, or biopsy, the usual first step in treatment is through conservative management. Techniques such as formula changes (when allergy is suspected), thickening of feeds, smaller feeding size, suggestions for burping techniques,

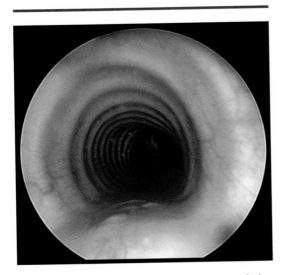

Fig 5–3. Cobblestone appearance of the tracheal mucosa is suggestive of aspiration.

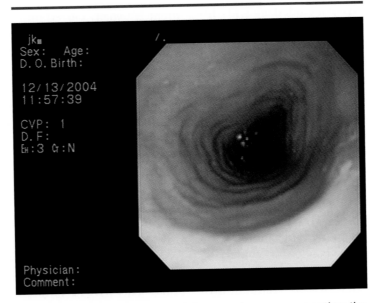

Fig 5–4. "Trachealization" of the esophagus suggesting the presence of eosinophilic esophagitis.

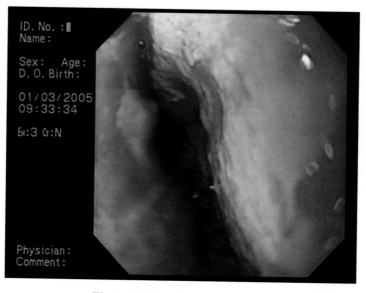

Fig 5–5. Erosive esophagitis.

and postcibal positioning therapy should all be entertained prior to beginning treatment with medications.[2,6,12] When necessary, medical treatment is successful in approximately 80% of cases.[15] Medications that have been used have included antacids, histamine receptor-2 (H_2) antagonists, proton-pump blockers, and prokinetic agents (Table 5–1).

MEDICAL MANAGEMENT

The use of antacids has been limited in the infant population due to the frequent feeding schedule and the potential risks from aluminum absorption. H_2 receptor anatagonists such as cimetidine and ranitidine, on the other hand, have been shown to be effective at treating both the clinical and histologic changes seen in children with GERD.[16-18] The prescribing physician should

be aware, however, that these drugs can rarely cause gynecomastia, diarrhea, and abnormalities in vitamin D or hepatic metabolism.[19] These risks seem to be less common with the use of ranitidine.[6] Treatment is usually carred on for 6 to 8 weeks for healing of mucosal irritation. Treatment can continue in order to prevent reinjury by reflux.

If more severe GERD is suspected, proton-pump blockers have become an important therapeutic option. These medications, which include omeprazole and lansoprazole, perform their action by inhibiting the proton-potassium ATPase enzyme system.[2] The common pediatric doses are listed in Table 5–1. Treatment with proton-pump inhibitors is generally 6 to 8 weeks minimum, as is the case for histamine receptor blockers. At one time there was a fear that long-term use of proton-pump blockers could lead to gastrinoma formation. This concern has not been proven to be true.[20]

Table 5–1. List of Commonly Prescribed Antireflux Medications and Doses

Medication	Dosage
Magnesium-aluminum hydroxide	0.5 ml/kg/dose PO before meals and qhs
Cimetidine	5-10 mg/kg/dose PO qid
Ranitidine	1-4 mg/kg/dose PO bid or tid
Metoclopramide	0.1 mg/kg/dose PO before meals and qhs
Omeprazole	1.0 mg/kg/dose, or 20 mg PO qd

Prokinetic agents are the last class of drugs to consider when treating clinically significant GERD. Otolaryngologists typically are hesitant to prescribe these drugs as the safety of both metoclopramide and cisapride has been questioned. The former has been associated with diarrhea, extrapyramidal symptoms, and dystonias. Cisapride, on the other hand, has been associated with serious cardiac arrhythmias, such as torsades de pointes and prolonged QT interval, and is no longer available in the United States.[6] It should be mentioned, however, that cisapride has been shown in a placebo-controlled, double-blind, 8-week trial to improve both pH scores and histologic changes in the esophagus.[21]

SURGICAL MANAGEMENT

Surgery is reserved for those children with diagnosed GERD who have failed medical management. The two most common operations are the Thal and Nissen fundoplications. The Thal is a 270-degree anterior wrap of the fundus of the stomach around the distal esophagus, whereas the Nissen is a 360-degree wrap. Indications for a wrap include failure to thrive, reflux-induced aspiration, peptic stricture, Barrett's esoph-

agus, and ALTE. Failure rates for the Nissen fundoplication vary from 3 to 40% after 4 to 9 years.[22]

CONCLUSION

Gastroesphageal reflux is very common during infancy. Often, this is not clinically significant and requires no further diagnostic studies or medical treatment. Most of these children can be managed by educating the parents on how to feed and by general reassurance. Occasionally changes to the type of formula the child is being given can be beneficial as well. However, children with a more worrisome history (failure to thrive, hematemesis, anemia, or recurrent pneumonia) require a more thorough evaluation.[2] The tests for GERD that are currently available to us all have advantages and disadvantages. A 24-hour pH probe with the addition of esophageal biopsies should be considered for the most severe cases. Bravo probes can be done if the child is an appropriate candidate. Addition of impedance testing may be beneficial in cases where nonacidic reflux is believed to be the causative agent. Once the diagnosis is made, 85% of children can be managed with medical therapy alone.

REFERENCES

1. Koufman JA. The otolaryngologic manifestations of gastroesophageal reflux disease (GERD): a clinical investigation of 225 patients using ambulatory 24-hour pH monitoring and an experimental investigation of the role of acid and pepsin in the development of laryngeal injury. *Laryngoscope.* 1991;101:1-78.

2. Tsou MV, Bishop PR. Gastroesophageal reflux in children. *Otolaryngol Clin North Am.* 1998;31:419-434.

3. Marino M, Assing E, Carbone M, et al. The incidence of gastroesophageal reflux in preterm infants. *J Perinatol.* 1995;15:369-371.

4. Khalaf MN, Porat R, Brodsky NL, Bhandari V. Clinical correlations in infants in the neonatal intensive care unit with varying severity of gastroesophageal reflux. *J Gastroenerol Nutr.* 2001;32:45-49.

5. Iacono G, Carroccio A, Cavataio F, et al. Gastroesopageal reflux and cow's milk allergy in infants: a prospective study. *J Allergy Clin Immunol.* 1996;97:822.

6. Sutphen JL. Pediatric gastroesophageal reflux disease. *Gastroenterol Clin North Am.* 1990;19:617-629.

7. Baer M, Maki M, Nurminen J, et al. Esophagitis and findings of long-term esophageal pH recording in children with repeated lower respiratory tract symptoms. *J Pediatr Gastroenterol Nutr.* 1986;5:187-190.

8. Vandenplas Y, Franckx-Goossens A, Pipeleers-Marichal M, et al. Area under pH 4: advantages of a new parameter in the interpretation of esophageal pH monitoring data in infants. *J Pediatr Gastroenterol Nutr.* 1989;9:34-39.

9. Contencin P, Narcy P. Gastropharyngeal reflux in infants and children. *Arch Otolaryngol Head Neck Surg.* 1992;118:1028-1030.

10. Little JP, Matthews BL, Glock MS, et al. Esophageal pediatric reflux: 24-hour double-probe pH monitoring of 222 children. *Ann Otol Rhinol Laryngol.* 1997;169:1-16.

11. Haase GM, Meagher DP, Goldson E, et al. A unique teletransmission system for extended four-channel esophageal pH monitoring in infants and children. *J Pediatr Surg.* 1987;22:68-74.

12. Malloy EJ, Fiore JM, Martin RJ. Does gastroesophageal reflux cause apnea in preterm infants? *Biol Neonate.* 2005;87:254-261.

13. Zalzal GH, Tran LP. Pediatric gastroesophageal reflux and laryngopharyngeal reflux. *Otolaryngol Clin North Am.* 2000;33:151-161.

14. Nussbaum E, Maggi JC, Mathis R, et al. Association of lipid-laden alveolar macrophages and gastroesophageal reflux in children. *J Pediatr.* 1987;110:190-194.

15. Andze GO, Brandt ML, Vil DS, et al. Diagnosis and treatment of gastroesophageal reflux in 500 children with respiratory symptoms: the value of pH monitoring. *J Pediatr Surg.* 1991;26:295-300.

16. Cucchiara S, Staiano A, Romaniello G, et al. Antacids and cimetidine treatment for gastroesophageal reflux and peptic oesophagitis. *Arch Dis Child.* 1984;59:842-847.

17. Cucchiara S, Gobio-Casali L, Balli F, et al. Cimetidine treatment of relux esophagitis in children: an Italian multicentric study. *J Pediatr Gastroenterol Nutr.* 1989;8:150-156.

18. Shepherd RW, Wren J, Evans S, et al. Gastroesophageal reflux in children. *Clin Pediatr.* 1987;26:55-60.

19. Hebra A, Hoffman MA. Gastroesophageal reflux in children. *Pediatr Clin North Am.* 1993;40:1233-1251.

20. Berlin R. Omeprazole: gastrin and gastric endocrine cell data from clinical studies. *Dig Dis Sci.* 1991;36:129.

21. Cucchiara S, Staiano A, Capozi C, et al. Cisapride for gastro-oesophageal reflux and peptic oesophagitis. *Arch Dis Child.* 1987;62:454-457.

22. Cilley R. Management of gastroesophageal reflux in children. *Curr Opin Pediatr.* 1991;27:260.

The Role of the Pediatric Pulmonologist

Kenan E. Haver

INTRODUCTION

Voice is generated by the modulation of airflow through the vocal folds. The production and maintenance of airflow requires the coordinated function of both the muscles of respiration and those muscles and structures involved in maintaining the caliber of both the large and small airways. Conditions that impair the function of the respiratory muscles, decrease the caliber by constricting the smooth muscle in the small airways, or affect the normal movements of the vocal folds can each affect the voice. This chapter discusses how pulmonary function studies may be useful in assessing respiratory muscle strength, detecting bronchoconstriction, and identifying inspiratory flow limitation[7] (Table 6-1).

ANATOMY AND PHYSIOLOGY OF THE UPPER AND LOWER AIRWAY

The vocal folds make complete contact with each other during phonation with each vibration transiently closing the gap between them which cuts off the escaping air.[1] When the air pressure in the trachea rises as a result of this closure, the folds are blown apart, while the vocal processes of the arytenoid cartilages remain in apposition. This creates an oval-shaped gap between the folds and some air escapes, lowering the pressure inside the trachea. Rhythmic repetition of this movement creates a pitched note. The pitch, volume, and timbre of the sound produced can be altered by the shape of chest and neck,

Table 6–1. Maximal Respiratory Pressures.[10]

	Maximal Inspiratory Pressure	Maximal Expiratory Pressure
Poor effort	Decreased	Decreased
Fatigue	Decreased	Decreased
Neuromuscular disease	Decreased	Decreased
Increased lung volume	Decreased	Normal
Decreased lung volume	Normal	Decreased

Conditions to consider in patients with decreased maximal respiratory pressures. Used with permission from Medical Algorithms Project, *Maximal Inspiratory and Maximal Expiratory Pressures*, Chapter 8, Pulmonary and Acid-Base, Copyright (©) 2006–2007, Institute for Algorithmic Medicine, Houston, Texas.

and the position of the lips, tongue, jaw, palate, and airway. The vocal folds themselves can loosen or tighten and change their thickness.

Airflow in the respiratory system begins with the active process of inhalation, which is principally dependent on the function of the diaphragm. With each contraction, the diaphragm flattens which enlarges the thoracic cavity. The diaphragm also elevates and stabilizes the lower rib cage.[2] During normal breathing, most of the accessory muscles are silent. However, these muscles may be recruited to stabilize the chest or abdominal wall to improve the efficiency of the diaphragm under certain conditions.

Airflow is increased during inspiration by negative pressure generated at the margins of the air column, a phenomenon referred to as the Bernoulli effect. The acceleration of flow as the air enters a narrowed passage, known as the Venturi effect, tends to reduce the diameter of the airways. These forces are resisted by the structural elements of the airway and the tone of the airway muscles. The upper airway must also be kept patent during inspiration and therefore the function of the alae nasi, phayngeal wall muscles, genioglossus, and arytenoid muscles also play an important role.[2]

Exhalation is generally a passive process. The lungs have a natural elasticity; as they recoil from the stretch of inhalation, air flows back out until the pressures in the chest and the atmosphere reach equilibrium. However, with active or forced exhalation, as when singing, the abdominal and internal intercostal muscles are used to generate abdominal and thoracic pressure which forces air out of the lungs.[3]

MEASURING RESPIRATORY MUSCLE STRENGTH

Muscle weakness needs to be considered in the evaluation of patients with voice-related problems. Muscle weakness, either congenital or acquired, can impair respiratory muscle function, decrease airflow, and subsequently affect the voice. Voice changes have been associated with a variety of diseases that affect the muscles of respiration, including Guillain-Barré syndrome, myasthenia gravis, muscular dystrophies, and poliomyelitis.[4] Spinal injuries can also directly impact the muscles of respiration. Finally, respiratory muscle strength can be affected by deconditioning, which can be caused by debilitating diseases, mechanical ventilation, malnutrition, or immobilization.

Establishing the cause for the weakness is important to select appropriate therapy. Even when specific therapy is not available to treat the disorder, inspiratory muscle training (IMT) may help patients strengthen and improve their voice. Additional benefits from IMT include decreased perception of exertional dyspnea, enhanced cough, and improved airway clearance.[5]

Measuring respiratory muscle strength is straightforward. Both the maximum inspiratory pressure (MIP—the highest pressure developed during inspiration) and maximum expiratory pressure (MEP—highest pressure developed during expiration) can be measured and compared to controls. Patients with disorders that affect respiratory muscle strength may have impaired MIPs and MEPs. These can be measured quite easily at the mouth using a pressure meter. Normal values have been published for both adults and children. Caution is needed in the interpretation of the studies as values in the lower quarter of the normal range are compatible both with normal strength and with mild to moderate weakness. A normal MEP with a low MIP suggests isolated diaphragmatic weakness. These tests are volitional and require full cooperation. Accordingly, an abnormal result may be due to lack of motivation and does not

necessarily indicate reduced inspiratory or expiratory muscle strength.[6]

Clinical Case

Jennifer is an 18-year-old young woman who is an aspiring singer with a history that included an interrupted aortic arch and ventricular septal defect who presented with a hoarse voice and chronic aspiration. She was found to have a paralyzed left vocal fold and underwent a left ansa cervicalis to recurrent laryngeal nerve anastomosis procedure with a fat graft injection laryngoplasty. Over the next year, she regained the ability to eat orally without evidence of aspiration and her conversational voice had markedly improved. However, as she was an avid singer, she still noted difficulty with sustaining notes. She asked if another procedure would help. Videostroboscopy suggested that she has good glottal closure with no significant glottal gap and no apparent mucosal wave abnormalities.

Her surgical options were reviewed which included a revision thyroplasty. Physical examination revealed her chest was clear to auscultation, but her breath sounds were diminished bilaterally. Her diaphragm moved appropriately by palpation. We measured her maximal inspiratory (MIP) and expiratory pressures (MEP) to evaluate the strength of her respiratory muscles. Her MIP was very low at 24 cm H_2O and her MEP was at the low end of the normal range at 85 cm H_2O. Her reduced respiratory muscle strength may have been due, at least in part, to deconditioning. She was referred to a respiratory muscle strength-training program, where she would breathe in and out against progressively increasing resistance. Her respiratory muscle strength increased significantly following her participation in the program. Her maximal respiratory pressures increased to a MIP of 32 (improved but still below the range of normal) and her MEP increased to 107. Along with the changes seen in her maximal respiratory pressures, she reported improvement in her ability to sing and no longer desires further surgical intervention. This case illustrates how pulmonary function studies helped establish the cause for her weak voice. With this information we were able to direct her to nonoperative therapy. We can continue to monitor her progress by regular reevaluation of her respiratory muscle strength.

Measuring Respiratory Muscle Strength Using the Sniff Test

Another test of muscle strength is the sniff test. This is a short, sharp voluntary inspiratory maneuver performed through one or both unoccluded nostrils. It involves contraction of the diaphragm and other inspiratory muscles. The sniffs need to be a maximal effort to be a useful test of respiratory muscle strength. This is relatively easy for most willing subjects, but may require some practice. Subjects should be instructed to sit or stand comfortably, and to make sniffs using maximal effort starting from relaxed end expiration. Detailed instruction on how to perform the maneuver are generally not necessary, and may, in fact, be counterproductive. However, subjects should be encouraged to make maximal efforts, with a rest between sniffs. Most subjects achieve a plateau of pressure values within 5 to 10 attempts. When done properly, the maneuver achieves rapid, fully coordinated recruitment of the inspiratory muscles.[6]

MEASURING SMALL AIRWAY OBSTRUCTION

The lower respiratory tract plays a key role in voice production by delivering airflow to the vocal folds. Airflow can be impaired by intrinsic or extrinsic compression of the airways. Asthma, which is characterized by chronic inflammation and smooth muscle dysfunction in the small airways, can present with both breathlessness and dyspnea. Asthma is the most common obstructive pulmonary disease in children and is characterized by reversible airway obstruction. Patients with asthma often present with dyspnea, but during a severe exacerbation may appear breathless and unable to complete sentences. Small airway obstruction can be detected by pulmonary function tests, even when the patient appears well and the chest is clear to auscultation.

Changes in pulmonary function that are insignificant with normal speech have been shown to lead to performance impairment for both amateur and professional singers. In a study of singers with voice problems (including vocal fatigue) who did not have causal laryngeal pathology, the investigators found that they had bronchodilator responsive airway obstruction. The singers, when treated for asthma, were shown to have improvement in their performance-related difficulties. The authors concluded that singers who present with complaints of impaired vocalization, such as vocal fatigue, decreased control, and excessive muscular tension, should be evaluated for increased airway reactivity as a possible cause of their complaints.[7]

Restrictive lung disease, which can be differentiated from obstructive lung diseases with spirometry and other tests of pulmonary function, can arise from interstitial lung disease or limitations to chest wall movement such as chest wall deformities. These deformities can include scoliosis, space-occupying intrathoracic processes (large bullae or congenital cysts), and alveolar filling defects (lobar pneumonia or pleural effusions).

Spirometry is the best method for documenting airflow obstruction. Spirometry measures the volume of air inspired and expired as a function of time, and is by far the most frequently performed test of pulmonary function in children. Pulmonary function tests enable clinicians to establish mechanical dysfunction in children with respiratory symptoms, quantify the degree of dysfunction, and define the nature of the dysfunction (Table 6–2).[8] Table 6–3 illustrates how spirometry can differentiate an obstructive from a restrictive process.

Figure 6–1 illustrates a normal flow-volume loop obtained during a respiratory maneuver that includes both inspiration and forced exhalation, whereas Figure 6–2 is a flow-volume loop of a patient with asthma for comparison. A reliable study requires patient effort and cooperation, accurate testing equipment, as well as a skilled and knowledgeable staff. Although the maneuvers needed to obtain measurements appear straightforward, studies are only valid if they reflect maximal effort and are reproducible. Children over the age of 6 can often perform adequately, although children as young as age 3 years have been shown to be able to perform spirometry with coaching. Each test needs to be repeated twice, and two studies need to have results within 5% of each other before the study can be reported as accurate.[9]

Table 6–2. Uses of Pulmonary Function Studies in Children

- To establish pulmonary mechanical abnormality in children with respiratory symptoms
- To quantify the degree of dysfunction
- To define the nature of pulmonary dysfunction (obstructive, restrictive, or mixed obstructive and restrictive)
- To aid in defining the site of airway obstruction as central or peripheral
- To differentiate fixed from variable and intrathoracic from extrathoracic central airway obstruction
- To follow the course of pulmonary disease process
- To assess the effect of therapeutic interventions and guide changes in therapy
- To detect increased airway reactivity
- To evaluate the risk of diagnostic and therapeutic procedures
- To monitor for pulmonary side effects of chemotherapy or radiation therapy
- To aid in prediction of the prognosis and quantitate pulmonary disability
- To investigate the effect of acute and chronic disease processes on lung growth

Modified with permission from Castile R, Pulmonary Function Testing in Children. In *Kendig's Disorders of the Respiratory Tract in Children*, 7th edition. Edited by Chernick V, Boat TF, Wilmott RW, and Bush A. Philadelphia, Pa: Saunders; 2006:168.[8]

Table 6–3. Characteristics of Obstructive and Restrictive Patterns of Lung Disease (FVC = forced vital capacity, FEV_1 = forced expiratory volume over 1 second)

Measurement	Obstructive	Restrictive
FVC	Normal/Decreased	Decreased
FEV_1	Decreased	Decreased
FEV_1/FVC	Decreased	Normal

Obstructive and restrictive lung diseases can be distinguished by expiratory flow measurements. FVC = forced vital capacity; FEV_1 = forced expiratory volume in the first second.

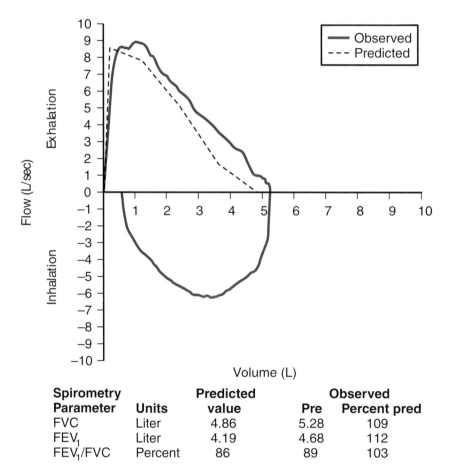

Spirometry Parameter	Units	Predicted value	Observed Pre	Observed Percent pred
FVC	Liter	4.86	5.28	109
FEV_1	Liter	4.19	4.68	112
FEV_1/FVC	Percent	86	89	103

Fig 6–1. Normal pulmonary function test. The normal flow-volume curve obtained during forced expiration rapidly ascends to the peak expiratory flow. Shortly after reaching the peak expiratory flow, the curve descends with decreasing volume following a reproducible shape that is independent of effort. In this normal flow-volume curve, the FEV_1/FVC, FEV_1, and FVC are all within the normal range for this patient's age group. The shapes of both the inspiratory and expiratory limbs are normal as well.

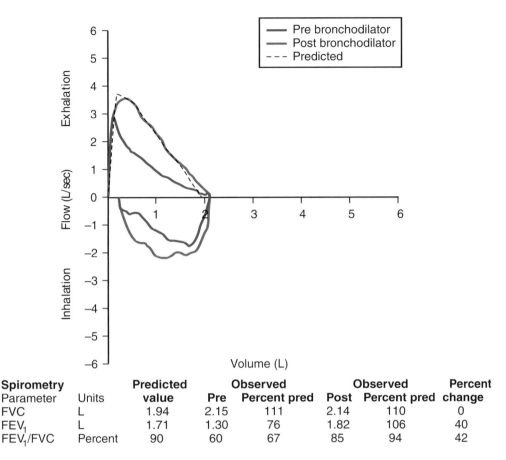

Spirometry Parameter	Units	Predicted value	Pre	Observed Percent pred	Post	Observed Percent pred	Percent change
FVC	L	1.94	2.15	111	2.14	110	0
FEV$_1$	L	1.71	1.30	76	1.82	106	40
FEV$_1$/FVC	Percent	90	60	67	85	94	42

Fig 6–2. Pulmonary function test demonstrating a reversible obstructive defect. The forced expiratory volume over one second (FEV$_1$) as a percentage of forced vital capacity (FVC) is decreased in patients with airway obstruction. The prebronchodilator curve shape (blue) is scooped. Following administration of a short-acting bronchodilator, the curve shape (brown) appears normal and there is an increase in both the FEV$_1$/FVC and FEV$_1$. This child has asthma and demonstrates a marked increase in FEV$_1$ after treatment with a short-acting bronchodilator. Reversible airflow obstruction is one of the hallmarks of asthma.

With a forced maneuver, the volume exhaled from full inhalation in the first second is referred to as the forced expiratory volume in the first second (FEV$_1$). The maneuver is completed when the subject has completed exhaling as fast as possible after a maximal inhalation. The maximal exhalation is referred to as the forced vital capacity (FVC). Normally, a child should be able to exhale more than 80% of the total lung volume in the first second of exhalation. Children with obstructive lung disease have a decreased ability to exhale. If the volume exhaled in the first second divided by the volume of full exhalation (FEV$_1$/FVC) is less than 80%, then airway obstruction is present (see Figure 6–2). The FEV_1 needs to be interpreted in the context of FVC as a low FEV_1 itself is not sufficient to make the diagnosis of airflow obstruction.

Spirometry cannot, however, provide data about absolute lung volumes because it measures the amount of air entering or leaving the lung, rather than the amount of air in the lung. Thus information about functional residual capacity (FRC) and lung volumes calculated from FRC (total lung capacity and residual volume) must be computed via different means. These tests include gas dilution and body plethysmography. Gas dilution is based on measuring the dilution of nitrogen or helium in a closed circuit connection to the lungs, whereas body plethysmography calculates lung gas volumes based on changes in thoracic pressures.

In addition to diagnostic uses, spirometry is used to assess the indication and efficacy of treatment. For example, the obstruction in those with asthma is usually reversible, either gradually without intervention or much more rapidly after treatment with a bronchodilator. An improvement in FEV_1 of 12% and 200 mL is considered a positive response.[9] In addition to confirming the diagnosis of asthma, the degree of airflow obstruction, as indicated by the FEV_1, is one indication of asthma control. A low FEV_1 or an acute decrease from baseline may reflect a child whose asthma is not under good control and therefore potentially at greater risk for an exacerbation.

Many children with a history strongly suggestive of asthma, even with a corroborating family history, may have a normal physical examination and normal spirometry when seen between exacerbations. Provocative testing can be used to induce bronchoconstriction in these patients. Cold air, exercise, and methacholine are commonly used to induce bronchoconstriction after a baseline study has been performed.[9] This can be reversed with the administration of a bronchodilator once the study has been completed.

CENTRAL AIRWAY OBSTRUCTION

One of the most common causes of central airway obstruction in children is due to paradoxical vocal fold motion (PVFM). PVFM involves excessive muscle tension that causes the vocal folds to involuntarily adduct during inhalation which restricts the airway opening. Often without a specific organic etiology, PVFM can masquerade as asthma, gastroesophageal reflux, vocal fold paralysis, or a functional voice disorder. PVFM may also be seen as a comorbid condition in these same patients. In some cases, PVFM may precipitate an apparent upper airway obstructive emergency, resulting in unnecessary endotracheal intubation, cardiopulmonary resuscitation, or tracheostomy. Other common presentations include laryngitis, hoarseness, choking, or stridor. Triggers include singing, shouting, exercise, and stress or anxiety. Exposure to cigarette smoke or viral infections may also trigger episodes of PVFM in the susceptible host.

The diagnosis of PVFM can be challenging. In addition to helping differentiate fixed from variable airway obstruction, spirometry may help to identify children with PVFM. This suggestive information can be gleaned from distinctive changes in the configuration of the graphic representation of inspiratory and expiratory flow volumes plotted against time or flow-volume loops. The flow-volume loop of a child with paradoxical vocal fold motion may appear normal between episodes, only taking on the characteristic shape on the flow-volume curve when the vocal cords are adducted. The observation that the obstruction is evident only intermittently helps establish the diagnosis and direct appropriate therapy.

A fixed central airway obstruction, such as tracheal stenosis, may obstruct both inspiration and expiration, flattening the flow-volume curve for each (Fig 6–3). Variable obstruction will tend to affect one part of the ventilatory cycle. When inhaling, the chest expands and draws the airways open. The chest and intrathoracic airways collapse during exhalation. Variable extrathoracic lesions tend to obstruct on inhalation more than exhalation, whereas intrathoracic lesions, such as tracheomalacia, will typically have a more pronounced effect on exhalation. Tracheomalacia will often produce both expiratory stridor, which may worsen with exercise and respiratory infections, and a characteristic truncation of the expiratory limb of the flow-volume curve.

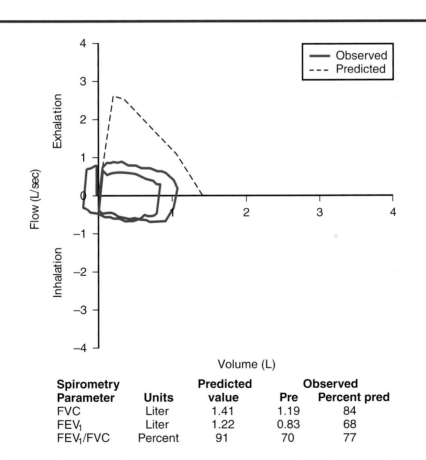

Spirometry Parameter	Units	Predicted value	Observed	
			Pre	Percent pred
FVC	Liter	1.41	1.19	84
FEV$_1$	Liter	1.22	0.83	68
FEV$_1$/FVC	Percent	91	70	77

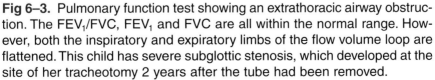

Fig 6–3. Pulmonary function test showing an extrathoracic airway obstruction. The FEV$_1$/FVC, FEV$_1$ and FVC are all within the normal range. However, both the inspiratory and expiratory limbs of the flow volume loop are flattened. This child has severe subglottic stenosis, which developed at the site of her tracheotomy 2 years after the tube had been removed.

CONCLUSION

Pulmonary function studies, including measurement of respiratory muscle strength and flow-volume curves, can be very useful for establishing the diagnosis in a variety of disorders that affect speech. In disorders where there is a question of muscle weakness, or where monitoring muscle strength is important, inspiratory and expiratory muscle strength can be easily measured. Spirometry not only can help establish the diagnosis of airflow obstruction, but also can help determine reversibility. Reversible airflow obstruction is characteristic of asthma, allowing the differentiation from other obstructive disorders. Careful review of the flow-volume loops can provide evidence of airflow obstruction that may not otherwise be appreciated.

REFERENCES

1. *The New Grove Dictionary of Music and Musicians.* In: Sadie S, Tyrrell J, eds. *Vol 6. Edmund to Fryklund*. Oxford: Oxford University Press;1980.
2. Chernick V, West JB. The functional basis of respiratory disease. In: Chernick V, Boat TF, Wilmott RW, Bush A, eds. *Kendig's Disorders of the Respiratory Tract in Children*. 7th ed. Philadelphia, Pa: Saunders Elsevier; 2006.
3. Forster RE, DuBois AB, Briscoe, WA, Fisher, AB. *The Lung, Physiologic Basis of Pulmonary Function Tests*. 3rd ed. Chicago, Ill: Year Book Medical Publishers, Inc; 1986.
4. Laghi F, Tobin MJ. Disorders of the respiratory muscles. *Am J Respir Crit Care Med.* 2003;168,10–48.
5. Koessler W, Wanke T, Winkler G, et al. Two years' experience with inspiratory muscle training in patients with neuromuscular disorders. *Chest.* 2001;120:765–769.
6. ATS/ERS Statement on Respiratory Muscle Testing. *Am J Resp Crit Care Med.* 2002; 166:518–624.
7. Cohn JR, Sataloff RT, Spiegel JR, Cohn JB. Airway reactivity induced reversible voice dysfunction in singers. *Allergy Asthma Proc.* 1997;18(1)1–5.
8. Castile R: Pulmonary function testing in children In: Chernick V, Boat TF, Wilmott RW, Bush A, eds. *Kendig's Disorders of the Respiratory Tract in Children*. 7th ed. Philadelphia, Pa: Saunders Elsevier; 2006.
9. National Asthma Education and Prevention Program. *Full Report of the Expert Panel: Guidelines for the Diagnosis and Management of Asthma* (EPR-3). 1st ed. Pending, National Heart, Lung, and Blood Institute, National Institutes of Health; 2007:1–6064.
10. Medical Algorithms Project. (Chapter 8), Pulmonary and acid-base. *Maximal Inspiratory and Maximal Expiratory Pressures*. Institute for Algorithmic Medicine: Houston, Tex: Copyright (©) 2006–2007.

Laryngeal Electromyography in Pediatric Patients

Al Hillel

The understanding of laryngeal disorders has been greatly advanced in recent years with the increasing use of laryngeal electromyography (LEMG). LEMG is the only test that can define the underlying neurophysiology of abnormal laryngeal function. Although vocal fold mobility can be assessed and described by video studies, paralysis and paresis can only be assessed by LEMG.

In the adult population diagnostic LEMG can be performed in almost all patients. Limited topical anesthetic, or even no anesthetic, is required. No sedation is needed. Patients are asked to perform various tasks during LEMG, and the patient's ability to cooperate with the examiner greatly enhances the quality of the information acquired during testing. A detailed LEMG can provide information about the degree of injury, the age of injury, the ongoing or stable nature of an injury, and the prognosis for recovery. The ability of a patient to tolerate needle insertion quietly and to perform various tasks when requested are both necessary requirements for a thorough LEMG study.

The pediatric population presents unique challenges for the laryngeal electromyographer. Children are generally frightened of needles, do not tolerate painful tests, and often are limited in their ability to cooperate with test procedures, especially if they are uncomfortable and performed by an unfamiliar adult.

This chapter attempts to address the complexities of LEMG in children. A brief description of LEMG is presented in order to outline the procedure as well as the patient tasks required.

LEMG

Electromyography is the study of the electrical activity of muscles. Based on the results of the recordings, many aspects of the condition of the muscle and the motor nerve can be deduced. Three general types of electromyography are commonly used.

Diagnostic electromyography closely examines the types of electrical waveforms while the muscle is at rest, mildly contracting, and maximally contracting.[1-4] Fine wire EMG uses indwelling hooked-wire electrodes to examine many muscles simultaneously to determine the degree and timing of participation of each muscle during a specific task.[5,6] Repetitive stimulation and nerve conduction velocity tests record the electrical activity in the muscle when the motor nerve is triggered by a nerve stimulator.[7,8]

To achieve accurate and in-depth results, all types of electromyography require the skills of an experienced electromyographer and, with laryngeal electromyography, require the skills of an otolaryngologist comfortable with laryngeal anatomy and management of airway issues. It is most important to understand that electromyography and, in particular, LEMG, is most effective when the clinical information from a thorough evaluation and exam is well known to both the electromyographer and otolaryngologist. It is a fallacy to regard electromyography as simply an isolated "test" that can report "test results."

Conceptually, LEMG should be considered an examination rather than a prescribed procedure.[9] A chest radiograph is a fairly standard procedure with an expected "product" that can be interpreted by standard criteria. However, with an ultrasound examination, the examiner needs to know what he is looking for, and needs to conduct the test until a result can be seen and interpreted. In this analogy, LEMG is closer to ultrasound. When the examiners know the clinical history and know what they are looking for, they can then examine the patient with EMG and can continue the testing until results are obtained. Also, the examiners have the option of changing test techniques as the testing proceeds.

Generally, the most useful type of electromyography in laryngeal evaluation is diagnostic EMG. Diagnostic EMG is usually performed with an insulated monopolar electrode that allows the examiner to search for the muscle by directing the needle. The position of the needle in the muscle can often be confirmed by a simple vocal task (confirmation test).[10] Once the needle is in the muscle, the examiner can sample multiple sites to look for the presence of a variety of waveforms.

A complete presentation of the possible findings with diagnostic EMG is not the purpose of this chapter, but a brief description of the terminology and of the types of results found with LEMG serves as a guide to some of the following discussions.

When the needle is inserted in a muscle at rest, it usually stimulates the motor units to fire briefly. The presence of this "insertional activity" is a sign that muscle fibers are present. The degree of the insertional activity is a clue about the state of the muscle. If there is brisk insertional activity, then one can assume that there is little fibrosis, and if further testing reveals no voluntary or stimulable activity, then this muscle might be a good candidate for reinnervation. If there is minimal or no insertional activity, then the muscle might be completely fibrosed. Insertional activity should be seen as a clue, and is one of the findings that can help develop an interpretation of LEMG.

With the needle in place in the muscle, the patient is instructed in a task to activate the muscle (generally an "eee" or a "sniff"). This response is called voluntary recruitment and is a sign of how well the patient can control the activity of the muscle. The pattern of voluntary recruitment can also give an indication whether the deficit is due to a peripheral nerve injury or a central nervous system process. The timing of the recruitment during a variety of tasks can also provide clues regarding the presence of synkinesis that can sometimes present as immobility on fiberoptic laryngoscopy.

With the muscle at rest, the needle is moved slowly through the muscle looking for diagnostic waveforms or motor unit action potentials (MUAPs). During voluntary recruitment, the MUAPs are also examined, and most EMG machines are able to capture individual motor units during the test. The types of MUAPs found offer clues about the age of a nerve injury, the maturity of the injury, whether the injury is ongoing, stable or recovering, and a general prognosis for further recovery.

The clinical interpretation with LEMG is based on the "normal" MUAP (Fig 7-1)

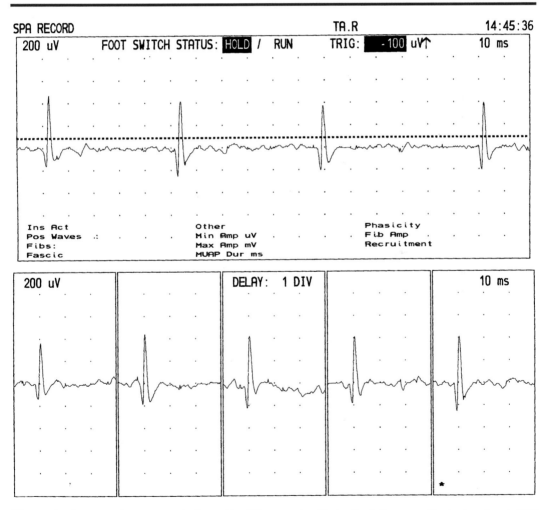

Fig 7–1. A normal motor unit from the TA muscle. Note that the amplitude is about 700 millivolts (200 mV/division) and the duration is about 7 milliseconds (10 ms/division).

which is the electrical signal generated by the muscle fibers controlled by one nerve fiber. A fibrillation potential (Fig 7–2) is a sign of ongoing denervation whereas a polyphasic potential (Fig 7–3) is a sign of ongoing regeneration. A large MUAP (Fig 7–4) is a matured polyphasic potential and signifies an older peripheral nerve injury that is now stable. When the patient is asked to phonate (voluntary recruitment), a full pat-

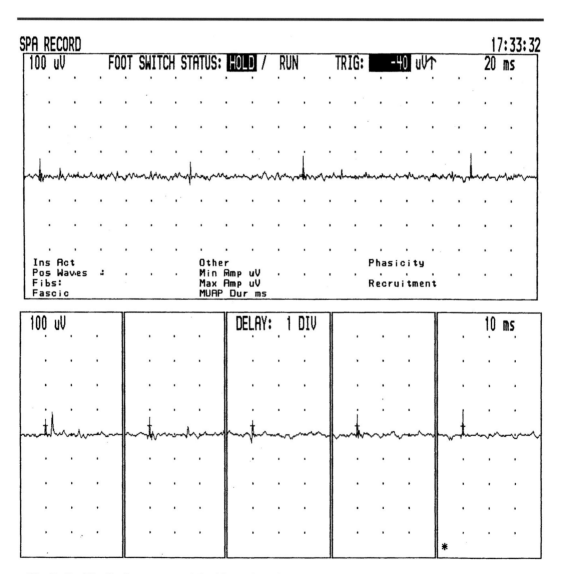

Fig 7–2. Fibrillations potentials. Note that the duration of this waveform is about 1 ms.

tern with many MUAPs is seen (Fig 7–5). The finding of few MUAPs firing fast (Fig 7–6) suggests that very few MUAPs are present and that they are being driven by the central nervous system to compensate by firing quickly. The presence of many MUAPs firing slowly (Fig 7–7) indicates that the initiating signal is at a deficit and is a sign of a central nervous system disorder.

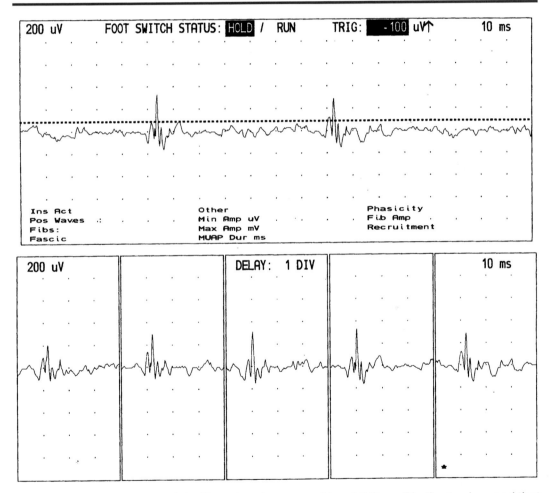

Fig 7–3. Polyphasic potentials. Note that there are at least 5 "turns" in the tracing, and that the duration is prolonged at about 12 ms.

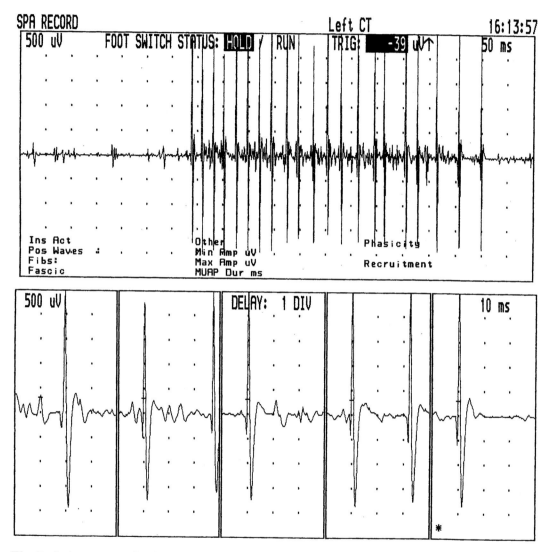

Fig 7–4. Large amplitude motor unit depicting an old but stable peripheral nerve injury. The amplitude is about 4 mV (200 mV/division) with under 2 mV being the normal range. Note that the waveform is triphasic and that the duration of the waveform is about 7 ms.

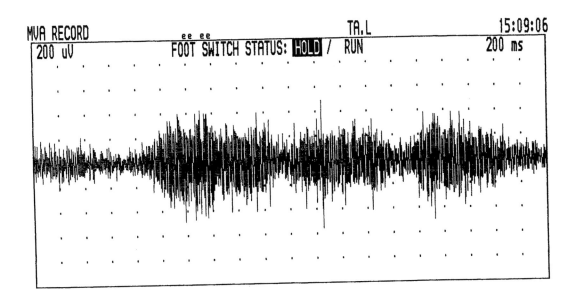

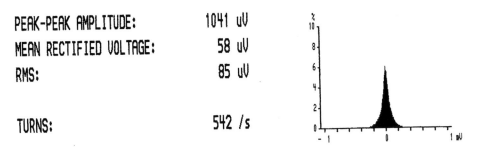

PEAK-PEAK AMPLITUDE: 1041 uV

MEAN RECTIFIED VOLTAGE: 58 uV

RMS: 85 uV

TURNS: 542 /s

Fig 7–5. Normal recruitment pattern during the phonation task of "eee,eee,eee" (/i,i,i/). Note the dense recruitment representing the firing of many motor units.

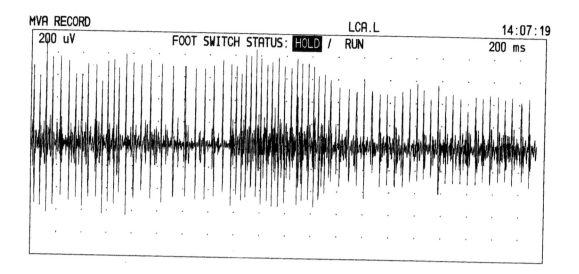

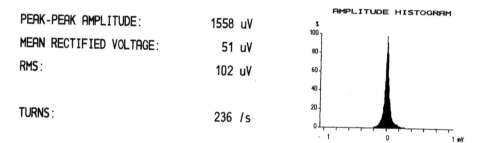

Fig 7–6. Few motor units firing fast indicating evidence of a peripheral nerve injury. Note that the recruitment pattern is less dense than in Figure 7–5. Also note that in contrast to Figure 7–5, individual motor units can be seen and are repetitive at a rate indicating fast firing. This condition is known as "few motor units firing fast."

CLINICAL INTERPRETATION OF LEMG

LEMG, as previously mentioned, is most useful when used with clinical history and physical examination. In many cases, LEMG can confirm a suspected diagnosis. In other cases, it can help the clinician decide among a number of reasonable treatment options. In some cases, the LEMG can be very direc-tive toward a clinical treatment pathway. Many of the benefits of LEMG are seen primarily in adults who can undergo a test while awake that allows an in-depth examination. These benefits are often less clear in the pediatric population due to the limitations of testing awake children.

The most classic use of LEMG is in the evaluation of unilateral vocal cord immobility.[11,12] Generally, the timing of the LEMG is just prior to intervention. If the clinical

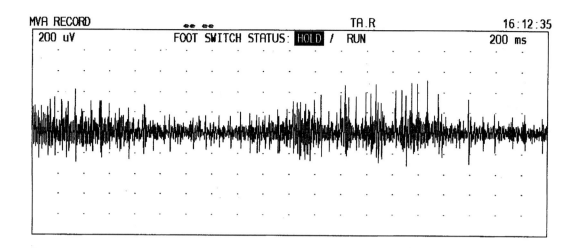

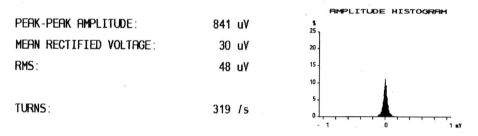

Fig 7–7. Many motor units firing slowly indicating concern for a central deficit. Note that the recruitment pattern is not as full as in Figure 7–5, and that the motor units do not seem to be rapidly repetitive as in Figure 7–5. This condition is characterized as "many motor units firing slowly."

decision is to wait the traditional one year to allow for spontaneous recovery, then the time to perform the LEMG is at one year, prior to surgical intervention. A partially innervated vocal fold, or a synkinnetic vocal fold, might be best treated with laryngeal framework surgery. If many polyphasic potentials are seen (a sign of ongoing recovery), it might be reasonable to delay treatment in the hopes of further spontaneous improvement. If little or no voluntary activity is seen (indicating a dense nerve injury), then a reinnervation procedure might be the ideal choice.

If early intervention is considered, due to the needs of the patient, whether temporary improvement is sought by injection medialization or permanent intervention is considered with framework medialization, then a LEMG should be considered. If there are vigorous signs of ongoing recovery, then the patient might choose to wait a little bit longer. If no clear signs of imminent recovery are seen, both the patient and surgeon might feel clearer in the decision to intervene.

Another valuable use of LEMG that can provide definitive clinical direction is with the patient who is suspected of having had an arytenoid dislocation. Classically, these patients have a general anesthetic with an attempt to "relocate" the arytenoid, often with forceful maneuvers. Unfortunately, rarely do these patients have the opportunity to have an LEMG prior to the decision to undergo this procedure. Many, or most, of these patients actually have a paralysis that presents with an arytenoid that is tipped forward, mimicking a dislocation. An LEMG that demonstrates paralysis would allow the patient to avoid a surgical procedure.

LEMG is also very valuable in the evaluation of patients who present with bilateral vocal fold immobility. In many cases, especially those who present without an iatrogenic etiology, the underlying disorder is cricoarytenoid joint fixation. The evaluation of the cricoarytenoid joint (CAJ) under general anesthetic is often difficult, and in this author's opinion, is one of the most underrated assessments undertaken during laryngoscopy. An accurate assessment requires deep paralysis, careful position of the laryngoscope so CAJ mobility is not impaired, and firm manual fixation of laryngeal movement during palpation of the CAJs. In addition, the examiner must be careful to avoid confusion between CAJ fixation and interarytenoid scarring. A suspicion of CAJ fixation can be greatly reinforced with an LEMG that demonstrates laryngeal innervation adequate to suggest vocal fold movement in the absence of CAJ fixation.

PATIENT SELECTION

In a cooperative patient, the LEMG results, along with the patient's history and physical examination, can guide the physician to a good understanding of the underlying pathophysiology, and in many cases can significantly influence recommendations for treatment options. To a certain degree, the "quality" of the LEMG is often based on the extent of the patient's ability to remain quiet during the waveform study, and their ability to perform assigned tasks on cue. Sedation is rarely used, and if needed is usually very mild. In the adult population, some test sessions are very limited due to patient anxiety whereas some test sessions are extraordinarily thorough due to the patient being calm during the examination. Almost all adult patients are able to tolerate LEMG well.

LEMG in the pediatric population is usually rather limited due to patient tolerance. LEMG is not a test that can be done without a patient's willingness to undergo the procedure. Standard awake-LEMG is rarely accomplished in children under 10 years old. A few children between 10 and 12 can be coaxed to have the procedure, but the LEMG usually needs to be halted after one or two needle insertions. Very little can be accomplished once the patient becomes anxious. Often children 13 and older will cooperate with at least a limited LEMG study if they are carefully prepared.

As LEMG is performed by a team of specialists, it is unusual for the physicians to know the child very well before the test. Whereas adults are accustomed to examination by strangers, children usually will not be able to cooperate with a painful procedure by someone they do not know. Our experience has led us to defer the LEMG to the second or third visit, and to spend a lot of time with the child before the test. Whereas an adult LEMG might take 20 minutes from the time the patient enters the room, an hour or more is typical for a limited awake-test in a child.

In an adult LEMG, there is great benefit to being somewhat systematic in the procedure. Examining the unaffected side is usually performed first to get familiar with the individual anatomy, and to get a baseline result. In an LEMG for a child, the procedure should be changed to examine the critical area first as study of only one or two areas might occur before the test is terminated.

Due to the difficulty of performing awake-LEMG in children, other options can be tried. Sedation can be used but confirmation tests to ensure accurate needle placement cannot be performed. Light sedation usually allows the examiner to begin the procedure easily, but usually results in a terminated study once the needle insertions begin.

Deep sedation with the help of an anesthesiologist is usually successful in allowing needle insertion, but the patient then is not able to initiate voluntary tasks. Some limited information can be obtained with needle insertion and by moving the needle through the muscle to look for abnormal MUAPs.

Another option for LEMG in children is in the operating room. In this scenario, the child is given a general anesthetic. Direct laryngoscopy is performed and either endoscopic or percutaneous wire electrodes are placed in the vocal cords (TA or thyroarytenoid muscle). With greater difficulty, fine wires can also be placed in the posterior cricoarytenoid (PCA) muscles. With the laryngoscope still in place, the anesthetic is stopped, and the vocal folds are observed by stimulating a cough to look at the TAs, or by obstructing the airway to stimulate abduction and the PCA muscles. Generally, the information gathered in this type of LEMG is limited to a gross evaluation of recruitment. The hooked-wire technique does not allow the electrode to be moved to sample different areas in the muscle.

Another indication for testing in the operating room, both in adults and children, is bilateral vocal fold immobility because of the concern that the LEMG could trigger an airway crisis. In our early experiences, we did electrode placement under a light general anesthetic and recorded responses as the patient awakened. However, as noted above, the results in these cases were difficult to interpret. Currently, if there is a concern about the airway, we do a limited awake-LEMG by testing just the LCA muscles to avoid the risk of vocal fold edema caused by needle insertions in the TA muscles.

INTERPRETATION OF LEMG IN CHILDREN

The limitations of voluntary needle studies in children make interpretation of LEMG difficult. As previously mentioned, LEMG is valuable in conjunction with the history and physical findings. The goal of an LEMG is to provide information that can further the understanding of the pathophysiology of the underlying disorder. The brief recordings that can be obtained in children are often not in depth enough to adequately sample diagnostic MUAPs. The gross recruitment gathered with hooked-wire electrodes as a child awakens from a general anesthetic does provide clues regarding the innervation of the muscles. However, when we compared the LEMGs obtained in a similar fashion in adults with the eventual clinical outcomes, we concluded that the gross recruitment sampled as patients awoke from anesthetic, although a positive sign of innervation, did not predict meaningful voluntary recruitment postoperatively. For the most part, we have abandoned this type of testing.

CASE REPORTS

Case 1

A 10-year-old girl presented in our clinic with a diagnosis of bilateral vocal fold paralysis since a colon interposition for esophageal reconstruction after a lye ingestion. The patient had a limited airway since the surgery, even after a posterior cricoid split with interposition graft 2 months prior to her visit. Laryngoscopy demonstrated a 1-mm glottic gap at rest with paradoxic movement during a sniff. A diagnosis of laryngeal synkinesis was considered but it was felt that she was too young for an LEMG. Empirically, an injection of 0.5 units of botulinum toxin to the LCA muscles was performed with EMG guidance under moderate sedation.

The patient returned to clinic 4 weeks later noting an improved airway and a breathy voice. On laryngeal exam, the glottic gap was 5 to 6 mm on inspiration with slight paradoxing. Over the next 3 years she had 8 more injections of botulinum toxin without sedation. She maintained a good airway until the last two injections. At that time, she was 13 years old and agreed to have awake-larygneal EMG testing to evaluate her presumed diagnosis of laryngeal synkinesis.

The LEMG results demonstrated bilateral innervation of the LCA muscles. The muscles were active during phonation and had less than 10% activity during inspiration. The PCA muscles were not tested due to stridor and patient tolerance. No evidence of abductor synkinesis was noted.

Further evaluation was undertaken in the operating room. Under sedation, an LEMG was attempted. Fine wire electrodes were placed in the TA muscles, the LCA, and PCA muscles. The TAs demonstrated an estimated 70 to 100% recruitment with a cough, the LCAs demonstrated reduced numbers of motor units firing fast, and the PCAs demonstrated large amplitude motor units but limited recruitment when the patient was stimulated to sniff. Again, no clear synkinesis was demonstrated and the innervation was felt to be adequate for good vocal fold movement.

Based on the LEMG results, a direct laryngoscopy was performed. Palpation of the cricoarytenoid joints showed a fixed joint on the right and a stiff joint on the left. These findings, along with the results of the LEMGs, led us to be confident that she would not likely benefit from any further botulinum toxin, and a right vocal cordotomy was performed.

The patient did well postoperatively, and 7 years later gave birth with a normal vaginal delivery without airway issues.

A review of this case raises a number of questions. It is not clear why the patient had 2 years of improved airway with botulinum toxin. Clearly, at the time the botulinum toxin stopped working, LEMG showed that the patient did not have synkinesis. It would have been interesting if she had been able to have an LEMG at initial presentation. The lack of vocal fold movement seen in clinic, along with the good recruitment seen in the intraoperative LEMG, predicted the finding of cricoarytenoid joint fixation which was confirmed during direct laryngoscopy. Although the finding of fixed joints alone would have been a good indication for cordotomy, the finding of innervation without movement offered confirmation of the clinical decision.

Case 2

A 12-year-old boy presented to our clinic with a history of inspiratory stridor. The patient was noted to have wheezing, shortness of breath, and poor exercise tolerance since birth. Examination showed a healthy appearing boy with inspiratory stridor and a barking cough. Laryngeal exam revealed essentially no abduction of either vocal fold, with slight adduction noted with phonation. The glottic gap was estimated at 1.5 mm.

His history included a reference to bilateral vocal fold paralysis and some type of nerve procedure to his larynx at age 7 which, by report, was felt to be unsuccessful. These records were not available.

The family history was notable for two preceding generations with inspiratory stridor. The patient's mother carried a diagnosis of bilateral vocal fold paralysis, diaphragmatic paralysis, heart failure, short stature, and diffuse muscle weakness. A tracheotomy maintained her airway. The grandmother was also reported as having bilateral vocal fold paralysis, short stature, and lower extremity weakness.

The patient had a formal neurologic evaluation which noted definite weakness in the small hand muscles, some absent deep tendon reflexes in the arms, and short stature. These findings, along with the history of bilateral vocal fold paralysis led to the conclusion that he suffered the familial disorder of his mother and grandmother.

The patient was taken to the OR to perform a laryngeal EMG under controlled conditions in the event the procedure triggered an airway crisis. Under anesthesia, fine wire electrodes were placed in both TA muscles, the IA, and the right PCA. EMG activity was monitored as the patient awakened. During early awakening, motor units in the TA muscles were noted to be firing fast (about 25 Hz), but when the endotracheal tube was clamped, periodic bursts in the TA muscles and right PCA appeared to be normal. The IA muscle had occasional motor unit potentials but had less activity than the other muscles.

Based on these findings, an examination under anesthesia was performed. A band was found between the arytenoids that appeared to restrict arytenoid movement. The band was cut and increased arytenoid mobility was noted. Due to vocal fold edema from the procedure, a tracheostomy was performed.

Three weeks after the procedure, examination showed a 2 to 3-mm glottic opening with good adduction. Six weeks after the procedure the glottic gap was estimated at 4 mm. The tracheostomy tube was removed. Five months after the surgery, the glottic gap was estimated at 3 mm and bilateral adduction/abduction was noted. At 9 months after his procedure, the glottic gap was estimated at 3.5 mm and complete glottic closure was achieved during phonation. The patient was able to run over a mile but did have some difficulty when wrestling in gym class.

The last visit by the patient was 3 years after the procedure. At that time he indicated that he continued to run and play basketball. He noted noisy breathing with significant activity. Examination showed that he had an estimated glottic gap of 2.5 to 3 mm on a sniff, which increased to about 5 mm on deep inspiration. Paradoxing of vocal fold movement was not noted during breathing tasks but was noted during deep inspiration while laughing.

The case shows the value of LEMG, even within the constraints of the setting of a general anesthetic. The LEMG results demonstrated that, in spite of the long history of assumed vocal fold paralysis, bilateral vocal fold innervation was present. Based on these results, further evaluation led to the interarytenoid lysis with a successful result of mobile, although limited, vocal fold function and the avoidance of a permanent tracheostomy.

Case 3

A 12-year-old boy presented to our clinic 2 years after a tracheal transection suffered from a water ski tow rope as he was crossing the wake in a personal watercraft. He had a tracheostomy for 5 months after the accident. Examination showed no left vocal fold movement and minimal right vocal fold movement.

The patient was taken to the operating room for an LEMG under controlled conditions. The left TA showed markedly reduced numbers of motor units firing fast (50 Hz). The right TA appeared normal. The left PCA showed rare motor units, whereas the right PCA showed decreased numbers of motor units with a few polyphasic potentials. Based on these results, an anterior/posterior cricoid split with interposition rib graft was performed with the hope that the residual innervation would be enough to allow for glottic closure.

When the laryngeal stent was removed, the rib graft was noted to have failed. Four months later, with the tracheostomy tube plugged, the airway was estimated at 2 to 3 mm with some movement of the right vocal fold and the tracheostomy tube was removed. Ten months after the procedure the patient had some increasing shortness of breath but was still active, noting stridor when running beyond two bases in baseball.

At 3 years after his surgery, the patient, now 15 years old, reported a poor airway. The patient was again taken to the OR for an LEMG. The left TA showed reduced motor unit action potentials active with phonation and with a sniff. The left PCA showed reduced numbers of large amplitude motor units active with a sniff. The right TA and right PCA did not demonstrate any crisp recruitment. In the hopes that the left side had enough innervation to allow for vocal fold movement, an anterior/posterior cricoid split with interposition rib graft was performed. Again the rib graft failed. Over the next months the patient did not tolerated decannulation, and a conservative left cordotomy was performed. The cordotomy was enlarged 4 months later and the tracheostomy was later removed.

The patient was last seen 4 years after his cordotomy at age 21. He reported that his voice was serviceable for his needs. He was able to run a mile and snowboard without difficulty unless the hill was steep with moguls. Audibly, he had a breathy voice with low volume with a large component of false fold phonation. His cordotomy remained open and there was no paradoxic movement with rapid respiration.

This case shows that the intraoperative LEMGs were used to make the decisions to proceed with anterior/posterior cricoid splits with the belief that the innervation was adequate to allow for glottic closure during phonation and swallowing. The outcomes of these surgeries are difficult to evaluate due to the failure of the rib grafts. In retrospect, when looking at the LEMG results, it is not convincing that the amount of innervation seen would have been adequate to achieve the movement needed. It is also notable that the two LEMGs performed 3 years apart did not have the same results. An awake-LEMG with controlled voluntary recruitment might have demonstrated less convincing signs of innervation than the results obtained during the "bursts" seen in the patient when his endotracheal tube was clamped. The results of this case, as well as a number of similar cases in adults with bilateral immobility, have led us to abandon concern of airway compromise as a key indication for intraoperative LEMG testing. Instead, we now do a limited awake-LEMG of the LCA muscles.

CONCLUSION

LEMG is a valuable tool to evaluate the abnormal larynx. LEMG is the only test that can confirm a suspected paresis or paralysis. All other evaluations, at best, can only strongly suggest a neurologic etiology for the dysmobility or immobility. In many instances, LEMG can be helpful in deciding the best treatment course for a patient. Admittedly, in the pediatric population, LEMG has the limitation imposed by the difficulty of performing the test in child.

Overall, laryngologists, both in the adult and the pediatric populations, are forced to make treatment choices with a limited understanding of the pathophysiology of patients' disorders. Although in many cases, an LEMG can contribute to the understanding of a disorder, and in some cases clearly direct the clinician, LEMG should be considered in all cases of disordered mobility in the larynx. Our understanding of the neurophysiology in these patients, even in those cases that are not influenced by the LEMG results, will make us better clinicians, and over the time of our careers, will further our ability to make wise choices and devise improved treatment options.

See Appendix for a description of a novel technique available to enable operative LEMG in children with vocal fold immobility.

REFERENCES

1. Faaborg-Andersen K. *Electromyography of Laryngeal Muscles in Humans: Technics and Results*. Vol. 3. Basel: S. Karger. 1965: 1–71.
2. Golseth JG. Diagnostic contributions of the electromyogram. *Calif Med.* 1950;73(4): 355–357.
3. Golseth JG. Electromyographic examination in the office. *Calif Med.* 1957;87(5): 298–300.
4. Faaborg-Andersen K, Buchthal F. Action potentials from internal laryngeal muscles during phonation. *Nature.* 1956;177: 340–341.
5. Hirano M, Ohala J. Use of hooked-wire electrodes for electromyography of the intrinsic laryngeal muscles. *J Speech Hear Sci.* 1969; 12:363–373.
6. Hillel AD. The study of laryngeal muscle activity in normal human subjects and in patients with laryngeal dystonia using multiple fine-wire electromyography. *Laryngoscope.* 2001;111(4 pt 2 suppl 97):1–47.
7. Petyz F, Rasmussen H, Buchtal F. Conduction time and velocity in human recurrent laryngeal nerve. *Dan Med Bull.* 1965;12: 125–127.
8. Atkins J. An electromyographic study of recurrent laryngeal nerve conduction and its clinical applications. *Laryngoscope.* 1973;83(5):796–807.
9. Sulica L, Blitzer A. Electromyography and the immobile vocal fold. *Otolaryngol Clin North Am.* 2004;37(1):59–74.
10. Hirose H, Gay T., Strome M. Electrode insertion techniques for laryngeal electromyography. *J Acoust Soc Am.* 1971;50: 1449–1450.
11. Hiroto I, Hirano M, Tomita H. Electromyographic investigation of human vocal cord paralysis. *Ann Otol.* 1968;77:296–304.
12. Kotby MN, Haugen LK. Clinical application of electromyography in vocal fold mobility disorders. *Acta Otolaryngol.* 1970;70: 28–437.

Pediatric Laryngeal Electromyography

Andrew R. Scott
Christopher J. Hartnick

CASE

DM was a 2-month-old ex 27-week premature infant who was intubated for respiratory distress shortly after birth and mechanically ventilated for 6 weeks in the neonatal intensive care unit. At 7 weeks of age she had persistent stridor and otolaryngology was consulted. Flexible laryngoscopy demonstrated bilateral vocal fold immobility. She underwent direct laryngoscopy, bronchoscopy, and suspension laryngoscopy with intraoperative laryngeal electromyography (LEMG) with the NIM 2 system. Findings were notable for vocal folds which were mobile to palpation. LEMG during spontaneous respiration demonstrated motor unit action potentials (MUAP) in the left thyroarytenoid (TA) muscle, but no activity in the right TA muscle (Fig 8–1A). The parents refused tracheotomy, and the child remained in the hospital under close observation for management of complications related to bronchopulmonary dysplasia.

Four weeks later the patient was again taken to the operating room. Direct laryngoscopy and bronchoscopy findings were unchanged, however intraoperative LEMG was now notable for the presence of MUAP in both TA muscles (Fig 8–1B). Repeat flexible laryngoscopy while the patient was awake demonstrated persistent right vocal fold paralysis; however, the left vocal fold was now mobile.

Over the next 4 weeks the child continued to improve clinically. Flexible laryngoscopy performed in the office at a one-month follow-up appointment confirmed return of function of both vocal folds with full and symmetric movement.

BACKGROUND

Chapter 7 clearly describes the limitations of electromyographic evaluation of children with laryngeal dysfunction. The utility of performing LEMG in patients under anesthesia

Left TA   Right TA

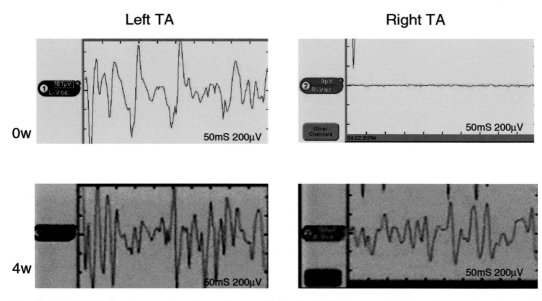

Fig 8–1. LEMG tracings at various time points. **A.** Initial presentation. LEMG tracings of the right and left TA muscles using monopolar paired electrodes and NIM 2 Response system; gain set to 200 μV with a sweep speed of 5 ms/division. Normal MUAP in the left TA muscle and electrical silence in the right TA muscle. **B.** 4-week follow-up. LEMG tracings of the right and left TA muscles using monopolar paired electrodes and the NIM 2 Response system set at a gain of 200 μV with a sweep speed of 5 ms/division. Normal MUAP in both TA muscles.

remains controversial. The significance of MUAPs produced during respiratory variation as this activity pertains to voluntary laryngeal function is still unknown. Often, however, children will not comply with office based, awake, volitional, task-focused laryngeal EMG and the question remains whether operative laryngeal EMG has any clinical role to play. Our institution and others continue to perform intraoperative LEMG in select cases, such as children with bilateral vocal fold immobility where any hint of recovery of function would have clinical utility or children with stable bilateral vocal fold immobility when a surgeon is deciding which side to perform a cordotomy. These procedures require the use of electromyography equipment in the operating room, which often must be further modified for use in the pediatric larynx.[1-5] Chapter 7 presents a brief review of a simplified technique for intraoperative LEMG in children using nerve monitoring equipment, which has made electromyography more accessible at our institution. This chapter introduces this simplified technique to the interested practitioner so as to spur more thought and research into developing modalities by which LEMG can best be performed in children.

TECHNIQUE

Anesthesia and Exposure

An IV is placed after mask-induction, and adequate general anesthesia is obtained using a remifentanil and propofol infusion. A single intraoperative dose of dexamethasone (0.5 mg/kg) is given. The glottis is exposed using a Lindholm laryngoscope (Fig 8–2A) and the child is placed in suspension. Anesthesia is lightened until the patient is breathing regularly and spontaneously.

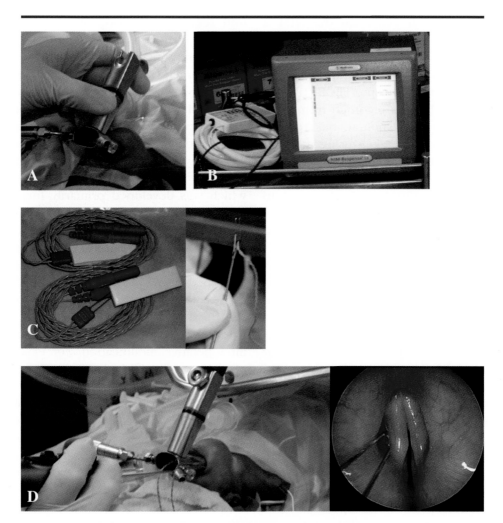

Fig 8–2. A. The pediatric Lindholm laryngoscope is used to expose the larynx. **B.** The NIM Response 2.0 monitor and attached "patient interface" cord. **C.** Paired subdermal electrodes, which are inserted using laryngeal alligator forceps. **D.** Endoscopic placement of electrodes into the TA muscle.

Technique of Laryngeal Electromyography

The NIM Response system (Medtronic ENT USA, Inc., Jacksonville, Fla) is used to perform laryngeal EMG (Fig 8–2B). A monopolar grounding electrode (Medtronic ENT USA, Inc., Jacksonville, Fla) is placed subcutaneously into the right shoulder. Paired, monopolar, subdermal monitoring needle electrodes (Fig 8–2C) from the NIM 2 Response kit (Medtronic ENT USA, Inc. Jacksonville, FL) are placed endoscopically into each thryoarytenoid (TA) muscle using laryngeal alligator forceps (Fig 8–2D). Intraoperative LEMG is recorded from both TA muscles during spontaneous respiration. Recordings are taken using the NIM 2 Response monitor (Factory settings: EMG display: 80 Hz–2 kHz (−6 +3 dB @ 500 Hz), EMG Audio: 120 Hz −1.7 kHz (−6 +3 dB @ 500 Hz), sweep speed 50 ms (5 ms per division), and gain values of 50 μV and 200 μV).

In order to capture data for later analysis by a consulting neurologist, video and audio recordings are made using a digital video recorder (Med X Change DRS2, Med X Change, Inc, Bradenton, Fla), which is connected to the NIM 2 Response monitor via audio and video outputs using a video converter (TView MicroXGA, Focus Enhancements, Inc, Campbell, Calif). The acoustic signal and video data are stored and later reviewed by a neurologist with electromyography training. Once recordings have been made, the child is taken out of suspension and allowed to recover from anesthesia.

Although pediatric intraoperative LEMG is not routinely performed at referral centers, the small body of literature on the subject and our own experience suggest that the technique is safe and can be performed as an outpatient procedure.[3,5]

CRITIQUES

Currently, pediatric LEMG remains primarily a research tool and no standard application has been widely accepted. Possible reasons for this relate to technical challenges in performing intraoperative LEMG as well as a lack of data in regard to the utility of electromyography in accurately predicting vocal fold recovery. Additionally, there is no accepted, standardized technique for performing intraoperative LEMG and no established normal values or outcome measures exist for pediatric patients. Issues relating to children that further complicate electromyographic evaluation of vocal fold paralysis (VFP) include understanding the pathophysiology behind congenital and idiopathic VFP and how the standard adult model, which was developed primarily for iatrogenic injury, may or may not be applicable to this disease process.

Our simplified method for intraoperative LEMG addresses many of the problems described above; however, some disadvantages remain. Improvements over previously-described protocols include the use of standardized equipment that does not require intraoperative modification. For example, placement of paired electrodes from the NIM Response 2 kit using laryngeal forceps is far less difficult than endoscopic placement of needle electrodes or hooked-wire electrodes described in prior studies. The paired, subdermal electrodes were chosen because the 2.5-mm spacing between the two monopolar electrodes allows thorough sampling across the length of the TA muscle. Additionally, the paired electrodes allow for two-point fixation within the muscle, resulting in less waveform variability with body motion than is observed with standard, single-needle electrodes. The electrodes are ready-made, requiring no further modification for use in the pediatric larynx.

Utilizing nerve monitoring equipment that is already present in most operating rooms obviates the need for obtaining commercial EMG equipment. The use of a digital video recorder allows for the storage of both audiovisual data for future viewing by a consulting neurologist, thereby negating the need for intraoperative interpretation of acoustic signals and electromyographic data.

The limitations of our technique should be noted as well. As with any intraoperative LEMG technique, the procedure requires general anesthesia and measures EMG activity that is nonvolitional, correlating with respiratory variation rather than phonatory effort. Additionally, the NIM 2 Response system uses a sweep speed of 50 ms, or 5 ms per division, which is different from the standard display setting for most laryngeal EMG protocols. This intraoperative LEMG protocol also only samples the TA muscles, as the paired electrodes are not optimally shaped for sampling the posterior cricoarytenoid (PCA) muscles. Finally, there are no established criteria for differentiating background noise from a true motor unit action potential using the NIM system. The waveform generated with the NIM system is lower in amplitude and has a "blunted" quality in comparison to waveforms recorded with concentric, monopolar electrodes (Fig 8–3).

FUTURE DIRECTIONS

One way around the conundrum of assessing voluntary RLN function under anesthesia is through the use of evoked laryngeal electromyography (ELEMG), in which a nerve stimulator is used to deliver a preset current to the RLN and laryngeal muscles.

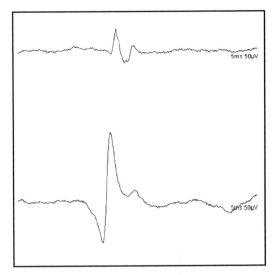

Fig 8–3. A side-by-side comparison of MUAP wave morphology using paired subdermal electrodes (*top*) and a standard concentric, monopolar electrode (*bottom*). Measurements were made simultaneously from the left deltoid muscle; both electrodes are sampling the same, single motor unit. Recording with the TECA system: sweep speed of 5 ms per division; gain set to 50 µV.

A technique for the use of ELEMG on awake adults was first described by Satoh in 1978 and had the added benefit of potentially localizing lesions along the course of the recurrent laryngeal nerve.[6] The method of delivering a standardized stimulus to the RLN rather than relying on volitional movement or respiratory variation allows for the possibility of quantifying the level of innervation of laryngeal muscles. ELEMG has many parallels to evoked EMG of facial muscles, or electroneurography (ENoG). In the same way that ENoG plays a role in predicting return of facial nerve function, ELEMG may hold promise for prognosticating RLN recovery. Investigation is already underway in the development of a practical and reproducible

ELEMG technique. Zealear et al performed an investigative study in 24 canines and determined that a relatively noninvasive technique was possible.[7] Both Zealear's technique and the original method described by Satoh require the use of a percutaneous needle stimulator, which may provoke anxiety in patients and cause some discomfort with repeated nerve stimulation. This technique may actually be better suited for children, who must be anesthetized for any form of LEMG. Furthermore, the simplified technique of intraoperative LEMG described herein involves modifying the use of a machine that is, in fact, designed primarily for recording evoked waveforms.

REFERENCES

1. Jacobs IN, Finkel RS. Laryngeal electromyography in the management of vocal cord mobility problems in children. *Laryngoscope*. 2002;112:1243-1248.

2. Koch BM, Milmoe G, Grundfast KM. Vocal cord paralysis in children studied by monopolar electromyography. *Pediatr Neurol.* 1987;3:288-293.

3. Gartlan MG, Peterson KL, Hoffman HT, Luschei ES, Smith RJH. Bipolar hooked-wire elctromyographic technique in the evaluation of pediatric vocal cord paralysis. *Ann Otol Rhinol Laryngol.* 1993;102:695-700.

4. Berkowitz RG. Laryngeal electromyographic findings in idiopathic congenital vocal cord paralysis. *Ann Otol Rhinol Laryngol.* 1996; 105:207-212.

5. Wohl DL, Kilpatrick JK, Leschner RT, Shaia WT. Intraoperative pediatric laryngeal electromyography: experience and caveats with monopolar electrodes. *Ann Otol Rhinol Laryngol.* 2001; 110:524-531.

6. Satoh I. Evoked electromyographic trest applied for recurrent laryngeal nerve paralysis. *Laryngoscope.* 1978;88:2022-2031.

7. Zealear DL, Swelstad MR, Fortune S, et al. Evoked electromyographic technique for quantitative assessment of the innervation status of laryngeal muscles. *Ann Otol Rhinol Laryngol.* 2005;114(7):563-572.

PART II

Treatment of a Child With a Voice Disorder

Voice Therapy for Children

Katherine Verdolini Abbott
Nicole Yee-Key Li
Rita Hersan
Leslie Kessler

Voice problems are common within the pediatric population. Their prevalence has been estimated to be anywhere between 11 to 36%, thus affecting over five million school-aged children in the United States.[1,2] Although most pediatric voice problems are not life threatening, they often result in negative consequences including a delay in the development of communication skills, difficulty participating in classroom discussions, problems with social interactions and psychosocial functioning, and loss of productivity, self-esteem, and well-being.[3] Pediatric voice disorders may also progress to voice problems in adulthood, ultimately requiring treatment and generating negative professional and personal consequences.[4] Because of the potentially disruptive consequences of voice disorders in children, federal mandates require that children with voice disorders affecting their educational performance receive services for them in the schools (Individuals with Disabilities Act). Most conservative estimates indicate several million children are appropriate for

such formal intervention annually and nearly one-third of speech language pathologists report they treat children specifically with voice/resonance disorders.[4]

The most common physical condition associated with pediatric dysphonia is thought to be vocal fold nodules.[5-7] As most clinicians are aware, vocal fold nodules are protuberances that develop on the free margins of the true vocal folds, usually at the midpoint of the membranous folds bilaterally (Fig 9–1). Both physical evidence and logic suggest the principal cause of nodules is perpendicular impact force between the vocal folds during phonation, for example.[8] The lesions are best distinguished on stroboscopic exam or, if needed, microsuspension laryngoscopy, given the inherent difficulties in accurately diagnosing lesions on single-view fiberoptic examination of hesitant children. Nodules are implicated in as many as 35 to 78% of cases of childhood dysphonia.[9-13] For example, in one recent report from the United Kingdom, case records were retrospectively reviewed for all children

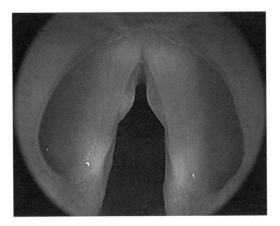

Fig 9–1. Bilateral vocal nodules in a child. These are protuberant lesions on the medial surface of the true vocal folds, located at the midpoint of the membranous vocal folds bilaterally.

presenting to a children's hospital with a primary complaint of dysphonia.[14] Results showed that 45% of 137 cases of children between birth to 16 years were diagnosed with "vocal abuse." Of those, 58% had nodules. Data also indicate there is a clear gender effect associated with nodules in children. The prevalence of vocal fold nodules has been reported to be as high as 21.6% in males and much lower, at 11.7%, in females in children 7 to 16 years of age,[5,15] the reverse of the gender bias for nodules in adults. Nodules are often associated with inferior quality of life and social function in children.[16,17] Children with nodules also tend to have significantly worse vocal function than normal children, as measured for example by voice range profiles and computer-assisted voice analyses.[18,19] Also, the severity of hoarseness, breathiness, straining, and lack of voice has been linked to the physical extent of nodules.[20]

Finally, clinical wisdom as well as data suggest children with nodules may be vocally exuberant and thus are predisposed to phonotrauma.[21] More troubling, some data imply many children with nodules have behavioral issues. According to one report, children with "hyperkinetic dysphonia" were more aggressive and immature than their healthy counterparts, based on results from a "picture frustration task."[22] A more recent report qualitatively echoes those findings, indicating children with nodules are more likely to act out, and have disturbed peer relations and immature behaviors as compared to age-matched children without nodules, based on results from the Walker Problem Behavior Identification Checklist for parents.[16] However, other findings run counter to these common notions. The most recent paper of which we are aware on the topic used the Childhood Behavior Checklist (CBCL/4-18)[23] to assess the behaviors of children with and without nodules, based on parental report.[21] Results failed to detect group differences for any of the scales reflecting behavior problem syndromes. Group differences were approached for the terms "screams a lot" and "teases a lot," with children with nodules showing higher scores. However, the group with nodules also obtained higher scores on the "Social scale," which encompasses a list of positive attributes of a child's social activity, contact with friends, behavior alone, and behavior with others. Results indicated children with nodules were "outgoing" or "extroverted." However, prior claims about aggression, attention problems, or impulsive behavior in children with nodules were not borne out. Thus, although some links may exist between personality and nodules on average, no a priori assumptions can be made about personality factors—especially factors related to behavioral problems—for any individual child with nodules.

Of course, numerous other conditions can affect children's voices besides nodules. However, given their prevalence and negative effects for children, the remainder of this chapter focuses on treatment of children with nodules. Many of the principles discussed here are applicable to many other conditions that affect children's voices, as well.

OVERVIEW OF VOICE THERAPY FOR CHILDREN WITH NODULES

Treatment of children with nodules may involve some combination of behavioral, pharmacologic, and surgical interventions. In this chapter, "voice therapy" refers to behavioral intervention. This type of therapy is the most commonly used first-line treatment for children with vocal fold nodules. According to one study, 95% of surveyed otolaryngologists chose this method of treatment first for children.[24] In another previously cited study, 74% of children diagnosed with so-called "vocal abuse" (of which 58% had nodules and 42% had simple "abuse" presumed by history but normal laryngeal exam) were enrolled in voice therapy.[14] The remaining children were not enrolled in voice therapy due to the clinician's impression—that many speech-language pathologists would not share—the children were too young to comply with it.

We return to the term "vocal abuse" toward the end of this chapter. At this juncture, discussion proceeds with an overview on the general rationale behind voice therapy for children with nodules. This approach is based on the theory that nodules are, as noted, primarily the result of phonation patterns. The traditional view is that nodules' origins are principally quantitative: an affected individual has phonated too much, too loudly—that is, has engaged in "vocal abuse".[25-27] However, recent thought emphasizes the idea that phonation *quality* is at least as important as phonation *quantity*

in the pathogenesis of nodules. Specifically, "pressed voice"—produced with strong medial compression of the folds—is thought to increase the risk of nodules due to the link between vocal fold adduction and perpendicular impact stress to the folds[28,29] and further between impact stress and tissue injury.[8] According to this view, children who speak with *pressed voice* may have increased risk of phonotrauma such as nodules, whether they speak or sing loudly or not. Children who phonate loudly, or extensively, with less forcefully adducted vocal folds may have less risk. Speculation also indicates genetic factors may be predisposing for nodules, assuming the presence of phonatory stresses that exceed some minimal threshold.[30-32]

In all approaches to voice therapy for children with nodules, the general goal is to address behaviorally factors believed to contribute to pathogenesis. In much of the traditional school, the focus generally is "indirect" voice therapy. This approach tends to employ "vocal hygiene" education to inform children about voice production mechanisms and injury, and guide them towards the identification and reduction of "vocal abuse" including loud phonation, the imitation of animal and machine noises, hard glottal stops, coughing, yelling across a distance, and similar behaviors.[33-37] An extension of the traditional school incorporates actual voice work, which generally focuses on a quiet, gentle voice as an antidote to phonotraumatic forces that may have contributed to onset and maintenance of pathology.

The traditional approach is conceptually reasonable. However, concerns are raised about its practicality. First, there are questions about the number of behaviors we ask children to monitor in the traditional approach to therapy. Data indicate that patient compliance is inversely related to the load placed on patients in treatment,[38,39] and thus children may adhere poorly to such programs. More cogently, there are questions about the extent to which it is feasible to get an inherently vocally exuberant child, whose exuberance may be causal in the disorder, to substantially reduce the amount and loudness of his phonation. In fact, vocal exuberance is likely related to personality traits that endure across the life span regardless of any interventions.[40,41] Recent thought emphasizes the notion that if children are predisposed to exuberant phonation due to personality traits or life situation, our job is not so much to try to limit their voice use to provide them with a way to produce voice often and loudly as *safely* as possible.[42,43] Specifically, this alternative "direct" approach attempts to train children to produce voice in a way that can be loud, while minimizing potential damage to the tissue as well as physical effort. The biomechanical setup needed to achieve this target is discussed shortly. In the interim, it is important to note that attempting to tame a child's vocal exuberance may not only be met with resistance by the child. If a child does comply with this directive, it would seem the child could have counterproductive reactions including hesitancy about oral communication and loss of communicative self-esteem.

VIEWS REGARDING THE BENEFITS AND COSTS OF VOICE THERAPY FOR CHILDREN

In spite of how commonly it is utilized, the impact of voice therapy for nodules and other voice problems in children has not been established in prospective controlled studies, and its actual benefit is controversial. In some quarters, voice therapists have argued that "screaming is an entirely normal behavior of children; a history of shouting may in fact be less common among children with nodules than among those without," and strenuously argue against the utility of voice therapy in the pediatric population.[44] In accordance with this opinion, some retrospective data show that 77% of children with nodules still exhibited abnormal larynges, even after 2 months of traditional voice therapy involving attention to breath flow and gentle vocal fold adduction, using humming exercises.[45] Against this opinion, however, prospective uncontrolled studies of voice therapy in children have shown that 68% of children had improved vocal function after 15 sessions of voice therapy that apparently involved some actual voice work (eg, breathing coordination and "voice emission" exercises).[46] Surveys confirm that opinion is mixed among those who actually provide voice therapy, with only 48% of speech-language pathologists reporting that voice therapy was the preferable treatment for children with nodules.[24]

Voice therapy is time consuming and has a clear opportunity cost. Many clinicians are reluctant to provide voice therapy in the school setting due to lack of confidence in their abilities in voice therapy, uncertainty over how therapy can be justified vis-à-vis the Individuals with Disabilities Education Act (IDEA), and other factors.[1] Thus, it is likely that much voice therapy for children is deferred to the outpatient setting. As a result, therapy often is associated with missed school and missed work for parents. Formal data are not available. However, anecdotal reports indicate students may miss as many as 75 classes over a 9-month academic period for therapy in the school setting, and up to 15 half-days of school (and thus an estimated 60 classes) over a 15-week period for outpatient therapy (American Speech-Language-Hearing Association Special Interest Division 3 Voice and Voice Disorders listserve survey, conducted by K. Verdolini Abbott, January 28–February 1, 2009). Thus, voice therapy has potential deleterious effects in the context of having unclear benefits. Furthermore, the time investment itself is a significant burden, as therapy requires missed school and the associated problems of absenteeism. Absence from school for more than 10% of the time is associated with lower academic performance in children as young as those in kindergarten through third grade, even if absences are excused.[47] School absenteeism is also a key risk factor for high-risk behaviors, psychiatric disorders, and economic deprivation[47,48] and has even been touted as a proxy measure of child health status.[49] Thus, although voice therapy is the most frequently utilized treatment for children with vocal nodules, at the time of this writing there are no prospective controlled data that have established its benefits outweigh the associated problems of its cost. Clearly, such data are badly needed and one hopes will be forthcoming in the next years, along with revised models of pediatric voice therapy itself.

REVIEW OF DATA ON VOICE THERAPY FOR CHILDREN

Individual Therapy

We have just noted contrasting opinions exist regarding the appropriateness and effectiveness of voice therapy for children with nodules. One previously cited retro-spective study pessimistically indicated 77% of children with nodules, who received 2 months of direct if not indirect voice therapy, demonstrated persistently abnormal larynges after treatment.[45] However, the seemingly negative interpretation of those findings may be tainted by the stance that laryngeal condition is the proper primary therapy outcome to assess, and within that stance, the conviction that nothing short of a normal larynx signals therapy success. Since the publication of that paper, emphasis has been placed on other parameters as indicators of therapy success, including voice quality, ease of phonation, and especially voice-related quality of life, which were not evaluated in the study in question.[17] Indeed, a more recent, prospective study already cited showed 68% of children with nodules, intracordal cyst, or fusiform mucous thickening had improved vocal function, especially as shown by improvements in various aspects of the phonetogram (vocal field) and perceptual ratings of roughness, breathiness, and overall grade of dysphonia, after 15 sessions of direct and indirect voice therapy.[46]

In addition to those studies, a few other scattered data sets have been reported in the literature on voice therapy for children, although none of them used prospective controlled designs. In one case study, a successful outcome of therapy was described for a 7-year-old girl with bilateral voice fold nodules following a combination of traditional ("indirect") and "direct" therapy.[50] Therapy involved seven sessions over 3 months. Indirect therapy targeted patient-family education including instructions to eliminate "vocal abuse," add recovery time following extensive voice use, and decrease caffeine and increase water intake. Direct therapy targeted "breath support," relaxed phonation, forward focus, and easy onset phonation. Specific exercises involved breathing, humming, and /h/ initial speech utterances. The report indicated that 3 months after therapy, the patient's vocal nodules were resolved and her voice quality was perceptually normal. Also, acoustic measures (jitter and shimmer) and aerodynamic measures (mean airflow rate and intraoral pressure) were improved compared to pretherapy and within normal limits for the child's age and gender. This case report is valuable for its illustration of principles of individual pediatric voice therapy discussed in the larger paper.

Other data are available from a somewhat larger retrospective study from Korea.[51] Eight boys (ages 4–12 years) who were diagnosed with nodules plus muscle tension dysphonia ($n = 7$) or muscle tension dysphonia alone ($n = 1$) received 30-minute individual voice therapy sessions once or twice weekly for up to 2.5 months. Therapy focused on: (1) enhancing the child's awareness of the voice problem and laryngeal tension, (2) producing easy-onset voice using sighing and humming techniques, and (3) self-monitoring and carryover. Following therapy, all of the children showed improvement in voice quality. Speaking fundamental frequencies improved from too high or too low before therapy to normal after therapy. Stroboscopic examinations, which were successfully performed in 4 children, showed reduced anterior-posterior suprgraglottic constriction or decreased nodule size in all of the children examined. This report has value due to the somewhat larger sample size and, again, its description of therapy. However, interpretation of the data is limited by the retrospective design and the lack of a control group.

Another study did use a prospective design in examining the outcome of voice therapy for a larger cohort of 28 children with isolated vocal (reporting on).[52,53] Of the full cohort, 26 children complied with voice therapy, and 77% of those children had resolution or improvement in their dysphonia. Only one child received microsurgical excision. In an additional group of 12 children with nodules and a second laryngeal diagnosis, only 40% showed improvement. Furthermore, for 7 children with cysts or polyps, voice therapy was entirely ineffective. Strengths of this report include its prospective design and the light it sheds on differential results of voice therapy that may be expected as a function of laryngeal diagnosis. However, interpretation of the data again is limited by the lack of a control group and, in this case, a lack of information about the type of therapy that actually was delivered.

Finally, a case study format was used to describe the results of a electromyographic (EMG) feedback program in the treatment of a 9-year-old boy with bilateral vocal nodules, who had been unresponsive to typical behavioral intervention.[54] Following a course of EMG biofeedback training in both nonspeaking and speaking conditions (treatment duration was not reported), laryngeal muscle tension was reduced, the vocal nodules were reportedly eliminated, and voice quality was grossly normal at 6-month follow-up. This report provides valuable information about the potential benefit of instrumented feedback in therapy for recalcitrant children. The ability to generalize the results is limited by the small subject number and the lack of an experimental design.

In sum, existing data are sparse and do not point to any firm conclusions about the value of voice therapy for children with nodules, in general. However, together, the data provide optimism that some combination of more or less traditional indirect and direct voice therapy may have value for some children with vocal fold nodules.

FAMILY AND SCHOOL-BASED INTERVENTIONS

Many clinicians who treat voice problems in children consider family and school support to be critical for the prevention and treatment of voice problems in children.[36,50,55-58] Several published reports are relevant.

In one study, a family program based on SYNGESTI ("Systemisch gestörte Stimme," ie, system-related voice disorders) model was tested in 9 German children, 7 boys and 2 girls, ages 6 to 10 years, and their families.[58] Six of the boys were diagnosed with nodules and the remainder were diagnosed with "functional" voice disorders. The program was conducted in five phases, involving a total of 28 one-hour sessions, delivered twice weekly. The phases targeted: (1) problem orientation, (2) exploration of the family system, (3) differentiated goal plan, (4) therapy program, and (5) evaluation. The important aspect of this study is that it emphasized interventions with family rather than direct voice therapy with the child. Parent questionnaires, consultation with parents, and parents' evenings were utilized throughout the program. Also, some voice activities, namely, listening games, movement games, role–playing, and voice games, were carried out along with the family interventions. Perceptual and acoustic measures of the affected children's voice in reading were compared before and after therapy. Significant improvements in voice quality were reported for hyperfunction, "gratings," and hard glottal attacks. For children who showed abnormal mean fundamental frequency before therapy, values achieved normal ranges following therapy. The authors suggested that SYNGESTI set itself apart from typical direct voice therapy for children because it focused on the family and thus took pressure off the child.

In terms of interventions within the school setting, two vocal hygiene studies were carried out as part of a classroom program for children grades 3 to 6[55] and grades 2 to 3.[36] In the study by Cook et al[55] the vocal hygiene program consisted of two half-hour classes weekly over three weeks, for a total of six sessions. Thirty-eight children identified as having hoarse voice participated in the program, which used cartoon illustrations presented by speech-language pathologists to small groups of 2 to 4 children. The program addressed the basic structure and function of the human vocal mechanism, voice quality, "proper" and "improper" use of the voice, and voice disorders. A 20-question test of vocal hygiene concepts was administered before and after therapy. Children showed significant improvement in test scores following the hygiene program. Results suggested that the children acquired knowledge about critical vocal hygiene principles. However, clinical outcome measures for voice were not reported.

In the second study, 155 children and their classroom teachers received an education program on vocal hygiene.[36] The program was presented by school speech-language pathologists and consisted of two half-hour sessions per week over 2 weeks, for a total of four sessions. A 10-item test of vocal hygiene concepts was administered to the children before (pretest) and after (posttest) the program, and again 5 months following termination of the program (retest). Significant differences in student test scores were found between pretest and posttest as well as between posttest and retest (all p <0.05). A voice screening was also performed before and after the program. Results indicated 7.7% and 5.8% of the students were judged having deviant voice quality before and after the program, respectively. Three children who were identified as having hoarse voice before the program were judged to have normal voice quality after the program. Last, teachers who underwent the program also showed improved knowledge useful for identifying and preventing voice disorders in students. Results from this study imply a voice education program may produce benefits for some children with dysphonia. However, due to the lack of a control group, it is unclear from the data whether improvements were due to maturation or other factors unrelated to the intervention.

Two further relevant reports addressed the frequency of direct voice therapy in the treatment of dysphonic children, and parents' and clinicians' views about the utility of a public school voice clinic program.[56,57] In a metropolitan school district, semiannual voice clinics were held for 10 years for children with dysphonia. Two hundred forty-nine (249) cases were reviewed for children in preschool through grade 12. Indirect laryngoscopy was performed on 90% of the children by attending otolaryngologists. (The remaining 10% could not be examined.) Of cases reviewed, 40% of the children showed nodules, whereas only 18% of the cases were judged to have normal larynges. Most of the remaining cases displayed chronic laryngitis or thick vocal folds. Contact ulcers and paralysis also were detected, but were infrequent. Four types of recommendations were made for the children: (1) direct voice therapy, (2) trial therapy or voice hygiene education, (3) voice monitoring, or (4) no intervention. Among these options, direct voice therapy was the most commonly utilized (65%). In a follow-up survey study, questionnaires were administered to both parents and clinicians to assess their views about whether the public school sponsored voice clinics were beneficial in the vocal rehabilitation process and, if so, how.[57] In general, parents and clinicians responded positively regarding the program's role in initial diagnosis, referral, and client education.

To summarize, a few data points are available indicating there may be value to family interventions and to school-based voice hygiene education for some children with vocal fold nodules. However, as for studies on individual voice therapy, the ability to interpret the data are hindered by limitations in the study designs.

GAPS IN THE DATA

As is clear from the foregoing review, data on the value of voice therapy for children with nodules are extremely limited. In sum: (1) there is a paucity of research; (2) the research that has been conducted has used largely observational designs; and (3) therapy approaches are rarely described in sufficient detail to allow for replication by other clinicians. Moreover, (4) cohesive conceptual frameworks for the interventions are lacking; and (5) reported approaches generally targeted reduction in voice use at some level. The lack of cohesive frameworks may reduce clinicians' enthusiasm for voice therapy, or their confidence in their ability to provide it. Questions also can be asked about the pragmatic utility of programs that target voice reduction in children, especially vocally exuberant children who are likely at the greatest risk for phonotrauma in the first place.

PROPOSAL AND FUTURE DIRECTIONS

A foundational proposal is that the further development of and inquiry into pediatric voice therapy ideally should be grounded in a cohesive conceptual framework, which generally is lacking in current, traditional approaches to therapy. Different frameworks can be envisioned. Ideas to consider follow.

Example of a General Framework for Pediatric Voice Therapy

One proposal is that, as for voice therapy in adults, potentially three broad parameters are necessary and arguably (in the extreme) sufficient to address in any training targeting motor behaviors: (1) the "what" of training, that is, what is the biomechanical goal of training? (2) the "how" of training, that is, how will an individual acquire the new behavior (motor learning)? And (3) the "if" of training, that is, what factors may influence the likelihood a patient will adhere to the training program (patient compliance)?[59]

These topics have been only dimly addressed in the pediatric literature in a way that is relevant for voice therapy. However, we can glean some possible ideas about them from corollary literature.

The "What" of Voice Therapy: Some Ideas About Biomechanical Goals

Relative to the "what" of therapy, there is general agreement that voice therapy usually should address both voice hygiene ("indirect therapy") and voice production ("direct therapy"). In a sense, voice hygiene can be considered under the rubric of "biomechanics" (the "what" of voice therapy) because most if not all hygiene recommendations aim at altering the vocal fold tissue substrate and thus its biomechanical properties. In the adult population, long "do" and "don't do" lists delivered to people with voice problems as hygiene instructions have not fared particularly well.[60-62] Possibly, shorter lists, especially ones that target

a specific individual's profile, might do better, as the compliance literature informs us that the more things we ask people to do the less likely it is they will do them, for example[39]. Thus, by targeting and tailoring voice hygiene instructions to a particular child, hygiene programs might have a greater likelihood of being followed and ultimately benefiting an individual patient as compared to generic programs that may be overwhelming and largely irrelevant to the individual.

In terms of a reasonable biomechanical goal for voice production itself, in the traditional approach, many clinicians target a widely abducted vocal fold configuration with small-amplitude oscillations during speech for the child with nodules. The resulting voice is quiet and breathy. That approach is based on the idea that this particular biomechanical setup should minimize intervocal fold impact stress during phonation, and thus attenuate the primary causal factor for the pathology. As noted, on the surface, the approach is sensible. However, there are two concerns with it. First, vocal fold contact can occur during breathy voice production, and contact is sometimes as forceful as with more adducted vocal folds.[28] Second, in terms of biomechanical goals, we need to consider not only the tissue but also a child's personality and life style. Where a vocally exuberant child is concerned, or a child who needs to speak loudly due to life circumstances, it would seem reasonable to identify a mode of phonation that allows functional communication to occur—loudly if needed—rather than trying to suppress it. Data from the adult literature indicate a barely ad/abducted vocal fold configuration, on the order of about 0.5 to 1.0-mm distance between the vocal processes, optimizes the relation of voice output intensity (large) to vocal fold impact intensity (relatively small; Fig 9–2) during phonation.[28] Stated differently, this

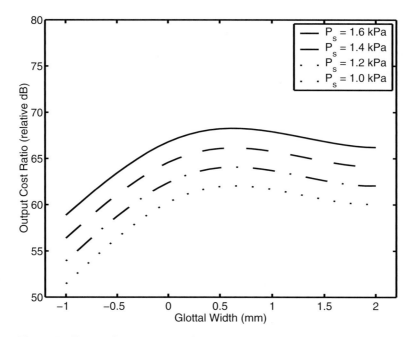

Fig 9–2. Ratio of voice output intensity divided by vocal fold impact intensity (unitless ratio) as a function of glottal width for 1.0, 1.2, 1.4, and 1.6 kPa at approximately 155 Hz, for combined excised canine and simulation data. From D Berry, K Verdolini, D Montequin, M Hess, R Chan, IR Titze. (2001). A quantitative output-cost ratio in voice production. *J Speech Lang Hear Res.* 44:29–37.[28]

configuration should allow people to speak quite loudly while relatively minimizing phonotrauma to the tissue—an ideal goal for vocal "activists" such as many children with nodules or at risk for them. Unpublished observations suggest this general laryngeal configuration is relevant for the pediatric situation as well (Berry, D. A., personal communication, March 2009).

In adults, the target posture corresponds to what is perceptually identified as "resonant voice," defined as voice produced with perceptible anterior oral vibrations and minimal perceived physical effort.[59,63,64] Preliminary observations suggest that the simple instruction to attend to "loud and easy" voice may be sufficient for children, without the need to invoke "resonant voice"

specifically. Cognitive literature as well as laws of practice to be discussed shortly imply it may be counterproductive to complicate voice therapy by addressing numerous additional targets, particularly when those targets are trained in isolation of each other. In other words, the typical approach of addressing breathing + easy onset + other phonatory parameters may be contraindicated in pediatric voice therapy. A ("loud")-easy target may be sufficient. Without a doubt, sometimes work on other parameters such as breathing may be necessary in order to achieve the target biomechanical configuration. For example, there may be coordination issues across respiratory and phonatory dynamics that limit a child's ability to obtain the laryngeal target. However, clinicians might want to consider the number of targets they address in therapy and keep them as lean as possible, at least as far as the *patient's* attention is concerned.

The "How" of Voice Therapy: Some Ideas About Motor Learning

Regarding the learning piece of voice therapy for children with nodules or other pathologies, information is not only limited in the literature. It is all but lacking. If we attempt to mine the pediatric motor learning literature to obtain some clues, we will find that most of it actually deals with motor *development* rather than motor learning. The developmental literature is divided across "representational" and "dynamical systems" camps. Deep discussion of the issues is beyond the scope of the present chapter. However, briefly, representational views tend to focus on higher order cognitive operations in motor behavior and learning.[65-67] In contrast, dynamical systems approaches strongly focus on interactions across tissue and environment to explain motor behavior and largely ignore learning in any explanatory sense.[68,69] Potentially, we might consult the pediatric cognitive literature in general to gain information about cognitive development across the pediatric cycle, to inform some of our choices about the best approach to motor training in pediatric voice therapy. Especially executive functions and attention may be relevant. However, at present, such consultation has not occurred in any systematic way relative to voice, of that we are aware, specifically.

Some speech motor learning literature is relevant. However, much of it is interweaved conceptually with literature on motor learning in adults. As a starting point, much literature in the adult domain suggests both motor performance and learning are facilitated by attention to gestures' *effects* rather than *biomechanics*.[70,71] We are not aware that there is any reason to think the situation would be different for children. If so, we would do best to direct our pediatric patients' attention to the sound and feel of their voice rather than the typical approach, which focuses children's attention on the *biomechanics* of voice production (eg, "Breathe in with a big belly," "Relax your shoulders," etc). An example would be to direct a child's attention to the *ease* and *clarity* of vocalization, rather than respiratory or other maneuvers believed to affect ease.

Discussion could be entertained about different aspects of attention, such as the ability to orient to a target, focally (consciously) process target information, and maintain vigilance on the target, see for example[72]. Again, detailed discussion is beyond the scope of this chapter. However, there is merit to the consideration that some children may have difficulty with one or more aspects of attention. Furthermore, some children may have difficulties with particular processing targets including audition and proprioception, both of which seem important for voice therapy. Clinicians may wish to focus on these issues during ongoing therapy with a child and address them as needed during the therapy program.

Another topic of interest relative to motor learning has to do with so-called "laws of practice" that have been established for adults, and may have at least partial applicability for children.[73] For example, variable practice—in the case of voice therapy referring to practice of the target voice in numerous phonetic, physical, social, and emotional contexts—should sharply increase generalization of the target behaviors to novel contexts compared to less variable practice. The value of variable practice for the generalization of motor behaviors has been robust for both children and adults.[73-77] In fact, in some clinicians' experience, variable practice in *naturalistic contexts* may be one of the most powerful tools with which we can arm ourselves in pediatric voice therapy, regardless of which biomechanical goals we are pursuing. Another factor pertinent to the "laws of practice" has to do with the relative merits of "part" versus "whole" practice. Literature on adults indicates that when component parts of a behavior ultimately are to be run off in parallel (at the same time), practice of the parts in isolation of each other may be harmful to learning, for discussion see ref. 73. There is no reason to suspect the situation should be different for children. In that case, it would indeed seem counterproductive to splinter voice therapy into pieces *separately* addressing different phonatory parameters that are integral parts of a whole production system such as breathing and phonation. Ideally, clinicians can find a way to train *coordination* across these production parameters, rather than training them in isolation. Exceptions can and do arise in some contemporary approaches to voice therapy (Kessler, L., personal communication, April 2009).

It also should be noted that some of the "laws of practice" established for adults may need to be softened for children, see review in ref. 78. In particular the "law" that says that infrequent augmented feedback about performance from a trainer or a device, which benefits long-term learning in adults, might reduce learning in children. Possibly, children need more feedback to optimize learning compared to adults. Similarly, children sometimes may benefit from blocked as opposed to random practice of targets. The suggested reason for both of these findings is that below a certain age, children's cognitive resources may be limited compared to resources for adults. Instituting some of the laws of practice, including infrequent augmented feedback and random practice, which increase cognitive demands, may

simply put the child over a resource "edge," at which point the child can no longer deal with learning effectively at all.[78-80]

Finally, the pediatric literature is clear that the child's ability to *discriminate* target from nontarget speech productions both receptively and productively constitutes a central foundation for speech learning, for example see refs. 81 and 82. Although this idea has not been tested in children with voice problems specifically, clinical experience as well as logic suggest discrimination should be key in pediatric voice therapy, as well.

The "If" of Voice Therapy: Some Ideas Regarding Patient Compliance

Again, systematic data pertinent to pediatric voice therapy are lacking as far as we know. However, the medical literature provides information that may be relevant. A first consideration is that adolescent children especially may be at risk for poor compliance with medical treatment recommendations. According to one study, noncompliance with medication use was four times greater in adolescents than in adults.[83] Therefore, some children may be at risk for poor compliance, increasing the importance of this variable for therapy outcome. In addition to adolescent age, among the most striking factors that appears to differentiate compliance in children versus adults is the perception of negative "cosmetic" effects of a treatment, which have been found to strongly reduce compliance with medical treatments in children, for example see refs. 84 and 85. In voice, a negative "cosmetic" effect might involve the child's perception that he is being made to sound different from his peers. Therefore, attention to the "cool" factor in voice training is appropriate, potentially as facilitated by *group* therapy delivered to a set of peers.

Additional factors specific to compliance in children have to do with parents. Some data indicate children's compliance with a treatment may be negatively affected by a critical as opposed to supportive parent.[86,87] Furthermore, regarding parental involvement in therapy, authors emphasize the importance of considering the load on parents when asking them to be involved in therapy activities, and to actively collaborate with parents in the development of a home program.[88] For example, it may be important to identify, with the parent, one or two daily activities during which the child will pay particular attention to voice use. As for adults, in children compliance with home programs decrease as the complexity and duration of the programs increase.[38,39] Additionally, clinician-patient rapport is considered crucial for compliance, as it is for adults, for example[89].

Summary on Proposals to Consider

The foregoing discussion provides a few ideas about broad factors that might be considered in the development of a conceptually cohesive framework for pediatric voice therapy. A rudimentary pediatric voice therapy program, Lessac-Madsen Resonant Voice Therapy—5 to 10, has been developed based on several of these principles. The program is currently undergoing revisions based on field testing. Extremely early findings for three pediatric patients with nodules, who received therapy based on an extended version of this program, are shown in Table 9–1 (Kessler & Verdolini, in progress).

Certainly, other options exist besides those briefly outlined here. Other, traditional approaches to voice therapy have been described in detail in the literature, some with attendant therapy materials. Examples include *The Boone Voice Therapy for Children*[34] and Andrews' approach to voice therapy for children and adolescents.[33] These approaches are appealing because they describe voice therapy for children in detail and are resources for many clinicians working with the pediatric population. Additional useful materials can be found in publications by Moran and Zylla-Jones,[35] Nilson and Schneiderman,[36] and Wilson.[37] Above and beyond the particular approach one takes,

Table 9–1. Pre- and Posttherapy Measures for Three Representative Pediatric Patients Receiving Voice Therapy for Nodules According to an Extended Version of *Lessac-Madsen Resonant Voice Therapy 5-10* (Kessler & Verdolini, in progress).

	MPT		Semitone Range		Voice Quality		Larynx	
Patient	Pre	Post	Pre	Post	Pre	Post	Pre	Post
01	4.0	8.4	8	32	G3	G0	BN	N/A
02	3.0	6.0	7	19	G3	G0	BN	NL
03	4.6	10.5	8	20	G2	GO	BN	NL

Maximum phonation time (MPT, seconds): Semitone pitch range (number of semitones): Voice quality (G3 = significant periods of aphonia, hoarseness, and strain; G2 = moderate hoarseness; G0 = clear, easy voice, normal): and Laryngeal appearance (larynx; BN = bilateral nodules; NL = normal larynx; N/A = data not available).

it is clear the field would benefit from systematic inquiry into the utility of any of the approaches to the treatment of nodules and other conditions affecting children's voices.

COROLLARY ISSUES

Laryngeal Exam: Necessary or Not Prior to Voice Therapy?

The question is: Is a laryngeal examination by an otolaryngologist necessary prior to initiating voice therapy for a child with dysphonia? This question is most pressing for voice therapy in the schools, where on-site laryngeal examinations are not available. Some clinicians feel that because the preponderance of cases of pediatric dysphonia involve benign pathologies or even no organic pathology at all, laryngeal examinations are not necessary before starting voice therapy with a child. This position is bolstered by the difficulties clinicians encounter in attempting to obtain such examination from a school-based platform. In contrast, other clinicians feel that even if a child with dysphonia is *likely* to have a benign condition, a medical evaluation is nonetheless required prior to embarking on voice therapy. These clinicians feel it is important to know the extent and nature of the underlying condition, which might affect the approach to treatment. For example, where isolated nodules without other findings are concerned, indirect and direct therapy might proceed normally. However, if a vocal fold hemorrhage is involved, complete voice rest may be indicated for a period. Alternatively, if a child is hoarse due to a cyst, voice therapy probably will be fairly useless, as least as far as lesion reduction is concerned. More gravely, some dysphonias in children are linked to serious medical conditions that should be identified. A classic case is recurrent respiratory papillomata. Clinicians concerned about these issues may routinely contact parents of children with dysphonia requesting their child undergo a laryngeal examination by an otolaryngologist prior to initiating voice therapy. However, clinicians pursuing this approach often are frustrated by the lack of parental response, or when a response is obtained, the medical evaluation may be thwarted by a lack of parental funds, insurance, or time. Finally, some parents are hesitant to subject their children to the procedure, which can be uncomfortable and frightening.

The challenges are real. We could discuss the issues philosophically. However, a professional issue of substantial proportions introjects itself. The American Speech-Language-Hearing Association (ASHA) Preferred Practice Patterns for the Profession of Speech-Language Pathology (1997)[90] states: "All patients/clients with voice disorders must be examined by a physician, preferably in a discipline appropriate to the presenting complaint. The physician's examination may occur before or after the voice evaluation by the speech-language pathologist.[90,91] Stated simply, the professional organization legally overseeing speech-language pathology practice mandates that individuals with voice problems be evaluated by a physician, preferably an otolaryngologist, before or after the speech-language pathology evaluation.

We thus find ourselves in a challenging situation. Not only may we have reticent clinicians. School policy may complicate matters. Specifically, some school administrators apparently instruct speech-language pathologists (SLPs) to indicate an otolaryngology consult is "preferred" rather than "recommended" for a child with dysphonia. The reason is that an official "recommendation" may put the school in the position of having to pay for the examination and administrators may prefer costs be passed on to parents. Legislation around these issues is unclear, and likely varies across school districts and states. However, SLPs who find themselves in this position encounter a "no-win" situation. They either violate their own code of ethics, based on ASHA dictates, or they violate school administration directives. We are not talking about issues of small numbers. We are talking about 60,000+ SLPs practicing in school settings in the United States.

How shall we proceed? To adhere to ASHA standards, some solution must be found. Initially, clinicians may find themselves in a position of having to argue the case one school district at a time. One possible model that has been proposed in the past has been the use of an on-site voice clinic, in which an otolaryngologist or otolaryngology resident travels to a school district to perform annual laryngeal examinations on children with dysphonia.[57,92] Funding may or may not be needed for this approach. Alternatively, perhaps an agreement can be reached with a given otolaryngology practice to refer all children with dysphonia, with a reduced fee schedule. In any event, we insist that despite the challenges, children with dysphonia must receive a laryngeal (and head and neck) examination by an otolaryngologist before a full course of voice therapy can be undertaken.

School-Based Versus Outpatient Voice Therapy

The approach to voice therapy may need to be modified considerably depending on whether it is provided in a school or outpatient setting. For example, clinicians in schools usually do not have sophisticated instrumentation to conduct exhaustive voice evaluations. Despite clinicians' frequent concerns around this question, the point actually is moot. As argued elsewhere, knowledge about pathologies affecting voice and measurement principles are more important than equipment for conducting a solid evaluation.[93] In fact, probably the only equipment that is strictly needed or strongly preferred for a good voice evaluation is a pitch pipe or keyboard and an inexpensive sound level meter.[93] More important, school clinicians may feel they are constrained to small working spaces that are inappropriate to address the type of voice activities most relevant for children in therapy. The counter to this concern is that clinicians working in the schools are housed in the very environment in which children spend a great deal of time. Thus, structuring things properly, clinicians have the opportunity to conduct highly ecologically valid therapy within the schools, *provided* they integrate therapy with the child's usual daily activities. Where better to conduct therapy than with the child's peers—on the playground, in gym class, and in other settings that not only *replicate* the child's typical environment, but actually *constitute* much of that environment? In fact, given children's general orientation to same-age peers, cogent arguments could be made that *group* therapy in the school setting has particular power to stimulate effective behavioral changes that are highly relevant to the child.

The advantages and disadvantages of voice therapy in the school setting generally are reversed for the outpatient clinical situation. In the latter setting, clinicians may have access to sophisticated instrumentation that can afford them an in-depth view of the child's phonatory situation. As well, the outpatient setting often will provide direct access to laryngeal examinations. However, although outpatient clinics may strongly facilitate the involvement of parents or caregivers in therapy because they are required for transportation at minimum, outpatient clinics do not spontaneously bring with them the child's peers or material that is relevant to a particular child. In such cases, it is important to collaborate with parents to gain as much information as possible about the child's school and home environment, favorite games and activities, and so forth, to incorporate them into therapy activities. Furthermore, some informal observations suggest that inviting the child's friends, siblings, or other children with voice problems to participate in therapy with the child in the outpatient setting may greatly facilitate learning and stabilization of target behaviors. It is recognized that billing issues may complicate matters particularly where group therapy is concerned. However, conceptually, there are important reasons to consider it.

"Vocal Abuse and Misuse"

A final issue has to do with the terms "vocal abuse and misuse." These terms are widely used in the care of both children and adults with voice problems. Vocal "abuse" is generally defined as a problem of phonation quantity: too much, too loud, too long. A definition of vocal "misuse" is more difficult to pin down in the literature, but it is generally described in terms of qualitative issues such as poor vocal "efficiency" (which itself is then usually not well defined).

It has been argued elsewhere that despite their nearly pervasive use in voice care, these terms are problematic.[94] First, they are conceptually circular. Take the case of vocal "abuse." An example is as follows. Hypothetically, Mrs. Smith takes her son, Johnny, to an ear, nose, and throat doctor because she is concerned about Johnny's hoarse voice. The physician, Dr. Jones, diagnoses vocal nodules. Mrs. Smith asks what causes nodules. Dr. Jones responds they are caused by vocal abuse. Mrs. Smith inquires, "What is vocal abuse?" Dr. Jones answers, "Oh, yelling and screaming. Does Johnny do a lot of that?" Mrs. Smith responds, "Yes, in fact he does." Then she thinks for a moment and says, "But the neighbor child yells and screams a lot too, but he doesn't appear to have nodules." Dr. Jones replies, "Oh, that's because yelling and screaming don't constitute vocal abuse for him." Mrs. Smith, an astute person, ponders for a moment and replies, "Wait a minute. What causes nodules? Vocal abuse. What's vocal abuse? A behavior that causes nodules?" In other words, we have conceptual circularity: a supposed cause of a phenomenon ("abuse") cannot be defined independently of its proposed effect (nodules). This situation is philosophically unacceptable and quickly can lead us down a slippery conceptual slope where we think we have defined a phenomenon when, in fact, we have not defined it at all. We can soon find ourselves in a position of conceptual unclarity without even knowing it. Similar considerations apply to the term "vocal misuse" as apply to "vocal abuse."

There are further concerns about these terms.[94] However, probably the most grave of them has to do with their potential effect on the therapy process and outcome. "Abuse" and "misuse" are not "nice" words. They are not compliments. The relevance to clinical practice is related to the concept of "self-efficacy." Self-efficacy is defined as one's belief in one's ability to carry out a given behavior.[95] Self-efficacy is not a pervasive personality trait such as "self-confidence." Instead, it is highly task specific.[96] Self-efficacy within a given domain is shown to be among the most potent factors influencing patients' compliance with treatment. As of 2009, nearly 20,000 citations emerge in a Pubmed search using the key term "self-efficacy." The corollary is that self-efficacy can be modulated with clinical language.[97] Within the voice domain, there is specific evidence from controlled, double-blinded data that the terms "vocal abuse" and "vocal misuse" harm self-efficacy for voice, in the sense that they interfere with normal increases in self-efficacy that usually are obtained with patient education, at least in adults.[98] Due to their potential to harm a patient's self-efficacy for voice, and self-efficacy's further influence on patient compliance and ultimate therapy outcome, a call has been made to discontinue their use in the clinical voice domain altogether.[94] Alternative terms can be used, such as those that simply describe potentially relevant behaviors without any judgmental overtones (yelling, screaming, grating, pressed voice, squeezed voice, or for adults, "phonotraumatic behaviors"). The decision about terminology use is a personal one for every clinician. However, it seems these issues should be considered in making that decision. The issues may be particularly cogent for the young and possibly impressionable children we dearly wish to serve in our voice therapy clinics.

CHAPTER SUMMARY

Voice problems in children are common. Often, they are associated with vocal fold nodules. Although these lesions are not life threatening, they can generate serious consequences for voice and quality of life. They matter. Many children with nodules may be vocally exuberant and socially oriented. However, claims about other, more negative personality characteristics that have been linked to children with nodules as a group,

such as aggression and impulsiveness, are dubious at best.

Although voice therapy generally is the preferred first treatment for vocal fold nodules in children, little systematic evidence is available to support or refute the approach. However, the sparse, cumulative data that do exist seem to point to several principles that are useful to consider in pediatric voice therapy. First, it appears that most clinicians feel that ideally, therapy should include both "indirect" (vocal hygiene education) and "direct" (voice work) elements. A caution is that it would seem wise to target indirect and direction interventions to an individual child, and to limit the number of parameters we ask a child to manipulate in daily life, rather than giving children uniform, nontargeted, and long lists of what may be annoying "do's" and "don'ts."

Second, although voice conservation would seem to make sense at some level for children with nodules, a concern is that our attempts to tame vocal exuberance in children who are predisposed to it may be met with resistance and less than perfect adherence by children. Moreover, possibly children who do adhere subsequently may develop hesitancy around oral communication, complicating not only communication but also personal psychology. An appealing alternative is to develop and implement approaches that teach children how to use loud voice safely, rather than attempting to remove loud voice from the table altogether. Recently, advances have been made in that direction.

Third, it is important to consider not only *what* the goal of voice therapy for children should be, but also *how* children can obtain the goal. Stated differently, clinicians' knowledge about motor learning is just as important as knowledge about biomechanics in coming to the therapy. Data from the general literature as well as clinical practice suggest variable practice of a target voice in numerous phonetic, physical, social, and emotional environments may be among the most potent tools to enhance generalization of a target voicing pattern to novel contexts the child has not encountered in therapy. The literature also suggests we would do well to direct the child's attention to the *outcome* of voice production maneuvers, such as vocal "ease" even with loud voice, rather than the *biomechanics* of voice instructions. Similarly, data suggest there is little value and there may even be harm to addressing component parts of voice production, such as breathing, voice onset, and overall phonatory mode, in *isolation* of each other. Although exceptions can occur, ultimately it is the global vocal "Gestalt" that seems to requires attention. Finally, it would seem central to build a discrimination component into as many therapy activities as possible, whereby an activity inherently requires the child to discriminate target from nontarget voice receptively and productively, if possible in game format. Ideally, it would seem the effectiveness of receptive and productive learning activities would be increased by a "functional" outcome built into the activities. That is, if "healthy" and "harmful" voice are correctly discriminated and produced, positive outcomes occur in the activity for the child (eg, the child gets a ball being tossed back and forth). If "healthy" and "harmful" voice are incorrectly discriminated or produced, the child might experience light-hearted disruptions or unwanted outcomes in the therapy game or activity.

Fourth, principles of compliance suggest we attend to the "cosmetic" aspects of a child's voice production. A voice that a child perceives as "different" (from his peers) may be unattractive to him and consequently reduce the likelihood he will adopt it in real life. Group treatment may allow clinicians to "therapize" a whole cohort of peers, thus instituting a new standard for what is vocally "cool." Parents also are important to consider in terms of compliance with voice therapy. Clinicians might want to help parents display a supportive rather than critical attitude around the child's voice productions. Additionally, although parental involvement in therapy may be important, we need to consider the load placed on parents by such involvement and collaborate with them in the development of a home program. The compliance literature also suggests we should limit the complexity and duration of what we ask of parents and children in any pediatric therapy program, and as for all types of interventions, clinician-patient rapport is critical.

Fifth, it seems clear that many clinicians indeed consider family and school support critical in the treatment of nodules and other voice-related conditions in children. Thus, integration of family, school, and we would add, peers within the therapy process would seem ideal. However, as noted, we need to be judicious in the load we place on parents in their participation in therapy, and also collaborate with them in establishing parental and child activities in therapy. In that light, perhaps the easiest and most effective route would involve the delivery of *group* voice therapy where possible, either within a group of children with voice problems or within a group of peers or siblings who then will acquire voicing patterns that can serve as good models for the affected child.

Sixth, the domain of voice therapy for children appears in need of a general "face-lift" involving the development of cohesive conceptual frameworks to guide it. Such frameworks would identify a key set of broad principles from which specific therapy goals and activities arise. Some recent developments are encouraging in this regard.

Finally, reading about information relevant to pediatric voice therapy is important, and clinicians should peruse new literature as it becomes available. However, also practical training and exposure to therapy techniques can strongly enhance clinicians' skills and confidence in their ability to provide children effective therapy for their voice problems.

REFERENCES

1. Sapienza CM, Ruddy BH, Baker S. Laryngeal structure and function in the pediatric larynx. *Lang Speech Hear Serv Sch.* 2004;35: 299-307.

2. State and County QuickFacts: Massachusetts (Publication 2009). United States Census Bureau Web site. http://quickfacts.census .gov/qfd/states/25000.html. Updated Sept 4, 2009. Accessed May 01, 2009.

3. Connor NP, Cohen SB, Theis SM, Thibeault SL, Heatley DG, Bless DM. Attitudes of children with dysphonia. *J Voice.* 2008;22(2): 197-209.

4. Incidence and Prevalence of Communication Disorders and Hearing Loss in Children. American Speech Language Hearing Association. http://www.nsslha.org/research/reports/ children.htm. Published 2008. Accessed October 17, 2009.

5. Akif Kilic M, Okur E, Yildirim I, Guzelsoy S. The prevalence of vocal fold nodules in school age children. *Int J Pediatr Otorhinolaryngol.* 2004;68(4):409-412.

6. Benjamin B, Croxson G. Vocal nodules in children. *Ann Otol Rhinol Laryngol.* 1987; 96(5):530-533.

7. Moran M, Pentz A. Otolaryngologists opinions of voice therapy for vocal nodules in children. *Lang Speech Hear Serv Sch.* 1987; (18):172-178.

8. Titze IR. *Principles of Voice Production.* Englewood Cliffs, NJ: Prentice-Hall; 1994.

9. De Bodt MS, Ketelslagers K, Peeters T, et al. Evolution of vocal fold nodules from childhood to adolescence. *J Voice.* 2007;21(2): 151-156.

10. Gray SD, Hammond E, Hanson DF. Benign pathologic responses of the larynx. *Ann Otol Rhinol Laryngol.* 1995;104(1):13-18.

11. Silverman EM. Incidence of chronic hoarseness among school-age children. *J Speech Hear Disord.* 1975;40(2):211-215.

12. Wetmore R. Management of pediatric voice disorders. *Arch Otolaryngol.* 2005;131:72.

13. Wohl DL. Nonsurgical management of pediatric vocal fold nodules. *Arch Otolaryngol Head Neck Surg.* 2005;131(1):68-70; discussion 71-62.

14. Connelly A, Clement WA, Kubba H. Management of dysphonia in children. *J Laryngol Otol.* 2009:1-6.

15. Mandell DL, Kay DJ, Dohar JE, Yellon RF. Lack of association between esophageal biopsy, bronchoalveolar lavage, and endoscopy findings in hoarse children. *Arch Otolaryngol Head Neck Surg.* 2004;130(11): 1293-1297.

16. Green G. Psycho-behavioral characteristics of children with vocal nodules: WPBIC ratings. *J Speech Hear Disord.* 1989;54(3): 306-312.

17. Merati AL, Keppel K, Braun NM, Blumin JH, Kerschner JE. Pediatric voice-related quality of life: findings in healthy children and in common laryngeal disorders. *Ann Otol Rhinol Laryngol.* 2008;117(4):259-262.

18. Campisi P, Tewfik TL, Pelland-Blais E, Husein M, Sadeghi N. MultiDimensional Voice Program analysis in children with vocal cord nodules. *J Otolaryngol.* 2000;29(5):302-308.

19. McAllister A, Sederholm E, Sundberg J, Gramming P. Relations between voice range profiles and physiological and perceptual voice characteristics in ten-year-old children. *J Voice.* 1994;8(3):230-239.

20. Shah RK, Woodnorth GH, Glynn A, Nuss RC. Pediatric vocal nodules: correlation with perceptual voice analysis. *Int J Pediatr Otorhinolaryngol.* 2005;69(7):903-909.

21. Roy N, Holt KI, Redmond S, Muntz H. Behavioral characteristics of children with vocal fold nodules. *J Voice.* 2007;21(2): 157-168.

22. Nemec J. The motivation background of hyperkinetic dysphonia in children: a contribution to psychologic research in phoniatry. *LOGOS*. 1961;4:28–31.

23. Achenbach TM. *Manual for the Child Behavior Checklist/4-18 and 1991 Profile.* Burlington, VT: University of Vermont Department of Psychiatry; 1991.

24. Allen MS, Pettit JM, Sherblom JC. Management of vocal nodules: a regional survey of otolaryngologists and speech-language pathologists. *J Speech Hear Res.* 1991; 34(2):229–235.

25. Hersan R, Behlau M. Behavioral management of pediatric dysphonia. *Otolaryngol Clin North Am.* 2000;33(5):1097–1110.

26. Maddern BR, Campbell TF, Stool S. Pediatric voice disorders. *Otolaryngol Clin North Am.* 1991;24(5):1125–1140.

27. Ramig LO, Verdolini, K. Treatment efficacy: voice disorders. *J Speech Lang Hear Res.* 1998;41(1):101S–116S.

28. Berry DA, Verdolini K, Montequin D, Hess MM, Chan R, Titze IR. A quantitative output-cost ratio in voice production. *J Speech Lang Hear Res.* 2001;44(1):29–37.

29. Jiang JJ, Titze IR. Measurement of vocal fold intraglottal pressure and impact stress. *J Voice.* 1994;8(2):132–144.

30. Gray SD, Pignatari SS, Harding P. Morphologic ultrastructure of anchoring fibers in normal vocal fold basement membrane zone. *J Voice.* 1994;8(1):48–52.

31. Gray SD, Thibeault SL. Diversity in voice characteristics—interaction between genes and environment, use of microarray analysis. *J Commun Disord.* 2002;35(4):347–354.

32. Roy N, Merrill R, Thibeault S, Parsa R, Gray S, Smith E. Prevalence of voice disorders in teachers and the general population. *J Speech Lang Hear Res.* 2004;47,281–293.

33. Andrews ML, Summers AC. *Voice Treatment for Children and Adolescents.* San Diego, CA: Singular; 2001.

34. Boone DR. The boone voice program for children. In: Cook JV, Palaski DJ, Hanson WR, eds. *A Vocal Hygiene Program for School Age Children.* Vol. 10. Austin, TX: Pro-Ed; 1993:21–26.

35. Moran MJ, Zylla-Jones E. *Vocal Hygeine Activities for Children: A Resource Manual.* San Diego, CA: Singular; 1998.

36. Nilson H, Schneiderman CR. Classroom program for the prevention of vocal abuses and hoarseness in elementary school children. *Lang Speech Hear Serv Sch.* 1983;14: 121–127.

37. Wilson DK. *Voice Problems of Children.* 3rd ed. Baltimore, MD: Williams and Wilkins; 1987.

38. Arguedas A, Loaiza C, Soley C. Single dose azithromycin for the treatment of uncomplicated otitis media. *Pediatr Infect Dis J.* 2004;23(suppl 2):S108–S114.

39. Gottlob I, Awan M, Proudlock F. The role of compliance in 2 vs 6 hours of patching in children with amblyopia. *Arch Ophthalmol.* 2004;122(3):422–423; author reply: 424–425.

40. Roy N, Bless DM. Personality traits and psychological factors in voice pathology: a foundation for future research. *J Speech Lang Hear Res.* 2000;43(3):737–748.

41. Roy N, Bless DM, Heisey D. Personality and voice disorders: a multitrait-multidisorder analysis. *J Voice.* 2000;14(4):521–548.

42. Verdolini K, Hersan R, Kessler K. *Clinician Manual: Lessac-Madsen Resonant Voice Therapy 5-10* [Unpublished training material]. 2009.

43. Verdolini K, Hersan R, Kessler K. *Parent-Child Manual: Lessac-Madsen Resonant Voice Therapy 5-10* [Unpublished clinical material]. 2009.

44. Sander EK. Arguments against agressive pursuit of voice therapy in children. *Lang Speech Hear Serv Sch.* 1989;20:94–101.

45. Deal RE, McClain B, Sudderth JF. Identification, evaluation, therapy, and follow-up for children with vocal nodules in a public school setting. *J Speech Hear Disord.* 1976; 41(3):390–397.

46. Trani M, Ghidini A, Bergamini G, Presutti L. Voice therapy in pediatric functional dysphonia: a prospective study. *Int J Pediatr Otorhinolaryngol.* 2007;71(3):379–384.

47. Kearney CA. School absenteeism and school refusal behavior in youth: a contemporary review. *Clin Psychol Rev.* 2008;28(3): 451–471.

48. Eaton DK, Brener N, Kann LK. Associations of health risk behaviors with school absenteeism. Does having permission for the absence make a difference? *J Sch Health.* 2008;78(4):223-229.

49. Houghton F, Gleeson M, Kelleher K. The use of primary/national school absenteeism as a proxy retrospective child health status measure in an environmental pollution investigation. *Public Health.* 2003;117(6):417-423.

50. Glaze LE. Treatment of voice hyperfunction in the pre-adolescent. *Lang Speech Hear Serv Sch.* 1996;27:244-250.

51. Lee EK, Son YI. Muscle tension dysphonia in children: voice characteristics and outcome of voice therapy. *Int J Pediatr Otorhinolaryngol.* 2005;69(7):911-917.

52. Emami AJ, Pizzuto MP, Simon D, Brodsky L. Management of voice disorders in children: a prospective analysis. Paper presented at: American Society of Pediatric Otolaryngology; May 1997; Scottsdale, AZ.

53. Pizzuto MP, Brodsky L. Management of voice disorders in children. *Curr Opin Otolaryngol Head Neck Surg.* 2000;8:479-484.

54. Allen KD, Bernstein B, Chait DH. EMG biofeedback treatment of pediatric hyperfunctional dysphonia. *J Behav Ther Exp Psychiatry.* 1991;22(2):97-101.

55. Cook JV, Palaski D, Hanson WR. A vocal hygiene program for school-age children. *Lang Speech Hear Serv Sch.* 1979;10:21-26.

56. Madison CL, Meadors DL, Miller SQ. A survey study of a public school voice clinic program. *Lang Speech Hear Serv Sch.* 1984;15: 276-280.

57. Miller SQ, Madison CL. Public school voice clinics, part II: diagnosis and recommendations, a 10-year review. *Lang Speech Hear Serv Sch.* 1984;15:58-64.

58. Nienkerke-Springer A, McAllister A, Sundberg J. Effects of family therapy on children's voices. *J Voice.* 2005;19(1):103-113.

59. Verdolini-Marston K, Burke MK, Lessac A, Glaze L, Caldwell E. Preliminary study of two methods of treatment for laryngeal nodules. *J Voice.* 1995;9(1):74-85.

60. Roy N, Gray SD, Simon M, Dove H, Corbin-Lewis K, Stemple JC. An evaluation of the effects of two treatment approaches for teachers with voice disorders: a prospective randomized clinical trial. *J Speech Lang Hear Res.* 2001;44:286-296.

61. Roy N, Weinrich B, Gray SD, Tanner K, Stemple JC, Sapienza CM. Three treatments for teachers with voice disorders: a randomized clinical trial. *J Speech Lang Hear Res.* 2003; 46(3):670-688.

62. Roy N, Weinrich B, Gray SD, et al. Voice amplification versus vocal hygiene instruction for teachers with voice disorders: a treatment outcomes study. *J Speech Lang Hear Res.* 2002;45:625-638.

63. Peterson KL, Verdolini-Marston K, Barkmeier JM, Hoffman HT. Comparison of aerodynamic and electroglottographic parameters in evaluating clinically relevant voicing patterns. *Ann Otol Rhinol Laryngol.* 1994; 103(5, pt 1):335-346.

64. Verdolini K, Druker DG, Palmer PM, Samawi H. Laryngeal adduction in resonant voice. *J Voice.* 1998;12(3):315-327.

65. Kuhl PK, Meltzoff AN. The bimodal perception of speech in infancy. *Science.* 1982; 218(4577):1138-1141.

66. Meltzoff AN, Borton RW. Intermodal matching by human neonates. *Nature.* 1979;282(5737): 403-404.

67. Meltzoff AN, Moore MK. Imitation of facial and manual gestures by human neonates. *Science.* 1977;198(4312):74-78.

68. Boliek CA, Lohmeier H. From the big ban to the brain. *J Commun Disord.* 1999;32(4): 271-276.

69. Thelen E. Motor development. A new synthesis. *Am Psychol.* 1995;50(2):79-95.

70. Wulf G, Lauterbach B, Toole T. The learning advantages of an external focus of attention in golf. *Res Q Exerc Sport.* 1999;70(2):120-126.

71. Wulf G, McNevin NH, Fuchs T, Ritter F, Toole T. Attentional focus in complex skill learning. *Res Q Exerc Sport.* 2000;71(3):229-239.

72. Posner MI, Petersen SE. The attention system of the human brain. *Ann Rev Neurosci.* 1990;13:25-42.

73. Schmidt R, Lee T., eds. *Motor Control and Learning: A Behavioral Emphasis.* Champaign, IL: Human Kinetics Publishers; 2005.

74. Aslin RN, Saffran JR, Newport EL. Statistical Learning in linguistic and nonlinguistic domains. In: B. MacWhinney, ed. *The Emergence of Language.* Mahwah, NJ: Lawrence Erlbaum; 1999.

75. Forrest K. Are oral-motor exercises useful in the treatment of phonological/articulatory disorders? *Semin Speech Lang.* 2002;23(1): 15-26.

76. Gierut JA. Phonological complexity and language learnability. *Am J Speech Lang Pathol.* 2007;16(1):6-17.

77. Kelly MH, Martin S. Domain-general abilities applied to domain-specific tasks: sensitivity to probabilities in perception, cognition, and language. *Lingua.* 1994;92:105-140.

78. Wulf G, Shea CH. Principles derived from the study of simple skills do not generalize to complex skill learning. *Psychon Bull Rev.* 2002;9(2):185-211.

79. Bjork RA, Linn MC. The science of learning and the learning of science: introducing desirable difficulties. *APS Observer.* 2006; 19:29-39.

80. Schmidt RA, Wulf G. Continuous concurrent feedback degrades skill learning: implications for training and simulation. *Hum Factors.* 1997;39(4):509-525.

81. Elbert M, McReynolds LV. Aspects of phonological acquisition during articulation training. *J Speech Hear Disord.* 1979;44(4):459-471.

82. Holt RF, Carney AE. Developmental effects of multiple looks in speech sound discrimination. *J Speech Lang Hear Res.* 2007;50(6): 1404-1424.

83. Rianthavorn P, Ettenger RB, Malekzadeh M, Marik JL, Struber M. Noncompliance with immunosuppressive medications in pediatric and adolescent patients receiving solid-organ transplants. *Transplantation.* 2004;77(5): 778-782.

84. Sergl HG, Klages U, Zentner A. Functional and social discomfort during orthodontic treatment—effects on compliance and prediction of patients' adaptation by personality variables. *Eur J Orthod.* 2000;22(3):307-315.

85. Willetts IE, Trompeter RS. Experience with cyclosporine in pediatric renal transplan-

tation. *Transplant Proc.* 2004;36(suppl 2): 211S-215S.

86. Schobinger R, Florin I, Reichbauer M, Lindemann H, Zimmer C. Childhood asthma: mothers' affective attitude, mother-child interaction and children's compliance with medical requirements. *J Psychosom Res.* 1993;37(7):697-707.

87. Wamboldt FS, Wamboldt MZ, Gavin LA, Roesler TA, Brugman SM. Parental criticism and treatment outcome in adolescents hospitalized for severe, chronic asthma. *J Psychosom Res.* 1995;39(8):995-1005.

88. Tetreault S, Parrot A, Trahan J. Home activity programs in families with children presenting with global developmental delays: evaluation and parental perceptions. *Int J Rehabil Res.* 2003;26(3):165-173.

89. Johnson PD, Cohen DA, Aiosa L, McGorray S, Wheeler T. Attitudes and compliance of pre-adolescent children during early treatment of Class II malocclusion. *Clin Orthod Res.* 1998;1(1):20-28.

90. American Speech-Language-Hearing Association. *Preferred Practice Patterns for the Profession of Speech-Language Pathology. (Section 12.7).* Rockville, MD: Author; 1997.

91. Lee L, Stemple JC, Glaze L, Kelchner LN. Quick screen for voice and supplementary documents for identifying pediatric voice disorders. *Lang Speech Hear Serv Sch.* 2004; 35(4):308-319.

92. Miller SQ, Madison CL. Public school voice clinics, part I: a working model. *Lang Speech Hear Serv Sch.* 1984;15:51-57.

93. Verdolini, K. Voice disorders. In: JB Tomblin, H Morris, D Spriesterbach, eds. *Diagnostic Methods in Speech-Language Pathology.* San Diego, CA: Singular Publishing Group; 1999.

94. Verdolini K. Critical analysis of common terminology in voice therapy. *Phonoscope.* 1999;2(1):1-8.

95. Bandura A. Self-efficacy: toward a unifying theory of behavioral change. *Percept Mot Skills.* 2002;94(3, pt 1):1056.

96. Kaplan RM, Atkins CJ, Reinsch S. Specific efficacy expectations mediate exercise com-

pliance in patients with COPD. *Health Psychol.* 1984;3(3):223–242.

97. McAuley E, Talbot HM, Martinez S. Manipulating self-efficacy in the exercise environment in women: influences on affective responses. *Health Psychol.* 1999;18(3):288–294.

98. Gillespie, A. *The Influence of Clinical Terminology on Self-Efficacy for Voice* [master thesis]. Pittsburgh: Communication Science and Disorders, University of Pittsburgh; 2005.

10

Working with the Pediatric Singer: A Holistic Approach

Robert Edwin

INTRODUCTION

Children sing. Whether it be nursery rhymes at home, songs in school choruses, show tunes on Broadway, or arias in opera, children sing. In my large private voice studio, over two-thirds of my students are under the age of 18. They represent but the tip of a very substantial "iceberg" of pediatric singers who want to study the art of singing. Add to that the many children who wish to sing better for amateur performance or for purely personal reasons, and the iceberg swells significantly. Yet, despite this large population so eager to be taught, the opinion still exists among many voice care providers and pedagogues that children should not study singing until after puberty.

This opinion, however, flouts the fact that no scientific, pedagogic, physiologic, or psychologic evidence exists indicating teaching children to sing is inherently harmful to their bodies, minds, or spirits. That is not to say children or others cannot do harmful things to the voice. Most voice care

professionals are well aware of the damage improper, ill-advised, or excessive voice use can inflict, but it will be argued here that properly trained young singers with age-appropriate vocal technique and repertoire are less likely than untrained singers to hurt themselves or allow themselves to be hurt by other people. For more support on this pedagogic point of view, please reference the American Academy of Teachers of Singing 2002 statement, "Teaching Children to Sing," at the end of this chapter (Appendix 10).

BEGINNING SINGERS

When do children start to sing? We know from numerous clinical studies that respiration and phonation begin at birth. Intonation (cooing, squealing, laughing) normally develops within the first 4 months of life. Articulation begins at around 4 months, with consonant-vowel alternations called babble following at 7 to 10 months. The first words with intentional accent and variation of pitch appear at 10 to 13 months. Before a child is 2 years old, two-word combinations are being used. It is important to note that after 7 or 8 months of age a child will stop using the sounds he does not hear on a regular basis and will use only those he hears most frequently.

An analysis of these data reveals that the necessary elements for singing—respiration, phonation, resonation, and articulation—are in place at a very early age. It follows then that the opportunity to teach children to sing can also occur at a very early age.

In this teacher's studio, such opportunities occur frequently. Like many of my colleagues in dance and instrumental music, I take great delight in introducing young children to a wonderful art form through the use of age-appropriate and voice-appropriate technique and repertoire that challenges but does not overly tax their minds and bodies.

A HOLISTIC PEDAGOGIC APPROACH

The voice does not exist in a vacuum. It is not like any other musical instrument. It issues forth from the very fiber of every human being, the result of the activity of flesh and blood, mind and body, psyche and soma. The voice is as individual as the individual who creates it.

A singing teacher's initial session with the pediatric singer can yield much information about that young person's uniqueness. As the singer sings a song or does a vocal exercise, we watch and listen and assess his or her voice technique including posture (slouched, rigid, or balanced), breathing (high or low in the body), phonation (breathy, pressed, or flow), resonation (nasal, covered, or balanced), and articula-

tion (sloppy, overpronounced, or clear). We evaluate acting skills and emotive qualities (passive, phony, or evocative), repertoire preferences (Bach to rock, and places in between), and personality traits (shy to brazen, defensive to vulnerable, nervous to confident, and more places in between).

As singing is both an intuitive, talent-based activity as well as a learned behavior capable of being taught, we evaluate what the singer has given us to work with and immediately begin to formulate strategies that may help the singer achieve a higher level of efficiency and expressiveness. In the initial session and in subsequent sessions, effective teachers of singing will establish rapport and maximize their effectiveness by acquainting themselves with the aspects of their young students' lives that affect their singing. That would include understanding and respecting the uniqueness and individuality of their pediatric singers: their hopes and dreams, their likes and dislikes, how they access information, what their learning modes are, and their medical history. The singing instructor might also want to learn more about their singers' friends and family, their personal habits such as diet, sleep patterns, and hygiene, as well as their musical heritage.

ROLE-PLAY AS VOCAL TECHNIQUE

It is not an oxymoron to say that instructing the pediatric singer should take the form of "serious play," as functional activities and creativity join forces to provide a comfortable, dynamic, and playful learning environment.

By making role-play or "characterization" a part of vocal technique, the mind and body are disciplined simultaneously.

Actor and singer are always working together in partnership. Student singers learn how to create appropriate mental environments and increase attention span so they can respond confidently and positively to technical and artistic demands. Furthermore, role-play or "storytelling" encourages the singer to create a character and scene and establish a context for singing each individual vocal exercise or song. Thus, the singer as storyteller can execute any task while retaining control of his environment even as outside influences such as voice teachers, conductors, choral directors, managers, agents, and parents are directing him.

BODY ALIGNMENT

Vocal instruction should begin with body alignment. In our very casual society, some of us have come to associate good posture with superiority or even arrogance. Children do not want to feel out of place, so they often stand as many of their peers stand— in a slouch. If students can understand good posture as both a storytelling issue as well as a primary component of vocal efficiency, they may be more willing to move from the reality of the peer pressure slouch to the created reality of the storyteller whose role requires them to have a more efficient and dynamic physical presence.

Exercises for Body Alignment

The simplest exercise to establish good individual body alignment is to have the singer fully extend her arms over her head while easily flexing the knees. That action lifts the rib cage (the primary player in posture), elevates the sternum, and lines up the rest of the body. Singers with poor posture

may experience discomfort when their bodies are placed in an unfamiliar position. They need to be reassured that, in time, their muscles will adjust to this new and more efficient position.

For the singer to better understand balanced posture, have her explore the extremes of posture in a role-play. Ask her to portray a girl who is shy or lacking in self- confidence. Most likely she will slouch over with a collapsed rib cage and rounded shoulders to model that hypoposture. Then, ask her to portray a girl who is over confident or "stuck up." Most likely she will exaggerate a lifted rib cage, pull back on the shoulders, and lock the knees to model hyper posture. Now repeat the initial exercise with the arms comfortably over the head and the knees slightly flexed to re-establish balanced posture and a sense of a confident individual. More intense and specific work on body alignment can be done through disciplines such as the Alexander technique and Feldenkrais method.

BREATH MANAGEMENT

The development of an "I'm-in-charge-and-having-fun" storyteller can also aid in breath management training. The singer need not be a shy, rib cage-dropping, shallow-breathing person; or a tense, rib cage-stretching, shoulder-raising person, but rather a confident, ribcage-elevated, lower torso-expanding, deeper breathing individual.

Exercises for Breath Management

First, have the singer take very shallow, small breaths as the shy boy with his upper torso collapsed. Then, have him take very high, big breaths raising his shoulders as if he were the "Big, Bad Wolf" in "The Three Little Pigs." Next, have the singer put his hands in a V shape on the lower part of his rib cage as Superman or Peter Pan would. Without taking a breath, have him pull in and tense his abdominal muscles ("tummy" to the younger students), then release them. Repeat this exercise a few times. Next, have him exhale while contracting his abs. Then, have him relax his abs as he inhales the next breath. Patience and numerous repetitions will eventually allow for a more spontaneous release of the abs that triggers the efficient intake of air.

Exhalation, the "support" part of the breath, can be easily demonstrated by hissing like a snake. The "hissssssss" will provide resistance so the singer feels the abs contracting and managing the airflow under pressure. The singer should eventually feel his hands on his sides move out as the rib cage, abs, and back all expand on inhalation. He then needs to learn to keep that expansion throughout the exhalation phase of the breath cycle so the air is used most efficiently.

PHONATION

Phonation, too, can be strongly influenced by the storytelling process. The extremes of singing span the traditional English Choir School use of exclusively upper register or "head voice" singing, to the so-called "Annie" school of singing where lower register or "chest voice" dominant belting is used exclusively.

It is, of course, necessary for the entire voice to be developed, strengthened, and coordinated to create a functionally healthy and efficient voice. The thyroarytenoid muscles (TA) and the cricothyroid muscles (CT) share responsibility for creating vocal fold thickening and stretching, respectively, and one isolated from the other is simply bad vocal pedagogy for any age group and any style of singing. The goal in phonation is to avoid the extremes of pressed and breathy, and create that balanced vocal fold posture called flow phonation.

Exercises for Phonation

The pediatric vocalist will usually have a preferred style of singing and, hence, a register preference. Once again, through storytelling techniques and characterization, the less preferred register can be engaged. For example, an Annie-type belter can be asked to imagine herself as a very young opera singer. As the child shifts from her dominant identity to that of the opera singer, her cricothyroid muscles ("head voice") will have a greater chance to participate more actively in phonation. Be aware that for her to achieve a CT-dominant vocal fold posture, it may be necessary to choose vocal exercises or songs that are above her normal belt range. C above middle C (C5) is a good starting point for triads (1-3-5-3-1 or, do-mi-sol-mi-do) and scales (1-2-3-4-5-4-3-2-1) with the "oo" [u] vowel, as in the word, "you," usually being the easiest vowel for a strong belter/weak soprano to produce.

For the boy or girl with a weak or nonexistent TA-dominant sound, a strongly, stubbornly, rudely, and loudly sung "no!" on middle C (C4) pitch or below will often trigger the dormant lower register or "chest voice."

As a warm-up or cool-down exercise, humming and chewing simultaneously on moderate pitches is one of the most beneficial. It is especially helpful for voices that have sung too long, too high, or too loud.

RESONATION

Yet another component of singing, resonation, can be addressed via storytelling. The three primary resonating cavities—the throat, the mouth, and the nose—provide almost inexhaustible combinations of sound textures as they amplify and reinforce frequencies created by the vocal folds. As the pediatric singer, to his or her detriment, often copies adult singers and adds too much thickness in vocal fold configuration and too much weight in resonance-coupling, finding the right balance or timbre for each child's voice should be a major goal of the voice instructor.

Exercises for Resonation

The full spectrum of resonance can be explored through characterization. For example, using triads, scales, or arpeggios, the pediatric singer can create a *Wizard of Oz* "Wicked Witch" storyteller to sing bright, treble-dominant, or even nasal sounds. Conversely, the "cowardly lion" character can create the dark, bass-dominant, covered sounds. Those two characters can then be given singing instruction to create a more balanced chiaroscuro, bright/dark sound, appropriate to the age and individual vocal instrument of the student.

Have the singer sing a triad (1-3-5-3-1) starting in a comfortable, medium to low pitch range (middle C) first as the "Wicked Witch" using the evil laugh, "heh, heh, heh, heh, heh." Ask the singer to sing it through her nose while scrunching up her face. (Pointing a crooked finger while singing is optional.) Move the triad up and down in half- steps to hear if such resonance can be kept consistent throughout the usable voice range. Make sure the sound is not pushed or pressed.

Next, have the singer create the "Cowardly Lion" character to sing the opposite extreme: a hollow, woofy sound with little or no treble or bright resonance. The same triad can be used, this time with the phrase, "Oh dear, Do-ro-thy." Once again, be on the alert for pushed or pressed phonation. The next step is to ask the singer to resing both phrases with a prettier sound, one that has a little of the Wicked Witch, a little of the Cowardly Lion, but mostly Dorothy. Experiment with the textures so the singer can hear the entire spectrum of her resonant voice.

ARTICULATION

Articulation also falls under the storytelling banner as sloppy, mumbled word formation, or crisp, clean pronunciation is assigned to specific characters. Actively and efficiently engaging the articulators—the lips, the teeth, the tongue, and the soft palate—will help the pediatric singer release excessive tensions as well as improve the intelligibility of both speech and song. Note that role-play may at times hit a bit too close to home so, initially, care must be taken to make the storyteller characters unthreatening to the student's core personality and behavior. For example, a child with a severe speech defect may react negatively to an exercise and character role-play that highlights her problem.

Exercises for Articulation

On a five-note diatonic scale (1-2-3-4-5-4-3-2-1), have the singer sing the alphabet with each letter being repeated on each note of the scale (a-a-a-a-a-a-a-a, b-b-b-b-b-b-b-b, etc). Listen and look for problems caused by malfunctioning articulators (lisps, tongue thrusts, retracted tongue, palatal rigidity). Do not take this exercise too high because the singer will begin to lose intelligibility as the notes go above the musical staff (G5). Next, ask the singer to repeat the exercise with two different characters, "Crisp," who overpronounces each letter, and "Sloppy," who underpronounces each letter. Once again, the extremes will help to define the middle or balanced position for each pediatric singer. This same exercise can be done with names, numbers, and food groups, and can serve a variety of pedagogic goals, such as phonation and resonation objectives. The exercises can also be interactive with the student providing input on the content such as names of friends or favorite foods.

MUTATION: THE "CHANGE OF VOICE"

One of the most rewarding pedagogic opportunities comes during the adolescent voice change as both the student's voice and psyche are guided through the turbulent waters of laryngeal growth. The instructor can use constantly changing storyteller modes and continual reinforcement of technique, especially the use of the upper register (falsetto or head voice) which acts as a counterbalance as the lower register (chest voice) heads "southward." One can play man's/woman's voice, boy's/girl's voice, and child's voice games exploring old and new timbres and vocal fold postures. Let the larynx dictate what it wants to do and in what range it wants to do it. Accept the narrowing of vocal range as a natural and temporary part of the transition process. Because of their ongoing singing through

mutation, male singers, especially, rarely experience the embarrassing register shifts and yodels of their untrained counterparts. For that alone, they seem forever grateful for singing lessons.

REPERTOIRE

Not all children aspire to be the next famous operatic or classical singer. Pavarotti, Hampson, Horne, or Battle may not be on any of their music listening devices, so the child voice pedagogue should be prepared to address and affirm, if they are willing and able, Contemporary Commercial Music (nonclassical) singing techniques and styles such as pop, rock, rhythm and blues, gospel, Tejano, jazz, and folk. Regardless of the style of singing, classical to CCM, teachers need to continually remind their young charges not to copy the adult voices they hear either live or on recordings. Student singers should be encouraged to develop voice techniques, styles, and repertoire that suit their age, their instrument, and their personality. For example, low-voiced, pediatric belters should avoid the temptation to try for a role in *Annie*. That show has been blamed for many a voice disorder, yet it is a very doable and vocally safe show for child singers with very high belt voices. Conversely, high-voiced singers should avoid repertoire whose pitch range stays in the low extreme of their vocal compass.

It is important to note here that no one voice technique can serve all the diverse styles of singing. Voice techniques are implemented to support the style and repertoire being sung. Just as a classically trained young soprano is not prepared to do the aforementioned *Annie* unless she is also simultaneously working on her belting and mixing voice technique, neither is an *Annie*-type belter prepared to sing in the opera, *The Magic Flute,* unless she, too, has developed a classical voice technique.

CONCLUDING THOUGHTS

Whether teaching the "Annie" and "Oliver" on Broadway, or the "Annie" and "Oliver" in the local synagogue show, a singing instructor needs to understand how to teach children and what to teach children. A basic knowledge of both child and adult psychology as well as vocal anatomy and physiology is essential. Critical is the recognition that children are not "miniature adults" to be trained with the same techniques and expectations.

The voice teacher needs to establish a child-friendly learning environment. The standard components of singing—posture, breath management, phonation, resonation, articulation, and interpretation—need to be addressed in a patient, creative, and playful manner. Also, the standard assortment of vocalises, lip and tongue trills, triads and scales need to be reshaped so that the exercises are perceived as games rather than dull, repetitive drills. Important, too, is the teacher's sensitivity to the ever changing bodies and minds of his or her student singers. As vocal and emotional limits expand and contract, the teacher must be able to adjust the lessons to keep the singer within these continually evolving boundaries.

On that same note, teachers should find out if the children will receive at home the kind of encouragement that will allow them to develop their own vocal identities. Even if parents or guardians are living out their own performing fantasies through the child, it is still possible for that child to grow independently as long as the child is allowed strong personal input in the learning process. The process tends to break down if an adult tries to dominate the child's musical will, or if the child is singing only to please the family.

The role of the pediatric voice pedagogue will not be a comfortable one for all teachers of singing. Teaching children to sing requires an even greater commitment beyond technique and repertoire. The child's constantly changing body and evolving mind challenge continuity with regard to predictability of either vocal or emotional stability. Every lesson should begin with, "where are you and your voice today?" The answer strongly influences the direction of the session. It is a wise and skillful teacher who looks, listens, and then begins the day's lesson.

On a personal note, my hope is that more singing teachers will join me in this fascinating and rewarding endeavor. Unfortunately, at this writing, there are simply too few of us willing and able to serve the needs of pediatric singers.

APPENDIX 10

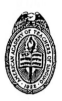

AMERICAN ACADEMY OF TEACHERS OF SINGING

www.voiceteachersacademy.org

Member
National Music Council

Chair
Robert C. White, Jr.
600 West 116th Street
New York, NY 10027-7042

Vice Chair
Jean Westerman Gregg
11 Old Quarry Road
Woodbridge, CT 06525-1005

Secretary
Jeannette L. LoVetri
317 West 93rd Street, #3B
New York, NY 10025-7236

Treaurer
Jan Eric Douglas
777 West End Avenue
New York, NY 10025-5551

Publications Officer
Robert Gartside
20 Loring Road
Lexington, MA 02421-6945

Adele Addison
Elaine Bonazzi
Claudia Catania
Lindsey Christiansen
Jan Eric Douglas
Robert Edwin
Shirlee Emmons
Robert Gartside
Jean Westerman Gregg
Katherine Hansel
Hilda Harris
Helen Hodam
Barbara Honn
Marvin Keenze
Paul Kiesgen
Antonia Lavanne
Jeannette LoVetri
Elizabeth Mannion
John McCollum
Joyce McLean
Klara Meyers
Richard Miller
Dale Moore
Gordon Myers
Louis Nicholas
Russell Oberlin
Chloe Owen
Julian Patrick
John B. Powell
George Shirley
Richard Sjoerdsma
Craig Timberlake
Robert C. White, Jr.
Beverly Wolff
Edward Zambara

TEACHING CHILDREN TO SING
A Statement by the American Academy of Teachers of Singing
November 2002

From their first cry at birth to their last sigh at death, human beings are sound-producing creatures. We know from numerous clinical studies that respiration and phonation occur at birth. Intonation (humming, cooing, squealing, laughing) normally develops in the first four months of life. Articulation and the first words occur at about one year of age. Before a child is two years old, two-word combinations are being used.

Analysis of such data reveals that the necessary elements for singing – respiration, phonation, resonation, and articulation – are in place at a very early age. It follows then that the opportunity to teach children to sing more efficiently and expressively can also occur at a very early age. There continues to this day, however, a controversy as to when, and even if, the training of young singers should begin. The **American Academy of Teachers of Singing** addresses the topic of teaching children to sing.

Acutely aware of the physical damage improper, excessive, or ill-advised singing can cause, the Academy in the past has recommended that children not engage in formal voice studies. However, upon further investigation, no scientific, pedagogical, or physiological evidence indicates that child voice pedagogy is inherently harmful to children's bodies, minds, or spirits.

The Academy now recognizes that there are benefits to teaching children to sing. In fact, well-trained singers of any age are less likely than untrained singers to hurt their vocal instruments or to allow their instruments to be hurt by others. Observing our fellow pedagogues in dance and instrumental music, we find they have identified and successfully acted on the potential to instruct interested and motivated young children in their respective disciplines. Clearly, these teachers have developed age-appropriate technical exercises and repertoire that challenge but do not overly tax the young body and mind. They are astutely aware that children are not "miniature adults," and should not be taught as such.

The Academy believes that teachers of singing should take their cue from the aforementioned colleagues to develop and utilize age-appropriate vocal exercises and repertoire that support the natural inclination of children to express themselves in singing and song. The quantity and quality of musical talent as well as the interest of each child, however, will vary greatly. Therefore, the Academy suggests three general categories of child singer:

Category one includes children for whom singing is but one activity to which they are exposed along with other disciplines such as mathematics, science, history, language, physical education, art, dance, and spirituality. For them, gaining an appreciation of and experience in the recreational joy of singing may be sufficient. Venues where this exposure occurs include home, school, and places of worship.

Category two includes children for whom singing is a recreational activity they wish to pursue more intensely. These children may express an interest in private voice lessons to improve basic vocal technique and develop repertoire. Venues include select choirs and choruses, and solo opportunities at school, clubs, sporting events, and places of worship.

2

Category three includes children for whom singing is a professional or pre-professional activity that subjects their vocal technique, performance skills, and repertoire to highly critical evaluation and scrutiny. For these children to deal successfully with the added physical and emotional demands a singing career requires, formal voice training should be considered a necessity. Venues include opera, music theater, recording, pageants, film, radio, and television.

Regardless of the categories of the singers, training should be in the hands of qualified teachers who understand both **how** to teach children and **what** to teach children. A basic knowledge of child vocal anatomy and physiology, age appropriate vocal technique and repertoire, and child psychology is essential for successful instruction. Teachers must know, for example, that a child's vocal instrument cannot sustain the larger and fuller tonal spectra adult vocal instruments are capable of producing. Teachers must also avoid repertoire that exceeds the physical, intellectual, and emotional understanding of the young student singer.

Critical to the pedagogical process is the establishment of a child-friendly learning environment. Elements such as posture, breath management, phonation, resonation, articulation, and interpretive skills need to be addressed in a patient, creative, and playful manner. Using standard pedagogical tools such as lip and tongue trills, scales, triads, and arpeggios, the singing teacher must endeavor to create exercises that resemble games rather than repetitive drills. For example, abdominal breathing activity can be explored by having the child "pant like a dog." Scales and other vocalises can be done using numbers, colors, names, or even items found in the studio. Role play and storytelling suggestions ("be a happy singer," or "pretend you are saying something very important") can help to focus the exercises by providing a context for their use. As lessons continue, the instructor must be sensitive to the growing and changing bodies and minds of the child singers, closely monitoring them to see if the students are singing within or beyond their vocal and emotional limitations. This is especially true during male puberty since rapid physical growth can radically alter and even temporarily destabilize the vocal instrument.

Important, too, is a willingness to work with the child's preference in music. Not all children wish or need to sing classical repertoire. Therefore, the teacher may need to address nonclassical singing styles such as music theater, pop, rock, jazz, gospel, Latino, country, rhythm and blues, and folk music, and provide vocal techniques to authentically support these and other vocal music categories. No matter what the vocal style, however, teachers need to remind their young students not to imitate the fuller, more mature adult voices they hear, but to develop a vocal sound that suits their own age, voice, and personality.

Since children are not independent beings, teachers must be able to effectively communicate with parents and guardians regarding their child's training, choice of repertoire, and potential for growth. Adults pushing unwilling young singers into training and performance environments need to be tactfully confronted and encouraged to let the children participate in the decision-making process.

In summary, singing is a natural and spontaneous activity for a majority of children. The **American Academy of Teachers of Singing** supports and encourages the teaching of children to sing. As in other activities in which youngsters are involved, singing can be accomplished on many levels from recreational to professional. At all levels, however, there should be qualified instructors willing and able to help young singers on their musical journeys.

Benign Lesions of the Pediatric Vocal Folds: Nodules, Webs, and Cysts

J. Scott McMurray

INTRODUCTION

The evaluation and management of hoarseness in children remains a highly controversial but also often speculative problem. Hoarseness in children is often neglected or overlooked as a transient and self-limiting problem. Many assume a stance of "benign" neglect to avoid potential iatrogenic aggravation of the laryngeal pathology. This attitude is often justified as a means to avoid potential life-lasting injury to the vocal folds. Common goals, however, for those who actively treat or use benign neglect for dysphonic children are their protection from harm and their improved quality of life. With advances in diagnostic tools, a better understanding of the developing layers of the vocal folds, better measures of the impact on quality of life, and refinements in surgical techniques and their indications, the treatment of hoarseness in children will dramatically change and the stance of

benign neglect will be determined as less than benign (Fig 11-1).

If we consider each dysphonic child as our own, we should worry about the worst, see what is there and treat what we find. Our experiences reinforce the need to visualize the larynx and accurately diagnose the cause of the dysphonia in the child. Too often, dysphonic children will be ignored as simply having something they will outgrow until they are found to have obstructing papillomata in severe respiratory distress (Fig 11-2). The psychological, social, and academic impact of dysphonia on a child is often underplayed as well. It has been shown that dysphonic children are often perceived as dirty, cruel, ugly, unfair, small, weak, slow, clumsy, or sick based solely on their vocal quality and no visual cues.[1] The assessment of the impact on perceptions of quality of life is also in its infancy. New tools are being designed to help determine the impact of dysphonia on children.[2] I believe that we will find that the dysphonic and

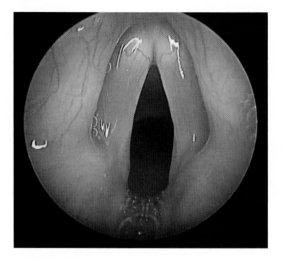

Fig 11–1. Endoscopic view of a normal 6-year-old larynx during direct micro-laryngoscopy. Note the relatively small membranous vocal fold to vocal process ratio when compared to an adult. This may concentrate vibratory trauma to a small area in the child than the adult.

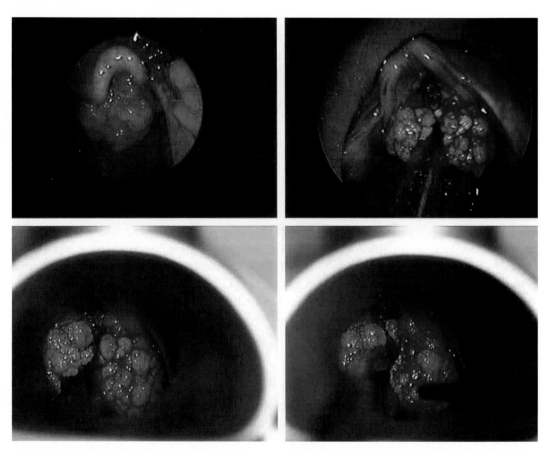

Fig 11–2. Young boy with severe papilloma. For 5 months he had been assumed to have a functional voice disorder until he began having breathing dificulties as well.

pressed voiced child perceives significant impairments to quality of life compared to the child with a normal voice. As better tools to measure perceived quality of life in children of all ages are developed, the true impact will be determined.

Recent review of the outcomes of children with nodules moving on to adolescence revealed that 29% of the nodules persisted and only 44% of children with nodules achieved a normal voice in adolescence.[3] All children were given vocal hygiene or voice therapy and only a few had surgery. This review suggests that a significant number of children do not improve simply with puberty and laryngeal maturation. The means for visualizing the vibrating pedi-

atric vocal fold are improving dramatically (Fig 11–3). Distal-chip cameras of smaller size, greater resolution, and brighter lighting will give the pediatric laryngologist the same capabilities of the adult laryngologists. It should be emphasized that if the diagnosis is uncertain or if what seems to be appropriate management is not demonstrating progress, direct microlaryngoscopy should be considered for a reassessment and perhaps more accurate diagnosis of the underlying pathology. As with any disease process, appropriate management relies on an accurate diagnosis.

This chapter addresses general overviews of benign glottic pathology. General approaches to each pathologic condition are

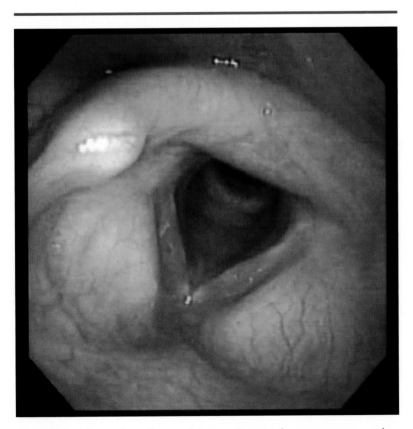

Fig 11–3. View of an 8-year larynx at nasopharyngoscopy using a distal-chip digital nasopharyngoscope.

outlined. Voice therapy, the main treatment paradigm for laryngeal disorders of adults and children is not specifically addressed in this chapter.

In the evaluation of the dysphonic child, many historical points need clarification. The duration and timing of the hoarseness is important. When did it start and who noticed it first. Was the hoarseness present since birth or did it come later? The severity and impact on the child's life must be assessed. Does the hoarseness wax and wane centered on a constant baseline of vocal quality or is the general baseline of the hoarseness progressively worsening? Are there associated breathing issues or swallowing concerns? Associated medical conditions such as asthma, environmental allergy,[3,4] chronic rhinosinusitis and cough, laryngopharyngeal reflux,[5-7] and snoring must be evaluated (Fig 11-4). A thorough voice use or abuse history should also be taken. Each of these historical points may lead us to a general idea of where inflammation or trauma to the vocal folds may be coming from. The appropriate management of concomitant medical conditions may be a prerequisite to successful management of the dysphonia.

VOCAL FOLD NODULES

Vocal nodules (Fig 11-5) are the most common cause of dysphonia in children. Although the incidence in the general pediatric population has not been extensively studied, one group from Turkey demonstrated that 36% of all school-aged children have some benign pathology of the vocal folds.[8] Dysphonia was found in the general population in 21.6% of boys and 11.7% of girls of school age.

Nodules are intense fibronectin deposits in the superficial layers of the vocal fold

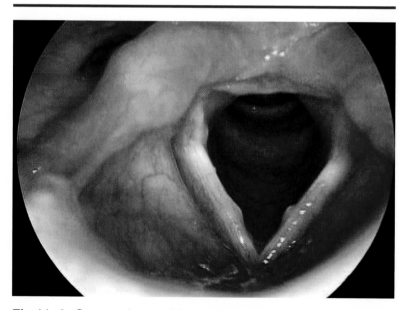

Fig 11–4. Symmetric vocal fold nodules during office rigid laryngoscopy with signs of laryngopharyngeal reflux.

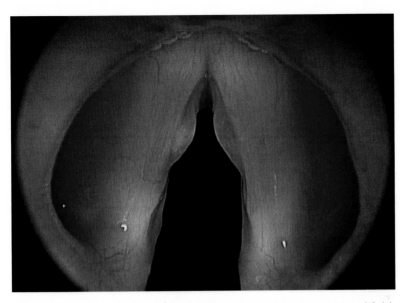

Fig 11–5. Symmetric nodules at the mid-membranous vocal fold.

often coupled with basement membrane zone injury as indicated by thick collagen type IV bands.[9] They are often centered in the mid-portion of the vibrating vocal fold and are generally symmetric to quasisymmetric (Fig 11-6). Although thought to come from vocal trauma or voice abuse, the exact inciting event leading to cyclic injury is not truly understood. Children with nodules often have a hard glottal attack and louder more pressed voices. The increased mass of the vocal folds caused by the nodules may incite a louder more strained voice. This may perpetuate the nodules but does not necessarily answer the question of their origin. Is the hard-pressed voice causing the nodules or are the nodules causing the hard pressed voice?

Further study will be required into the underlying ultrastructure and development of the layers of the vocal fold before a definitive cause will be determined. There is some controversy regarding the age when the layers of the superficial lamina propria

begin and complete their differentiation. The latest studies by Boseley and Hartnick indicate that the lamina propria may have the same ultrastructure of an adult by the age of 7 years.[10] This may be important for surgical considerations. It is not known if surgery prior to complete development of the layers of the superficial lamina propria will cause abnormal maturation and scarring or if the active differentiation and development of these layers will be protective and aid in healing. Furthermore, molecular and genetic differences in the vocal folds of hoarse and normal voicing children may play a more important role than presently understood.[11-14]

Vocal nodules generally affect boys more often than girls.[7] There is a bimodal presentation in age around 3 to 5 years and then again at 8 to 10 years. After the age of 13, dysphonia from vocal nodules becomes primarily a problem of young women. In a longitudinal study, 21% of children with prepubescent vocal nodules continued to have

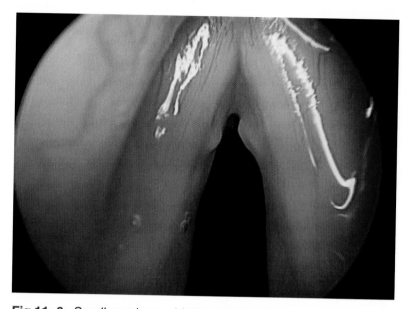

Fig 11–6. Small rough vocal fold nodules at the mid-membranous portion of the vocal fold.

dysphonia into adolescents despite voice therapy.[3] It is important, then, to discover if treating nodules at an earlier age may decrease the dysphonia seen after puberty. There is currently no widely accepted rating scale for vocal nodules in children. It is difficult to compare treatment strategies without a consistent grading scale. Shah and Nuss have recently reviewed their experience and have proposed a grading scale.[15] Their scale uses a three-point system determined by the configuration of the larynx, which is modified as "d" or "s," depending on whether the nodules are discrete or sessile. The grade 1 to 3 defines the laryngeal configuration, with 1 having a normal contour, 2 having an anterior glottic chink, and 3 having an hourglass appearance and glottic gap. Further study is required to determine the utility of their scale.

Shah and Nuss in another paper found that 75% of the children they evaluated with vocal nodules exhibited significant muscle tension disorder. This hyperfunction or muscular tension disorder correlated with nodules size.[7] It is unclear if the hyperfunction was a result of the nodule size or if the nodule size caused the increased vocal tension. They also found that 25% of the children with nodules had signs of laryngopharyngeal reflux. The presence of reflux did not correlate with nodule size, however. Their series of over 600 children illustrates the notion that not all nodules are the same (Figs 11–7 through 11–15). There may be several interrelated causes for the dense fibronectin and collagen deposition at the basement membrane and therefore treatment paradigms may need to vary depending on the cause and distribution of the nodule.

The typical history of a child with nodules consists of intermittent hoarseness that worsens with voice use and improves with voice rest. The baseline of vocal clarity generally does not worsen with time: however, the frequency of hoarseness and the duration

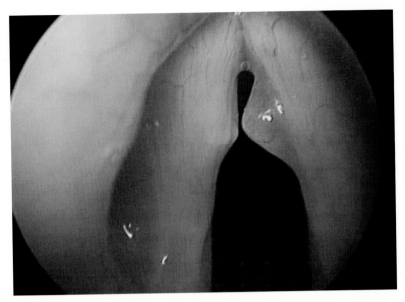

Fig 11–7. Right vocal fold polyp with left vocal fold nodule.

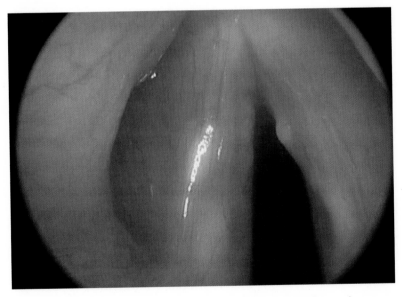

Fig 11–8. Small quasisymmetric nodules in the mid-membranous vocal fold.

with hoarseness may increase. It would be considered very unusual to have associated dysphagia. Aphonia may be experienced, symptoms of associated larygopharyngeal reflux, allergy, and chronic cough should also be noted.

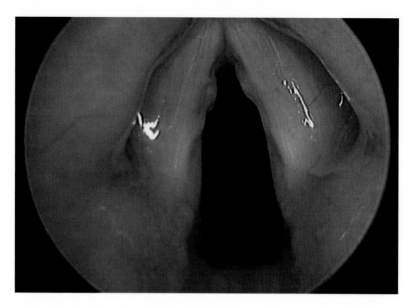

Fig 11–9. Vocal nodules at the mid-membranous vocal fold.

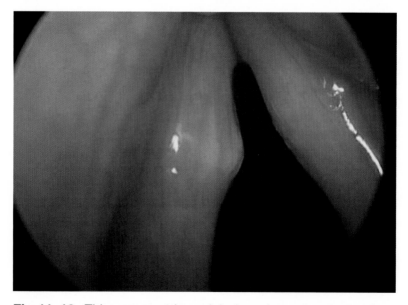

Fig 11–10. This asymmetric nodule has the appearance of an intracordal cyst.

The diagnosis is confirmed with indirect laryngoscopy. Either fiberoptic or rigid laryngoscopy should be performed to visualize the larynx. Stroboscopy may be helpful to distinguish subtle pathologies of the vocal folds such as the differentiation of

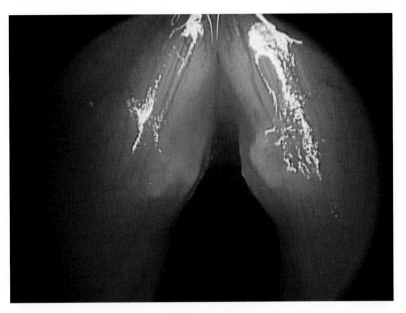

Fig 11–11. Rough appearing nodules.

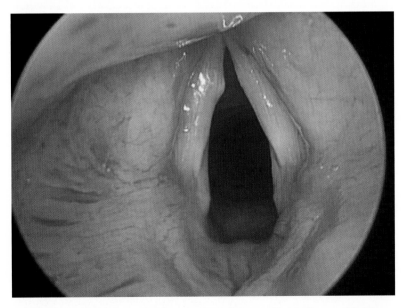

Fig 11–12. Asymmetric vocal nodule on the left vocal fold.

vocal nodules from intracordal cysts. If this cannot be determined, a trial of voice therapy and adjuvant medical therapy may be indicated with a follow-up examination. Nodules generally improve with voice therapy. In the case of a unilateral intracordal

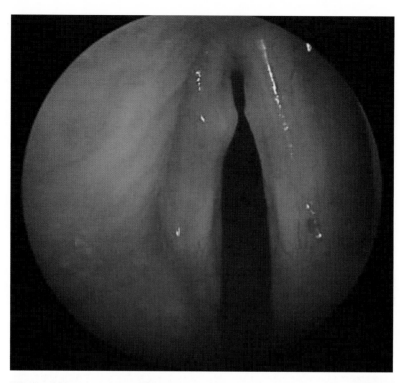

Fig 11–13. Vocal nodules at the mid-membranous vocal fold. The left nodule is slighter larger than the right nodule.

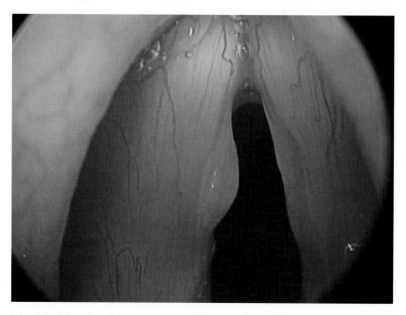

Fig 11–14. This is an asymmetric vocal nodule on the left vocal fold.

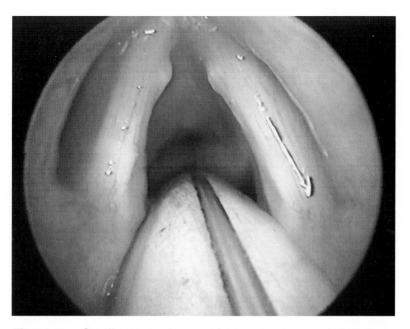

Fig 11–15. Small symmetric vocal fold nodules seen during direct microlaryngoscopy.

cyst with a contralateral nodule, the nodule and the surrounding edema of the vocal fold may improve with conservative management allowing the intracordal cyst to become more defined and easier to diagnose. If the diagnosis is still in question, direct microlaryngoscopy should be considered with palpation of the vocal folds. Proper management always relies on an accurate diagnosis (Fig 11-16).

Typically, treatment of vocal fold nodules consists of vocal hygiene, voice therapy, and behavioral management for possible reflux. Occasionally if signs and symptoms are significant for laryngopharnygeal reflux, proton-pump inhibitors are used over 3 to 4 months as an empiric antireflux therapy trial. There are currently no hard data regarding the efficacy of reflux management in the treatment of vocal nodules in children.

Other sources for potential laryngeal irritation or causes for laryngeal injury such as chronic throat clearing should be sought and treated if present. Postnasal drip from chronic adenoidal hypertrophy, chronic sinusitis, or environmental allergy may be another source for sticky mucus on the vocal folds. Environmental allergy treatment, nasal saline lavage, or surgical treatment for adenoidal or adenotonsillar hypertrophy for chronic sinusitis may be beneficial to the child with vocal nodules. The association has been made with these disease entities contributing to hoarseness but the efficacy of their treatment has not been studied.

Surgery has nearly been abandoned for the treatment of vocal nodules. This, in part, has come from the adage that the nodules will disappear with the onset of puberty. Previous surgical techniques may also have resulted in vocal fold scarring which may be lifelong. Overzealous removal of vocal fold mucosa or deep thermal injury from lasers may have contributed to these poor

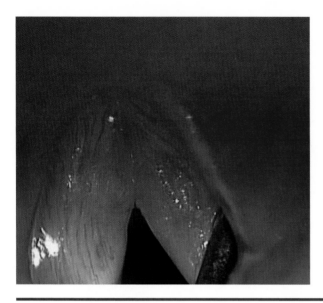

Fig 11–16. This boy had dysphonia from what looked like vocal nodules. When he failed voice therapy and medical management, direct microlaryngoscopy was performed. A sulcus vocalis was identified. This required surgical excision due to the severity of his dyphonia.

outcomes. Finally, many surgeons who have removed vocal nodules have been frustrated when some return. Successful surgical management requires proper patient selection and the development of proper surgical techniques. There are currently no reliable data on which to base the decision of when or how to remove nodules in children. It is not always an easy task to determine if a child has mastered proper voice use techniques. As with adults, good voice use may deteriorate into poor voice use depending on the circumstances. Surgical techniques for the management of vocal fold nodules will need to be developed to remove the fibrous scarring at the basement membrane zone while saving the overlaying epithelium and not disturbing the developing layers of the lamina propria. The latest techniques for removal of nodules include a superficial mucosal incision adjacent to the lesion with a dissection toward the nodule in the most superficial layers of the lamina propria. The underlying fibrous tissue is then dissected off the overlaying mucosa either with microsurgical

techniques or powered microresection. Care is taken to preserve the mucosa. Voice rest followed by proper voice use is prescribed in the postoperative period.

Proper patient selection is the key to successful surgical outcomes. Adequate mastery and adherence to voice therapy and a desire for vocal improvement are required from the patient at a minimum. There are a number of children who are motivated and are experts at proper voice use, who continue to have significant hoarseness due to the mass effect and stiffening of their vocal folds by their vocal nodules. These children are prime candidates for surgical intervention.

As for treatment modalities, Kazunori Mori followed 259 children with hoarseness.[16] Presented as retrospective case reports, his patients received four different modalities; (1) vocal hygiene, (2) voice therapy, (3) surgery and voice therapy, and (4) no treatment except reassurance. As a retrospective review, the severity of the voice disorder in each group was not controlled and may have been stratified unevenly into the different treatment groups. Sixteen percent in the vocal hygiene group improved, 52% percent in the voice therapy group improved, 56% percent in the reassurance group improved, and 89% in the surgery group improved. Regardless of the treatment modality, there was a dramatic improvement in voice after puberty that did not differ among the groups. He reiterated, however, that 12% of his patients continued to have dysphonia after puberty. He concluded that surgery was helpful in motivated patients who needed immediate help from their voice disorder. If immediate help was not required, voice therapy could be attempted, but the outcome was generally based on motivation. Although much of the dysphonia will resolve after puberty, dysphonic patients deserve close follow-up and individually tailored management.

Many treating physicians are concerned about the age at which interventions are appropriate. We give each child the benefit of the doubt regarding their ability to fol-low and adhere to voice therapy. The sessions are tailored to the child's age. Rest periods between groups of therapy sessions are given so that the child does not become bored or overburdened with the therapy. If a child is too young or immature and does not grasp the concepts or is incapable of performing the task, it is revisited after a break to reinforce what has been learned and assess the readiness of the child to proceed. Overall, the treatment of the dysphonic child is tremendously rewarding.

VOCAL FOLD CYSTS

Vocal fold cysts may also cause hoarseness in children. Cysts seen on the vocal folds are either congenital or acquired. Congenital cysts are either mucus-retention cysts filled with thick mucus such as that seen in a mucocele (Fig 11-17) or epidermal cyst filled with keratinous material (Fig 11-18).

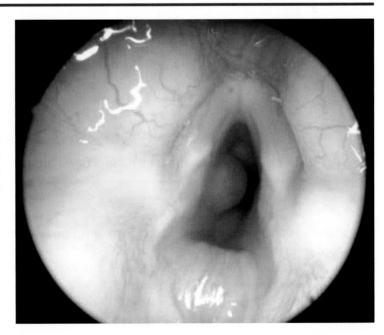

Fig 11–17. Large submucosal cyst in the immediate subglottis causing airway and voice disturbance.

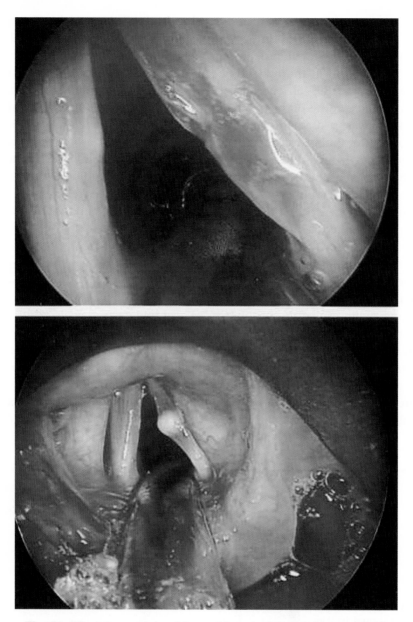

Fig 11–18. Intracordal epidermoid cyst of the right vocal fold.

Surgical excision is generally required for intracordal cysts. Careful dissection is required using microlaryngeal surgical techniques. Care is taken to completely remove the intracordal cyst as residual cyst wall will cause a recurrence. Rupture of the cyst during removal does not portend failure but careful inspection and complete removal of the cyst wall is still required.

As stated in the section on nodules, sometimes the diagnosis of an intracordal cyst is difficult to make, especially with mucus-retention cysts as they may mimic vocal nodules in appearance. Intracordal vocal fold cysts generally are unilateral, however. Epidermal cysts have a whitish appearance as they are filled with keratinous debris. If the diagnosis is in question, initial voice therapy may decrease the edema surrounding the intracordal cyst as well as decrease the contralateral nodule caused by the trauma of the cyst on the opposite vocal fold. This may make the diagnosis more clear and surgical management may proceed. If an accurate diagnosis is not possible with indirect laryngeal visualization, direct microlarygoscopy with palpation and possible vocal fold exploration should be considered.

Occasionally, acquired mucus-retention cysts of the subglottis may cause hoarseness or airway embarrassment. When recognized, these cysts are generally amenable to marsupialization with sharp instruments, electrocautery, or laser.

ANTERIOR GLOTTIC WEBS

Anterior glottic webs may be congenital or acquired. They cause dysphonia by changing the portion of the vocal fold allowed to vibrate and generate sound. As a band spanning from leading edge to leading edge of the true vocal fold they do not allow airflow across the membranous vocal fold and prevent the mucosal wave from propagating (Fig 11–19). Acquired glottic webs are generally iatrogenic (Fig 11–20). Repeated microsurgical resection of recurrent respiratory papillomata may result in the formation of an anterior glottic web (Fig 11–21). These webs are still difficult to treat but are generally thinner than congenital webs and are contained to the glottis without extension into the subglottis.

Congenital glottic webs, however, are causes by a problem of recannulization of the glottis during fetal development. They

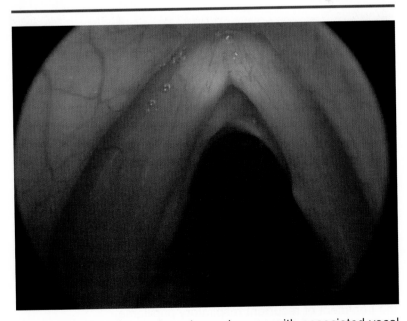

Fig 11–19. Small complex microweb seen with associated vocal fold nodule

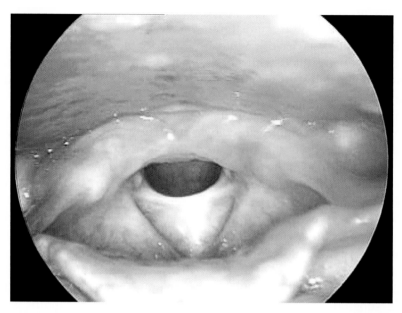

Fig 11–20. Severe glottic web caused by carbon dioxide laser treatments of recurrent respiratory papilloma.

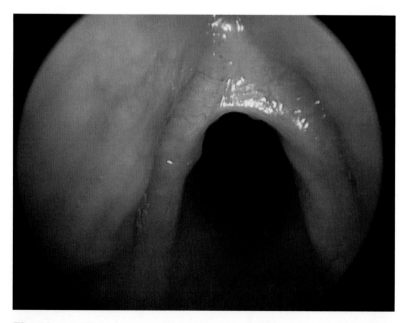

Fig 11–21. This is a small iatrogenic glottic web resulting from the treatment of recurrent respiratory papilloma.

may present with variable severity but often include thickening of the anterior cricoid cartilage (Fig 11–22). This may be seen as a "sail" sign in the subglottis on lateral neck radiographs. Treatment of congenital glottic webs generally requires treatment of the narrowed cricoid as well (Fig 11–23). An association with velocardiofacial syndrome (deletion of 22q) has been reported and children with congenital webs of the glottis should also have a genetic workup.[17]

The goal of surgical correction of an anterior glottic web is restoration of the vibrating vocal folds. A sharp anterior commissure is difficult to obtain without the placement of a keel to keep the edges of the anterior vocal fold from healing together. Keels may be placed externally with a laryn-gofissure or internally via an endoscopic approach. As surgical techniques advance, the endoscopic placement of a laryngeal keel has become more commonplace.

Treatment of the narrowed cricoid relies on the same principles of laryngotracheal reconstruction with augmentation of the cartilage framework with an autologous cartilage graft. In severe cases with cricoid involvement, the subglottic component is addressed initially with expansion laryngotracheoplasty and a keel is placed secondarily to resolve any residual webbing of the glottis. There are anecdotal reports of endoscopic repair of glottic webs with cricoid narrowing via endoscopic approach with an endoscopic anterior cricoid split using a sickle knife and primary endoscopic

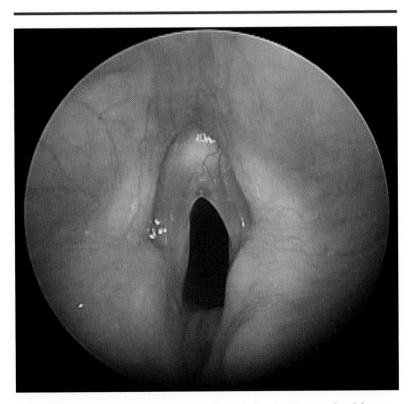

Fig 11–22. Small congenital glottic web in an 18-month-old causing mild stridor and dysphonia.

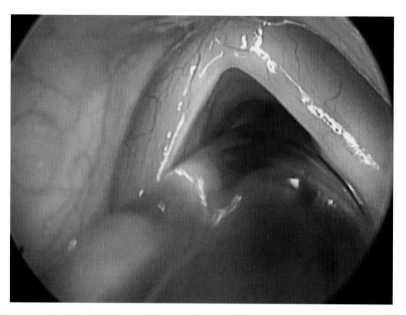

Fig 11–23. Result of congenital glottic web repair using an anterior costal cartilage laryngotracheoplasty.

placement of a keel. This technique sounds promising but larger case series will be needed to determine the indications and limitations of the technique.

CONCLUSION

Common laryngeal pathology in children fortunately is often benign. The appropriate treatment of some of these pediatric vocal fold lesions remains to be determined as the subspecialty of pediatric voice is still in its infancy. Above all, no lifelong irreparable harm should come to the developing vocal folds of the child. It should be pointed out, however, that significant prejudice is imparted on the child with dysphonia and so these children should not be ignored. As tools to measure perception of quality of life are developed, I believe significance impair-

ments will be discerned in the dysphonic child. Continued study of the differentiating layers of the vocal fold will help direct us as to when surgical interventions are possible to achieve positive benefits. Overall, evaluating and managing dysphonic children is a rewarding and gratifying part of the pediatric otolaryngology practice.

REFERENCES

1. Ruscello DM, Lass NJ, Podbesek J. Listeners' perceptions of normal and voice-disordered children. *Folia Phoniatr (Basel)*. 1988; 40(6):290–296.
2. Boseley ME, Cunningham MJ, Volk MS, Hartnick CJ. Validation of the Pediatric Voice-Related Quality-of-Life survey. *Arch Otolaryngol Head Neck Surg.* 2006;132(7): 717–720.

3. De Bodt MS, Ketelslagers K, Peeters T, et al. Evolution of vocal fold nodules from childhood to adolescence. *J Voice.* 2007;21(2): 151-156.

4. Hocevar-Boltezar I, Radsel Z, Zargi M. The role of allergy in the etiopathogenesis of laryngeal mucosal lesions. *Acta Otolaryngol Suppl.* 1997;527:134-137.

5. Halstead LA. Role of gastroesophageal reflux in pediatric upper airway disorders. *Otolaryngol Head Neck Surg.* 1999;120(2):208-214.

6. Mandell DL, Kay DJ, Dohar JE, Yellon RF. Lack of association between esophageal biopsy, bronchoalveolar lavage, and endoscopy findings in hoarse children. *Arch Otolaryngol Head Neck Surg.* 2004;130(11): 1293-1297.

7. Shah RK, Woodnorth GH, Glynn A, Nuss RC. Pediatric vocal nodules: correlation with perceptual voice analysis. *Int J Pediatr Otorhinolaryngol.* 2005;69(7):903-909.

8. Akif Kilic M, Okur E, Yildirim I, Guzelsoy S. The prevalence of vocal fold nodules in school age children. *Int J Pediatr Otorhinolaryngol.* 2004;68(4):409-412.

9. Gray SD, Hammond E, Hanson DF. Benign pathologic responses of the larynx. *Ann Otol Rhinol Laryngol.* 1995;104(1):13-18.

10. Boseley ME, Hartnick CJ. Development of the human true vocal fold: depth of cell layers and quantifying cell types within the lamina propria. *Ann Otol Rhinol Laryngol.* 2006;115(10):784-788.

11. Gray SD. Cellular physiology of the vocal folds. *Otolaryngol Clin North Am.* 2000; 33(4):679-698.

12. Gray SD, Chan KJ, Turner B. Dissection plane of the human vocal fold lamina propria and elastin fibre concentration. *Acta Otolaryngol.* 2000;120(1):87-91.

13. Gray SD, Titze IR, Alipour F, Hammond TH. Biomechanical and histologic observations of vocal fold fibrous proteins. *Ann Otol Rhinol Laryngol.* 2000;109(1):77-85.

14. Hammond TH, Gray SD, Butler JE. Age- and gender-related collagen distribution in human vocal folds. *Ann Otol Rhinol Laryngol.* 2000;109(10 pt 1):913-920.

15. Shah RK, Feldman HA, Nuss RC. A grading scale for pediatric vocal fold nodules. *Otolaryngol Head Neck Surg.* 2007;136(2): 193-197.

16. Mori K. Vocal fold nodules in children: preferable therapy. *Int J Pediatr Otorhinolaryngol.* 1999;49(suppl 1):S303-S306.

17. Miyamoto RC, Cotton RT, Rope AF, et al. Association of anterior glottic webs with velocardiofacial syndrome (chromosome 22q11.2 deletion). *Otolaryngol Head Neck Surg.* 2004;130(4):415-417.

Juvenile Onset Recurrent Respiratory Papillomatosis

Matthew T. Brigger
Christopher J. Hartnick

CASE PRESENTATION

A 15-month-old child is brought to the emergency room for increasing work of breathing and mild respiratory distress. Over the past several weeks, the child has experienced progressive dysphonia and stridor. He was started on empiric antibiotic therapy by his pediatrician and continued to experience progressive symptoms. Evaluation demonstrates the child to be in mild respiratory distress with biphasic stridor and minimal subcostal and suprasternal retractions. The child is essentially aphonic. Flexible fiberoptic endoscopy demonstrates the presence of an obstructing glottic lesion and associated ball valving effect with respiration. Subsequently, the child was taken to the operating room where a direct laryngoscopy and bronchoscopy confirmed the presence of a large obstructing glottic papilloma (Fig 12–1). At that time, the initial bulk of the disease was removed with a powered microdebrider. A significant degree

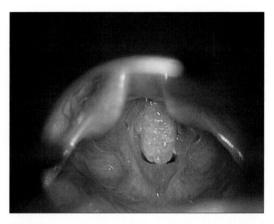

Fig 12–1. Preoperative endoscopic view of obstructing papilloma.

of residual disease was noted to be involving the anterior commissure of the true vocal folds. This region was treated with the 585-nm pulsed dye laser (PDL) (Fig 12–2). The child subsequently has done well and currently undergoes debridements at approximately 4-month intervals primarily with the PDL.

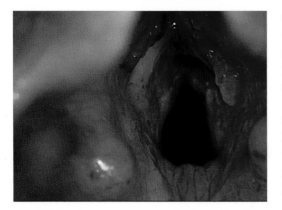

Fig 12–2. Postoperative endoscopic view of larynx after debulking of papilloma with a microdebrider followed by pulsed dye laser therapy to papilloma of the vocal fold anterior commissure.

INTRODUCTION

Recurrent respiratory papillomatosis (RRP) represents the most common neoplasm of the pediatric airway and often presents as airway obstruction.[1] As such, management of RRP represents a significant health care issue. RRP exists as two entities. The adult onset form (AORRP) tends to be of an indolent nature that rarely progresses to a debilitating condition. In contrast, juvenile onset recurrent respiratory papillomatosis (JORRP) is associated with a significantly more aggressive clinical course. Surgical intervention is the mainstay of therapy to prevent the morbidity of this disease as there is currently no effective medical treatment.

The course of JORRP adversely affects all functions of the human larynx. Specifically JORRP impacts the functional "laryngeal triad" of airway patency, voice production, and swallowing. Because complete eradication has yet to be realized, palliative surgical intervention serves to provide children

affected with JORRP the best quality of life despite inevitable recurrence. Goals of surgical therapy are as follows: improve airway, preserve voice, avoid aspiration, and operate as rarely as possible.

In JORRP, an aggressive disease course is associated with rapid regrowth of papillomas. This has led to the development of and search for adjuvant therapies to augment surgical intervention. Although results have been promising, many adjuvant therapies have marginally improved efficacy. Such adjuvant therapies also have both theoretical and known risks. A primary problem with conventional surgical methods involves the difficulty of precisely treating specific regions of the larynx such as the anterior commissure, the laryngeal ventricle, and the interarytenoid space, which are at particular risk for postoperative scarring and web formation. The recent development and use of angiolytic lasers has shown great promise in addressing glottic papillomas in both adults and children without increasing such scarification risk.[2-6]

EPIDEMIOLOGY

Despite recent advances, JORRP continues to be a source of significant morbidity for affected children; 75% of children diagnosed with JORRP present prior to age 5.[7] Arbitrarily, the term JORRP has been used to classify children diagnosed prior to age 12.[7] This age is based on the fact that JORRP tends to show a less aggressive course as adolescence is reached and individuals diagnosed during the teenage years tend to follow the less aggressive course associated with AORRP. The Multidisciplinary Task Force on RRP estimated a yearly pediatric incidence of 4.3 per 100,000 children with a surgical cost of approximately $109 million.[8]

PATHOPHYSIOLOGY

Human papilloma virus (HPV) has been definitively linked to the development of JORRP.[7] Although, more than 98 HPV serotypes have been defined, HPV-6 and HPV-11 are most commonly implicated.[9] In Wiatrak's 10 year longitudinal study, a more aggressive disease course was observed in patients infected with HPV-11.[9] Infection is associated with vertical transmission from mother to child via the birth canal. Clearly, control of HPV infection is the key to success in prevention. The association of cervical cancer in women with HPV has driven the development of HPV vaccines.[10] A quadrivalent vaccine for HPV serotypes 6,11,16, and 18 has displayed promising results and has recently been approved by the FDA for clinical use in females between the ages of 9 and 26.[7,10] However, until such a vaccine demonstrates clinical utility toward eradication of HPV, therapy for JORRP will remain a significant health care burden.

Papillomas generally occur in regions where ciliated and squamous epithelium are juxtaposed or regions of trauma or surgical manipulation such as tracheotomy.[11] Common regions affected by JORRP include the upper and lower ventricle margins, the undersurface of the vocal folds, the laryngeal surface of the epiglottis, the carina, the nasal limen vestibule, and the nasopharyngeal surface of the soft palate.[12] Histologically, papillomas are composed of a highly vascularized fibrous core covered by nonkeratinizing squamous epithelium.[1] The epithelial basal layer may demonstrate hyperplasia and there appears to be a disorder of cellular differentiation.[7]

Perhaps the most salient point regarding the pathophysiology of JORRP is the latent nature of HPV infection. The failure of all current treatment modalities rests on the fact that the HPV virus remains inactive in normal tissues until a period on reactivation. The pathways of reactivation are unclear at this time, but clearly some form of interaction with the immune system is related.

CLINICAL PRESENTATION AND EVALUATION

Respiratory obstruction and dysphonia are the hallmarks of JORRP. Hoarseness is most often the initial complaint, and is often associated with a delay in diagnosis greater than one year from the onset of symptoms. The progression during that time is generally associated with the onset of stridor or respiratory distress prompting endoscopic evaluation and thus confirming the diagnosis. Many children are initially treated for croup, asthma, allergies, or vocal nodules. Rarely, a patient will present with failure to thrive, recurrent pneumonias, or an acute life-threatening airway event.

A comprehensive history of a child with hoarseness is critical to establish the diagnosis of JORRP from other causes. The nature and timing of the symptoms, prior airway trauma or intubation, congenital anomalies, significant comorbidities, and associated symptoms must be addressed. Maternal history of vaginal or cervical condylomata should be assessed and follow-up recommended. A slowly progressive inspiratory or biphasic stridor is suggestive of a glottic or subglottic lesion that requires visualization. Attention to pulmonary compromise or nasal obstruction symptoms may provide clues to extension beyond the glottis.

A complete physical examination with visualization of the pharynx and larynx is generally sufficient to make a presumptive diagnosis. In the stable child without acute airway compromise, awake flexible nasolaryngoscopy is performed to assess anatomy, presence of lesions, and laryngeal function. Patients presenting with acute respiratory distress associated with tachypnea, cervical hyperextension, air hunger or hypoxia are evaluated in the operating room by direct laryngoscopy with surgical intervention or endotracheal intubation as necessary. Tracheostomy is avoided in all but the most acute cases of impending respiratory arrest. Most children will ultimately undergo direct laryngoscopy and bronchoscopy in a nonemergent fashion allowing complete evaluation of the aerodigestive tract.

Papilloma can range from small sessile lesions to bulky gross disease (Fig 12-3). Due to the range of presentations, Derkay et al[13] proposed a laryngoscopic staging system for assessing and tracking JORRP. The proposed staging system has subsequently become a commonly utilized tool within the otolaryngology literature when reporting JORRP outcomes. The system is based the anatomic breakdown of the upper aerodigestive tract into 25 subsites. Each subsite is assigned a score of 0, 1, 2 or 3. "0" represents no lesion, "1" represents a surface lesion, "2" represents a raised lesion, and "3" representing a bulky lesion. A composite anatomic score is then generated with a

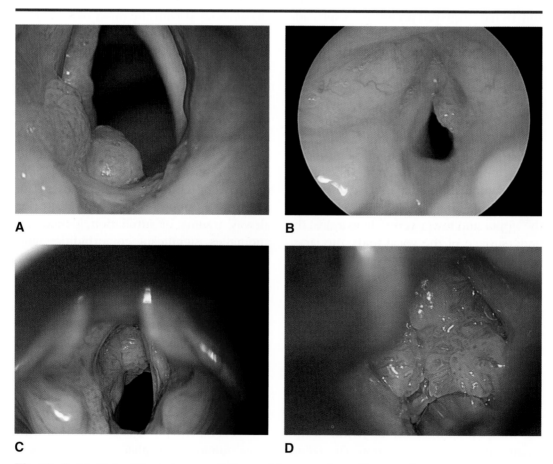

A **B** **C** **D**

Fig 12–3. Multiple different presentations of laryngeal papillomatosis.

maximum of 75. This is added to a clinical symptom score that consists of 4 graded questions for a total laryngoscopic staging and severity score.

In most children, few additional studies are requisite beyond clinical history and direct examination. A computed tomographic evaluation of the chest may be useful in children with extensive disease to assess pulmonary involvement. It is important to ensure that despite characteristic appearance all children with JORRP require histopathologic confirmation of the diagnosis and should undergo HPV typing. In children requiring frequent therapy, interval histopathologic evaluation is recommended to potentially identify malignant transformation.

TREATMENT

Surgical Therapy

JORRP has long been considered a surgical disease. Management has traditionally entailed operative debulking of symptomatic lesions. Balancing the laryngeal triad of airway patency, voice production, and swallowing to provide the best quality of life is the cornerstone of palliative laryngeal surgery. Microlaryngeal dissection with cold instruments was supplanted by CO_2 laser debulking as the preferred modality in the 1990s.[14] In more recent years, debulking with a powered microdebrider has been rapidly adopted and now represents the most common surgical method in use by members of the American Society of Pediatric Otolaryngology (ASPO).[15] Several studies have demonstrated improved functional outcomes, operative time and cost when microdebrider excision has been compared to CO_2 laser vaporization.[14,16,17] Other purported benefits of the microdebrider include

the elimination of the risk of intraoperative laser ignition fire and the lack of a smoke plume with potentially infectious particles that may lead to distal seeding or present danger to the operating room staff.[16,18] As the microdebrider has gained acceptance and widespread use, several limitations have been realized. The most troublesome limitation involves the removal of papilloma in so-called "difficult to treat areas" such as the anterior commissure, interarytenoid space, and laryngeal ventricle. The anterior commissure, in particular, requires staged resections as epithelial injury caused by the microdebrider can promote secondary webbing and scarring of the larynx.

Effective communication and cooperation with the anesthesiologist prior to and during laryngeal surgery for papilloma is critical. The bulk and location of disease along with the desired treatment modality will determine the appropriate method of ventilation. The presence of a pediatric anesthesiologist familiar and comfortable with spontaneous ventilation anesthesia techniques is desired. This anesthetic technique provides the best view of the larynx and extent of disease while allowing adequate access for debulking. Endotracheal intubation may be required initially for excessive disease and at times jet ventilation or apneic techniques are indicated.

Selective Angiolytic Laser Therapy

The above described surgical methods excise or ablate papillomas and directly debulk the burden of disease. As discussed, the inability to aggressively surgically address "difficult to treat" areas due to the potential for secondary epithelial damage is the primary limitation in debulking surgery. In theory, if these areas could be grossly cleared of disease, patients may experience an increase in time between surgeries and potentially improved voice during surgical intervals. The selective angiolytic lasers, of which the pulsed dye laser (PDL) is most commonly cited, are based on a concept where the laser is designed to be absorbed by intraluminal blood and result in coagulation of microvascularity without epithelial damage.[19] Loss of blood supply should therefore lead to involution of lesions. The highly vascular core of papillomas is a good match for the selective photothermolysis model. Initial data are promising and a multicenter trial is currently underway.

Adjuvant Therapy

As stated, all current surgical procedures serve to remove clinically significant lesions, but are not curative in nature. Due to the shortcomings of surgical debulking, a variety of adjuvant therapies have been explored. Currently accepted indications for adjuvant therapy include children requiring more than four surgical interventions per year, the presence of distal spread of disease, or rapid papilloma regrowth with resultant airway compromise.[7] It is estimated that as may as 20% of children with JORRP meet such indications.[15]

In a recent survey of ASPO members, the most commonly employed adjuvant therapy is intralesional cidofovir injections.[15] Cidofovir is a cytosine nucleotide analogue that is FDA approved for cytomegaloviral retinitis in the setting of HIV.[20] Although the mechanism of activity against HPV is unclear, cidofovir has demonstrated efficacy in a number of uncontrolled case series.[21-23] A variety of dosing regimens and outcome measures have been utilized. There is controversy concerning long-term efficacy and studies have shown a variable number of

nonresponders.[24,25] Additionally there has been a report of vocal scarring after cidofovir use.[26] Perhaps of greater importance is the issue of carcinogenesis. Wemer et al[27] recently presented the case of an adult with progressive dysplasia associated with cidofovir use. The Task Force on RRP issued a cautionary position statement regarding risk assessment in using cidofvir.[25] Several findings were cited including the known carcinogenicity in animals and the lack of long-term data in humans.[25] Although promising, there remains uncertainty regarding the routine use of cidofovir.

Other current adjuvant therapies include systemic interferon alpha, indole-3-carbinol (I3C), retinoic acid, photodynamic therapy, acyclovir, and heat shock protein (HSP) E7. Interferon-alpha has demonstrated efficacy that is often lost after discontinuation of therapy and is frequently limited by side effects.[20] I3C has not demonstrated deleterious side effects but has limited established utility.[28] Retinoic acid, photodynamic therapy, and acyclovir suffer from a small pool of variable data. Recently, a well-conceived single-arm multicenter trial of systemic HSP E7 demonstrated an increased intersurgical interval compared to baseline. Interestingly, this effect was more pronounced in females.[29] Unfortunately, further investigations of HSP E7 are currently delayed. Current studies assessing the roles of celecoxib, 3,3-diindolylmethane, and intralesional mumps virus vaccine as adjuvant therapies are underway.

Vaccination

As in all diseases, prevention serves as the best form of therapy. As suggested above, the FDA has approved a quadrivalent vaccine (Gardasil®) indicated for the prevention of disease caused by HPV types 6, 11,

16, and 18. Results of the phase 3 reports demonstrated the vaccine to confer excellent protection from developing anogenital condyloma in females.[30] Thus, Gardasil has been approved for use in girls and women 9 to 26 years of age, is currently recommended in the vaccine schedule published by the American Academy of Pediatrics. No clear data regarding therapeutic vaccination for JORRP are currently available. Clearly, the overall impact of the vaccine will take many years to realize, although cautious optimism exists regarding greatly reducing the disease burden or perhaps even eradication of JORRP in the future.

CONCLUSION

Although relatively rare, JORRP is a potentially devastating disease that causes significant morbidity to affected children and their families while presenting a significant burden on the health care system. Although there is no known cure, current efforts to improve the quality of life through new treatment modalities and the hope provided by the development of the HPV vaccine suggest that the burden on both affected children and society may be lessened in the future. A keen awareness combined with a fundamental knowledge of the current state of JORRP is requisite of all providers who treat children with aerodigestive disorders.

REFERENCES

1. Wiatrak BJ. Overview of recurrent respiratory papillomatosis. *Curr Opin Otolaryngol Head Neck Surg*. 2003;11:433–441.
2. Zeitels SM, Akst LM, Burns JA, et al. Office-based 532-nm pulsed KTP laser treatment of glottal papillomatosis and dysplasia. *Ann Otol Rhinol Laryngol*. 2006;115:679–685.
3. Zeitels SM, Burns JA. Laser applications in laryngology: past, present, and future. *Otolaryngol Clin North Am*. 2006;39:159–172.
4. Zeitels SM, Franco RA Jr, Dailey SH, et al. Office-based treatment of glottal dysplasia and papillomatosis with the 585-nm pulsed dye laser and local anesthesia. *Ann Otol Rhinol Laryngol*. 2004;113:265–276.
5. Bower CM, Waner M, Flock S, et al. Flash pump dye laser treatment of laryngeal papillomas. *Ann Otol Rhinol Laryngol*. 1998;107:1001–1005.
6. Franco RA Jr, Zeitels SM, Farinelli WA, et al. 585-nm pulsed dye laser treatment of glottal papillomatosis. *Ann Otol Rhinol Laryngol*. 2002;111:486–492.
7. Derkay CS, Darrow DH. Recurrent respiratory papillomatosis. *Ann Otol Rhinol Laryngol*. 2006;115:1–11.
8. Derkay CS. Task force on recurrent respiratory papillomas. A preliminary report. *Arch Otolaryngol Head Neck Surg*. 1995;121:1386–1391.
9. Wiatrak BJ, Wiatrak DW, Broker TR, et al. Recurrent respiratory papillomatosis: a longitudinal study comparing severity associated with human papilloma viral types 6 and 11 and other risk factors in a large pediatric population. *Laryngoscope*. 2004;114:1–23.
10. Freed GL, Derkay CS. Prevention of recurrent respiratory papillomatosis: role of HPV vaccination. *Int J Pediatr Otorhinolaryngol*. 2006;70:1799–1803.
11. Kashima H, Mounts P, Leventhal B, et al. Sites of predilection in recurrent respiratory papillomatosis. *Ann Otol Rhinol Laryngol*. 1993;102:580–583.
12. Kashima HK, Shah F, Lyles A, et al. A comparison of risk factors in juvenile-onset and adult-onset recurrent respiratory papillomatosis. *Laryngoscope*. 1992;102:9–13.
13. Derkay CS, Malis DJ, Zalzal G, et al. A staging system for assessing severity of disease and response to therapy in recurrent respiratory papillomatosis. *Laryngoscope*. 1998;108:935–937.

14. Pasquale K, Wiatrak B, Woolley A, et al. Microdebrider versus CO_2 laser removal of recurrent respiratory papillomas: a prospective analysis. *Laryngoscope.* 2003;113: 139–143.

15. Schraff S, Derkay CS, Burke B, et al. American Society of Pediatric Otolaryngology members' experience with recurrent respiratory papillomatosis and the use of adjuvant therapy. *Arch Otolaryngol Head Neck Surg.* 2004;130:1039–1042.

16. El-Bitar MA, Zalzal GH. Powered instrumentation in the treatment of recurrent respiratory papillomatosis: an alternative to the carbon dioxide laser. *Arch Otolaryngol Head Neck Surg.* 2002;128:425–428.

17. Patel N, Rowe M, Tunkel D. Treatment of recurrent respiratory papillomatosis in children with the microdebrider. *Ann Otol Rhinol Laryngol.* 2003;112:7–10.

18. Kashima HK, Kessis T, Mounts P, et al. Polymerase chain reaction identification of human papillomavirus DNA in CO_2 laser plume from recurrent respiratory papillomatosis. *Otolaryngol Head Neck Surg.* 1991;104: 191–195.

19. Zeitels SM, Akst LM, Bums JA, et al. Pulsed angiolytic laser treatment of ectasias and varices in singers. *Ann Otol Rhinol Laryngol.* 2006;115:571–580.

20. Lee JH, Smith RJ. Recurrent respiratory papillomatosis: pathogenesis to treatment. *Curr Opin Otolaryngol Head Neck Surg.* 2005;13:354–359.

21. Pransky SM, Albright JT, Magit AE. Long-term follow-up of pediatric recurrent respiratory papillomatosis managed with intralesional cidofovir. *Laryngoscope.* 2003;113: 1583–1587.

22. Pransky SM, Magit AE, Kearns DB, et al. Intralesional cidofovir for recurrent respiratory papillomatosis in children. *Arch Otolaryngol Head Neck Surg.* 1999;125: 1143–1148.

23. Peyton Shirley W, Wiatrak B. Is cidofovir a useful adjunctive therapy for recurrent respiratory papillomatosis in children? *Int J Pediatr Otorhinolaryngol.* 2004;68:413–418.

24. Milczuk HA. Intralesional cidofovir for the treatment of severe juvenile recurrent respiratory papillomatosis: long-term results in 4 children. *Otolaryngol Head Neck Surg.* 2003;128:788–794.

25. Derkay C. Cidofovir for recurrent respiratory papillomatosis (RRP): a re-assessment of risks. *Int J Pediatr Otorhinolaryngol.* 2005;69:1465–1467.

26. Lee AS, Rosen CA. Efficacy of cidofovir injection for the treatment of recurrent respiratory papillomatosis. *J Voice.* 2004;18: 551–556.

27. Wemer RD, Lee JH, Hoffman HT, et al. Case of progressive dysplasia concomitant with intralesional cidofovir administration for recurrent respiratory papillomatosis. *Ann Otol Rhinol Laryngol.* 2005;114:836–839.

28. Rosen CA, Bryson PC. Indole-3-carbinol for recurrent respiratory papillomatosis: long-term results. *J Voice.* 2004;18:248–253.

29. Derkay CS, Smith RJ, McClay J, et al. HspE7 treatment of pediatric recurrent respiratory papillomatosis: final results of an open-label trial. *Ann Otol Rhinol Laryngol.* 2005;114: 730–737.

30. Garland SM, Hernandez-Avila M, Wheeler CM, et al. Quadrivalent vaccine against human papillomavirus to prevent anogenital diseases. *N Engl J Med.* 2007;356:1928–1943.

Vocal Fold Immobility

Matthew T. Brigger
Christopher J. Hartnick

CASE PRESENTATION

A 14-year-old male presents with a long-standing history of poor vocal projection and rapid vocal fatigue. As a neonate, he underwent ligation of a patent ductus arteriosus that left him with long standing left-sided vocal fold immobility. Despite this history, currently he is a vocal student and is seeking to improve his voice beyond the gains that he has attained in speech therapy alone. He has never experienced swallowing difficulties or evidence of aspiration. He previously underwent medialization of his vocal fold with an endoscopic injection of fat into the paraglottic space from which he temporarily experienced excellent results. He now desires a more permanent solution. Surgical options offered included repeat injection laryngoplasty, medialization thyroplasty, and recurrent laryngeal nerve reinnervation. Subsequently, he and his parents elected to undergo recurrent laryngeal nerve reinnervation with the ipsilateral ansa cervicalis nerve branch. An absorbable gelatin injection laryngoplasty was performed simultaneously. He immediately noted significant improvement in his voice as a result of the injection laryngoplasty and began aggressive voice therapy. His vocal quality steadily declined over the first several months as the gelatin was resorbed. However, 5 months postoperatively he noted a significant improvement in his voice. During the course of his recovery, the position and bulk of his left vocal fold improved significantly, ultimately allowing approximation with the right vocal fold and decreased vibratory flaccidity. He currently has a much stronger voice and is satisfied with the result.

INTRODUCTION

Vocal fold immobility (VFI) has been reported to be the second most common etiology of stridor in infants and accounts for 5 to 10% of pediatric tracheostomies.[1-3] Central to a discussion of VFI in children is specific identification and recognition of the similarities and differences between unilateral vocal fold immobility (UFVI) and bilateral vocal fold immobility (BVFI). The importance lies in the associated manifestations of each entity, which are in direct relation to the functional anatomy of the larynx. Although the clinical features and the evaluation of each entity often overlap, treatment is individually based on the therapeutic goals for each patient.

ANATOMIC CONSIDERATIONS

Dysfunction of laryngeal movement can result from an insult at any point between the laryngeal motor nuclei and the intrinsic laryngeal musculature. This includes the entire length of the vagus and recurrent laryngeal nerves. Additionally, delineation between true neurologic dysfunction versus mechanical dysfunction secondary to cricoarytenoid joint pathology is necessary and may be difficult to differentiate. Cricoarytenoid arthritis or fibrosis often manifests as an immobile vocal fold.

The motor nuclei of the vagus nerve are located in the medulla oblongata within the nucleus ambiguus. Lower motor neurons subsequently exit the brainstem as 8 to 10 rootlets, which coalesce to form the vagus nerve. The vagus subsequently leaves the skull through the jugular foramen. The neural fibers innervating the intrinsic laryngeal musculature are of branchial motor origin. Glottic sensation is via the visceral afferent fibers within the laryngeal nerves.

In the neck, the vagus nerve travels within the carotid sheath and supplies the superior laryngeal nerve (SLN) and recurrent laryngeal nerve (RLN) (Fig 13–1A). The SLN descends along the pharynx to innervate the cricothyroid muscle. On the right, the RLN descends inferiorly and subse-quently wraps under the subclavian artery and ascends posteriorly within the tracheoesophageal groove to enter the larynx and innervate the remainder of the intrinsic laryngeal muscles. On the left, the nerve loops posteriorly under the aortic arch to ascend within the tracheoesophageal groove, thus placing the left nerve at significant risk during mediastinal procedures, particularly cardiac surgery.

From an anatomic standpoint, the RLN innervates all of the intrinsic muscles of the larynx except for the cricothyroid muscle (Fig 13–1B). The RLN therefore innervates the primary adductors (paired lateral cricoarytenoid and unpaired interarytenoid muscles) and the only abductor (posterior cricoarytenoid muscle), thus controlling closing (adduction) and opening (abduction) of the glottis. Additionally, the RLN innervates the thyroarytenoid muscle, which serves as a tensor of the vocal fold. The motor action of the SLN is through the cricothyroid muscle, which serves to add tension to the vocal folds by exerting motion about the cricothyroid joint leading to a downward visor effect of the thyroid cartilage on the cricoid cartilage.

Any discussion of the human laryngeal anatomy, particularly concerning vocal fold motion, must address the unique nature of the cricoarytenoid joint. On initial inspection, the diarthroidal joints appear to be characterized by a simple rotating motion that provides vocal fold apposition. In reality, the motion is a complex three-dimensional pattern that results in precise approximation of the vocal folds despite what often appears to be asymmetry in arytenoid movement.[4] The cricoarytenoid joint is an often overlooked cause of VFI as any cause of fibrosis, arthritis, or inflammation can limit articulation of the joint and on direct visualization can be indistinguishable from immobility secondary to lack of neural stimulation.

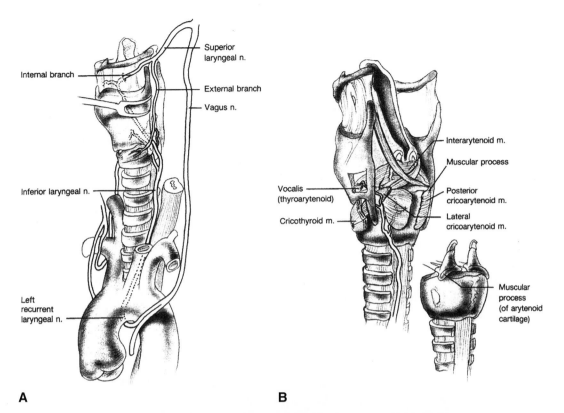

Fig 13–1. A. Course of the vagus and laryngeal nerves within the neck. **B.** Laryngeal musculature and relation to innervation by the recurrent laryngeal nerve. From: Bailey BJ, ed. *Head and Neck Surgery-Otolaryngology.* Vol 2. 3rd ed. Philadelphia, Pa; 2001. (Used with permission from Lippincott Williams & Wilkins.)

From a functional standpoint, the larynx serves first to provide an airway for ventilation and to separate the trachea from the esophagus during degluition. Secondarily, the larynx provides a mechanism for vocalization. Compromise of the laryngeal motion can result in clinical and subclinical disturbances in all functions of the larynx. The position of the immobile fold in relation to glottic opening directly correlates with the symptoms. Bilateral abductor paralysis with close approximation of the vocal folds in the midline results in airway obstruction that manifests as stridor and

exertional dyspnea, whereas unilateral paralysis tends to manifest primarily as soft vocalization due to the inability to approximate the vocal folds. These generalized statements refer to the common clinical manifestations often seen in older children; however, the small neonatal larynx may manifest similar symptoms in both BVFI and UVFI.

Although most cases of VFI are a combination of immobility both in adduction and abduction, the descriptive terms abductor versus adductor paralysis have come into common usage referring to the position of the vocal folds primarily in the setting of bilateral immobility. Vocal folds that approach midline and result in airway obstruction are referred to as abductor paralysis and those that are more lateralized are referred to as the much less common adductor paralysis.

ETIOLOGY

VFI can be congenital or acquired. Etiologies are generally attributed to one of several classifications: neurogenic, birth trauma, cardiovascular, iatrogenic, or idiopathic causes. Determining the true incidence of VFI and associated etiologies is limited by variable reporting between centers, which can be attributed to referral patterns and specifics of how VFI is classified.

In most series, neurogenic etiologies account for 12 to 30% of cases, most commonly bilateral.[5-9] Central neurogenic causes include structural anomalies, cerebral palsy, leukodystrophy, tumors, and spastic or hypotonia conditions.[10] One of the most common neurogenic etiologies is the Arnold-Chiari malformation. The condition is associated with varying degrees of inferior displacement of the cerebellar tonsils through the foramen magnum (Figure 13–2). The proposed, yet unproven, mechanism is traction on the vagal rootlets secondary to herniation of the brainstem through the foramen magnum. However, other proposed mechanisms of injury including altered vascular

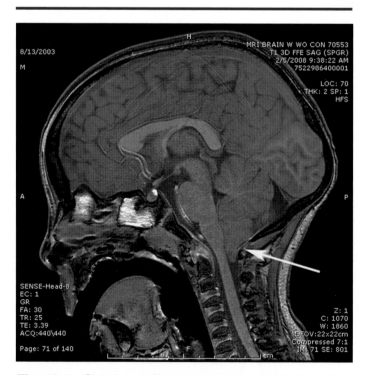

Fig 13–2. Chiari I malformation. Note the inferior displacement of the cerebellum through the foramen magnum.

supply have been forwarded.[3,11] Although generally presenting with BVFI, UFVI has been reported secondary to Arnold-Chiari malformations.[5] Neurosurgical procedures to release Arnold-Chiari malformations may result in improvement in VFI; however, in many children the VFI persists.[9] Peripheral nervous disorders including Charcot-Marie-Tooth disease have been associated with both UFVI and BVFI.[12,13]

VFI secondary to birth trauma is commonly associated with forceps delivery and has widely variable rates of UVFI versus BVFI accounting for 5 to 21% of cases.[5-7,9] Injury may be the result of compression or traction.

Cardiovascular anomalies including tetrology of Fallot, ventricular septal defect, patent ductus arteriosus, and vascular rings have been associated with VFI.[14] However, it is the repair of such anomalies that often leads to VFI. In a recent review, 33 cases of VFI were reported in a cohort of 2,255 children who underwent cardiac surgery. Of these children, 30 cases of unilateral immobility and 3 cases of bilateral immobility were reported. The most common associated procedure was coarctation repair in 10 children. PDA ligation resulted in 8 cases of UFVI. A series of 109 children undergoing cardiac surgery reported a 35% rate of VFI with the vast majority manifesting left-sided UVFI. Of note, however, 6 children had right UVFI and 1 child had BVFI.[15]

VFI has also been attributed to infectious agents including West Nile virus, Epstein-Barr virus, poliomyelitis, tuberculosis, pneumococcus meningitis, Lyme disease, and non-specific viral infection.[16-22] Other reports have suggested intubation, esophageal foreign bodies and chemotherapy to be associated with VFI.[23-25] Genetic transmission of BVFI has been documented in both autosomal dominant and X-linked fashion.[26,27]

Although often equated, VFI is not synonymous nor does it unequivocally imply RLN paralysis. As stated above, VFI can be a manifestation of a cricoarytenoid joint that is fused secondary to fibrosis. Additionally, VFI may be due to interarytenoid scarring or posterior glottic stenosis most often resulting from intubation injury. Autoimmune disease, gastroesophageal reflux, and cricoarytenoid arthritis have been implicated etiologic factors.[28]

Of primary importance is the fact that VFI is determined to be idiopathic in 7 to 41% of children.[7,8] In many series, this represents the most common etiology.[5,8] Both BVFI and UVFI are reported as idiopathic in variable proportions.

ASSOCIATED AIRWAY DISORDERS

Children with VFI often have other associated airway lesions. In Daya's review, 46 of 102 children had additional airway findings in which 10 had more than one additional lesion.[6] Laryngomalacia and tracheobronchomalacia are the most common associated associated airway findings. Other findings include subglottic stenosis, intubation granulomas, and supra- and subglottic cysts.[6,29]

NATURAL COURSE

The natural course of VFI is highly dependent on the etiology and clinical manifestations. Cases in which the nerve was iatrogenically severed generally will not regain function without intervention. High rates of spontaneous recovery (52–100%) have been reported when the etiology is idiopathic or secondary to neurologic dysfunction.[5,8]

In adults, 6 to 12 months of observation for return of function prior to surgical intervention have been advocated.[30] However, in children, most centers advocate observation of 12 months at a minimum prior to surgical intervention due to high rates of spontaneous recovery combined with conservative approaches to airway surgery.[31] Of note and perhaps arguing for a longer period of observation, the experience at Great Ormond Street demonstrated that over half of the children who recovered function, did so after 1 year and as late as 11 years after diagnosis.[6]

EVALUATION OF THE PEDIATRIC PATIENT WITH VFI

History

VFI has a wide range of presentations from acute airway obstruction requiring tracheostomy to subtle vocal abnormalities. A comprehensive history including a complete birth and family history is imperative in evaluating children with suspected VFI. A thorough review of systems is necessary. Details concerning the child's respiratory pattern, particularly the presence of stridor, cyanosis, or vocalization may give important clues. Stridor is more common in BVFI and generally biphasic; however, UVFI has been associated with stridor in as high as 77% of children.[6] The stridor of UVFI often has been reported to be primarily inspiratory in nature.[10] A history of exertional dyspnea is commonly elicited. A feeding history often reveals evidence of dysphagia particularly in children with UVFI. Feeding difficulties may be associated with either the inability to adequately close the glottis or sensory deficiencies at the laryngeal inlet. The presence of GERD has been associated with decreased laryngeal sensation, which may contribute to associated feeding difficulties.[32] Children with BVFI generally have fewer vocal difficulties given the lack of laryngeal abduction, whereas UVFI often manifests as a quiet cry or breathy voice. However, it must be reiterated that in the neonate, vocal qualities and stridor alone are insufficient to differentiate BVFI from UVFI.

Fifty-eight percent of cases of BVFI present within the first 12 hours after birth. Persistent symptoms of BVFI center on the associated lack of abduction, thus resulting in airway obstruction manifesting as stridor or exertional dyspnea. Airway patency is determined by the size of the posterior or respiratory glottis. Tracheostomy rates vary from 0 to 73% based on the series.[7,8]

UVFI in the neonate will often present as stridor. However, in older children the symptoms are similar to adults with dysphonia being the most common presentation. A breathy voice with decreased projection and rapid fatigue is the common presentation. Subtle or overt signs of aspiration may be present.

Examination

A comprehensive physical exam with attention to respiration is performed. Stridor should be assessed and correlated with respiratory phase. The presence of significant supra or substernal retractions often correlates with the degree of obstruction. Assessment of any craniofacial dysmorphisms as well as palpation of fontanelles in a neonate may give clues to potential underlying causes. Prior surgical scars are noted. A detailed neurologic exam with attention to the cranial nerves is performed. A neck exam is performed to potentially identify any mass lesion.

Endoscopic Examination

Awake fiberoptic endoscopy has become indispensable in diagnosing and monitoring VFI in children. A true dynamic vocal fold assessment is essential. Although fiberoptic endoscopy allows a view of the decreased supraglottic sensation and associated frank aspiration, a keen awareness of the difficulties in evaluating the larynx of a small child needs to be appreciated. The infant larynx, particularly when associated with laryngomalacia, is characterized by a floppy epiglottis and redundant aryepiglottic folds. Often, it can be difficult to clearly visualize the vocal folds. Additionally, the assured crying and agitation that accompanies an infant exam may allow only brief glimpses of the larynx. An important distinction is not to equate arytenoid movement with neuromuscular integrity of the vocal fold as small movement can be seen with respiratory variation or swallowing.[3]

In children who will not tolerate an awake exam or in whom a definitive diagnosis cannot be made, rigid laryngoscopy under anesthesia is indicated. An attempt is made to assess vocal fold mobility during emergence from anesthesia. Information concerning vocal fold mobility gained from an exam under anesthesia must be viewed cautiously as the effects of anesthesia are variable on laryngeal motion. The additional benefit is the ability to palpate the cricoarytenoid joint in an attempt to rule out associated fixation. As stated above, a significant number of children with VFI have associated airway anomalies suggesting a role for rigid laryngoscopy and bronchoscopy under anesthesia in many children with VFI.

Swallowing Evaluation

Swallowing dysfunction manifested as feeding difficulties or aspiration is often seen in children with VFI, particularly those with UVFI.[6,7] Adult series have documented aspiration rates of 23 to 44% in UVFI.[33,34] Subtle signs of feeding difficulty may be evident in a comprehensive feeding history. Any child with potential feeding concerns should undergo a swallowing evaluation. A videofluoroscopic swallowing study, also known as a modified barium swallow, is performed in conjunction with a speech and language pathologist in a fluoroscopy suite. In some patients, a fiberoptic endoscopic evaluation of swallowing (FEES) done at the time of nasal endoscopy may provide an adequate assessment at the time of initial evaluation. Additionally, the ability to add sensory testing of the supraglottis during a FEES study can give an assessment of compromised sensation often contributing to penetration and aspiration events.

Imaging

In the absence of a clear iatrogenic etiology of VFI, all children should undergo imaging of the central nervous system to rule out the presence of neurologic causes particularly Arnold-Chiari malformation. Additionally, at the time of imaging, it is prudent to consider imaging of the neck and chest to rule out compressive mass lesions or cardiovascular anomalies that may be associated with VFI. A chest radiograph may be indicated based on the child's symptoms. Although direct imaging of the larynx is frequently of low utility given the need for a dynamic assessment, laryngeal ultrasound has been reported to be of some utility.[35]

Laryngeal EMG

In adults, laryngeal electromyography (LEMG) has become a commonly used tool in the evaluation of VFI. In adults, it serves both as a diagnostic tool and a potential prognostic tool. LEMG allows a differentiation between cricoarytenoid fixation and denervation of the recurrent laryngeal nerve. Additionally, the prognostic value of LEMG has become increasingly described. The greatest utility appears to be in predicting poor functional outcome, perhaps allowing a shorter interval between injury and surgical intervention to be realized.[36-38]

In adults, LEMG is performed on an awake patient through the percutaneous placement of electrodes. This requires a considerable level of cooperation that is difficult to obtain in most children. Several reports have demonstrated the feasibility of LEMG under general anesthesia in children.[28,39,40] The described technique involves the placement of electrodes directly into intrinsic laryngeal musculature with the child under general anesthesia and following the LEMG tracing during emergence (Fig 13–3). Difficulties include cumbersome electrode placement in the small pediatric larynx, the development of edema, and the requirement for a neurologist with specialized EMG equipment to be present in the operating room.[41] A simplified method of LEMG using standard operating room equipment without the physical presence of a neurologist in the operating room, while still facilitating postoperative review, has been proposed.[41] The technique that we employ involves placing electrodes from a widely available intraoperative nerve monitor routinely used by otolaryngologists for ear surgery and recording the output digitally, which is then forwarded to an EMG trained neurologist who subsequently interprets the

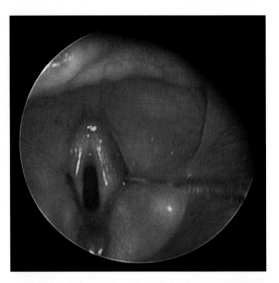

Fig 13–3. Endoscopic placement of EMG needle electrode into thyroarytenoid muscle.

study. This has allowed us to greatly facilitate the routine use of LEMG in the evaluation of children with VFI.

TREATMENT

Therapy for VFI is dictated by clinical manifestations, etiology, and the goals of the child and caretaker. In many cases, observation alone may be sufficient. As described above, aside from cases where a known transection has occurred, any surgical intervention should be delayed to allow spontaneous return of function. Most importantly, a frank discussion of options and expectations is necessary between the surgeon, the caregiver, and possibly the child. Additionally, the need for close cooperation and treatment with a speech pathologist, particularly when the therapy is directed at vocal outcomes, is necessary.

An understanding of the different issues caused by BVFI versus UVFI is imperative to understand the potential therapeutic interventions. Most cases of BVFI are difficulties in abduction with resultant airway obstruction. Therefore, the goal of establishing improved airway patency results in procedures that often lateralize fixed vocal folds to increase the glottic aperture. Unfortunately, this has led to a focus on decannulation of tracheostomy-dependent children and limited reporting of voice outcomes in the setting of BVFI. The goals of lateralization procedures for BVFI are quire different from the goals of medialization procedures designed to treat the breathy dysphonia or aspiration of UVFI secondary to incompetent glottal closure. A special case is in the setting of BVFI when the vocal folds are in a position of abduction and the child suffers from marked aspiration or dysphonia. These children require medialization of their vocal folds.

Surgical Therapy for UVFI

Injection Laryngoplasty

Injection laryngoplasty involves surgical medialization of the immobile vocal fold with an injectable material placed into the paraglottic space. First conceived by Bruning in the early 1900s, the procedure entails visualization of the vocal fold and subsequent delivery of material to be injected through a needle.[42] Figure 13–4 demonstrates the medialization obtained by injection laryngoplasty. A variety of substances have been used over time with variable degrees of success and long-term outcomes.[42] Widely used injectables include autologous fat, micronized acellular dermis, hyroxylapatite, and absorbable gelatin foam. Polytetrafluoroethylene (Teflon) was used for many years until the long-term complication of granuloma formation was realized, leading to its rare use now.[42] Choice of injectable material depends on the desired duration and overall goal of the procedure. Favorable results have been shown in children.[43] The fact that many of the injectable materials resorb over time may offer advantages in terms of immediate improvement while allowing additional time for recovery of motion.

Medialization Thyroplasty

Although initially described in 1915, the concept of laryngeal framework manipulation to treat VFI did not become widespread until 1974 when Isshiki described a series of phonosurgical procedures.[44,45] Among them, he described the type 1 medialization thyroplasty as a method of cutting a window within the thyroid cartilage and placing an implant (autologous cartilage in his initial description) within the paraglottic space to medialize an immobile vocal fold.[45] Over the years, various descriptions and implant materials have been championed including cartilage, Silastic, and expanded polytetrafluoroethylene (Gore-Tex).[46,47] Unlike injectable Teflon, Gore-Tex is not associated with severe granuloma reactions. The addition of arytenoid procedures, cricothyroid subluxation, or even reinnervation procedures to medialization thyroplasty has been advocated.[48,49] Safety and feasibility have been demonstrated in children.[43,50] Additionally, it has been realized that the pediatric vocal folds sit at a relatively lower region of the thyroid cartilage when compared to adults.[50] Thus, a combined endoscopic visualization of externally placed needles to define the appropriate location to create the thyroid cartilage

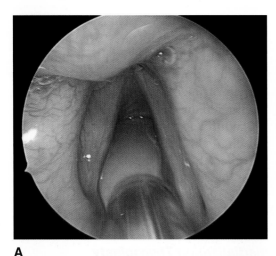

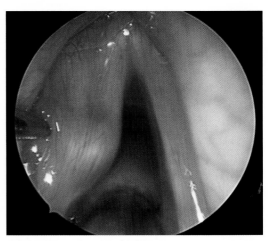

A

B

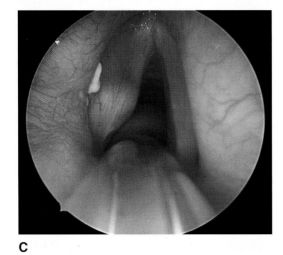

C

Fig 13–4. A. Immobile left vocal fold prior to injection laryngoplasty with calcium hydroxylapatite. **B.** Calcium hydroxylapatite being injected into left vocal fold. **C.** Immobile left vocal fold after calcium hydroxylapatite injection. Note significant bulking and medialization of vocal fold.

window for implant placement in children has been described.[50] In our experience, the use of Gore-Tex as a medialization implant serves to allow precise intraoperative placement and adjustment.

In adults, medialization thyroplasty is typically accomplished under local anesthesia and the voice is "tuned" to desired effect. Unfortunately, most children will not tolerate such a procedure and require general anesthesia and such intraoperative tuning will not be possible. In our experience, placement of a small endotracheal tube and endoscopic visualization allows adequate medialization. Additionally, the use of a laryngeal mask airway and flexible endoscopic visualization has been described.[51]

Laryngeal Reinnervation

When a known transection of the recurrent laryngeal nerve occurs, most authors advocate a primary neurorraphy. However, the role of attempts at reinnervation in the absence of clear transection or trauma has been a subject of controversy that has gained support over time, particularly in the setting of UVFI. Multiple methods have been described using various donors (phrenic nerve and ansa cervicalis) and various configurations (direct nerve anastamosis, nerve stump placed into laryngeal musculature, strap muscle pedicle placed into laryngeal muscle belly) both unilaterally and bilaterally.[52] Most reports describe the use of the ansa cervicalis anastamosed to a stump of recurrent laryngeal nerve or directly to the thyroarytenoid muscle belly. In the setting of UVFI, the primary goal is not to achieve active motion, but to improve the tone and bulk of the immobile vocal fold to allow better approximation and generation of phonation. Several series report on sustained voice outcomes, overall better approximation of the vocal folds postoperatively, and some even report the presence of active adduction.[53-55] Although most series involve adults, recently the feasibility and safety in children has been described.[43] Tucker reports the utility of reinnervation at the time of medialization laryngoplasty primarily focusing on maintaining vocal fold bulk by avoiding atrophy over time.[54] Results typically are not realized for several months and often injection laryngoplasty is performed at the time of intervention to provide immediate relief.

Surgical Therapy for BVFI

Tracheostomy

The development of acute airway obstruction in the neonate as a presentation of BVFI may necessitate a tracheostomy. In Cohen's 1982 review at the Children's Hospital of Los Angeles, 45 of 62 (73%) children underwent tracheostomy placement at a mean age of 34 days.[7] Daya's 2000 review of the Great Ormond Street experience noted that 28 of 49 (57%) children with BVFI required tracheostomy.[6] In most patients, further interventions as described below can be undertaken toward a goal of decannulation.

Endoscopic Procedures

A number of endoscopic procedures have been proposed for management of BVFI in children. All serve to increase the glottic aperture generally with the use of the CO_2 laser to perform a posterior cordotomy or arytenoidectomy.[31,56,57] Figure 13-5 demonstrates a left vocal fold cordotomy performed with a CO_2 laser. Note that the posterior airway is opened while preserving the anterior phonatory aspect of the vocal fold. Outcomes of endoscopic procedures demonstrate various degrees of success. Although primary decannulation rates for endoscopic procedures tend to be below 50%, when multiple procedures are considered overall decannulation rates are over 80%.[31] Although initial success may be limited, the low associated morbidity and lack of external incisions often make endoscopic procedures an attractive initial intervention or as a revision adjunct.

External Lateralization Procedures

The initial descriptions of external lateralization procedures involved open arytenoidectomies either through a window in the thyroid ala, removing the posterior half of the thyroid ala, or by a posterior approach of releasing and rotating the thyroid cartilage to provide access to the arytenoid.[58-60] The procedure involved removing most of the arytenoid cartilage while preserving the vocal process to which the vocal fold is attached. Subsequently, the vocal process was secured laterally to the thyroid ala. Priest first applied the procedure to

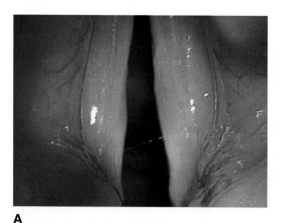

A

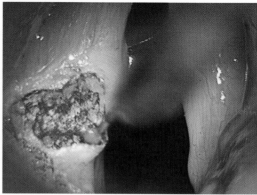

B

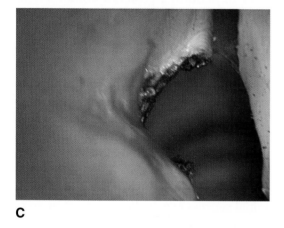

C

Fig 13–5. A. Bilateral immobile vocal folds prior to endoscopic laser cordotomy. **B.** Thulium laser fiber being used to remove posterior aspect of left vocal fold. **C.** Immediate postoperative result.

children in 1960.[61] Over time additional solutions came into favor including access via a laryngofissure and cartilage-preserving suture lateralization arytenoidopexy techniques.[31,62] Reported decannulation rates demonstrate greater than 70% success with poorly defined voice outcomes.[62,63]

Expansion Laryngotracheoplasty

Expansion laryngotracheoplasty (LTP) involves the placement of a cartilage graft into the posterior glottis effectively expanding the respiratory airway with a goal toward decannulation (Fig 13-6). Although LTP may represent a more complex surgical procedure and recovery period secondary to the harvest of a costal cartilage graft and the necessity of splitting the cricoid cartilage, decannulation rates have been reported to be quite favorable.[31,56,63,64] In recent years, endoscopic approaches have been well described and spare the child the morbidity of an open laryngofissure.[64] Posterior LTP is often best suited for children with a significant degree of interarytenoid scarring resulting in posterior glottic stenosis or children that have associated subglottic stenosis. Although, the theoretical risk of aspiration is certainly a concern in significantly opening the posterior glottis, most series have demonstrated a low incidence.[31,64]

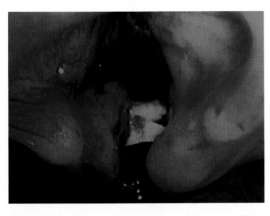

Fig 13–6. Posterior costal cartilage graft in situ immediately after placement.

Laryngeal Reinnervation

Abductor reinnervation in the setting of BVFI has been described. However, the results are not as promising as those published in the setting of UVFI. The goal is an attempt to restore active abduction. The unpredictable effects of synkinesis despite reinnervation directed at specific muscle groups may contribute to the known limitations. Although excellent results have been reported, reproducibility and concerns about sustained outcomes have limited the widespread utility of this procedure in BVFI.[52,55]

Medialization Thyroplasty

Bilateral medialization thyroplasty has been rarely described in children with adductor BVFI leading to aspiration and breathy dysphonia.[43,50] The glottal incompetence in these children is in contrast to the tracheostomy-dependent airway obstruction that is often the hallmark of BVFI. The few descriptions in the literature concerning bilateral thyroplasties in children report both staged (unilateral followed by the contralateral side at a separate anesthetic)

and simultaneous procedures. The procedure represents a directed solution to a difficult problem that is not commonly encountered. However, in our experience, when performed in a properly selected child with appropriate informed consent and expectations the results can be quite satisfying.

CONCLUSIONS

VFI is a condition with a variety of manifestations. The associated disability of untreated VFI can range from minimal dysphonia to devastating airway obstruction or intractable aspiration. Proper evaluation and examination are requisite to formulate an individual treatment plan. With proper management, the associate morbidity of VFI can be minimized and excellent outcomes can be expected in most children.

REFERENCES

1. Corbett HJ, Mann KS, Mitra I, et al. Tracheostomy—a 10-year experience from a UK pediatric surgical center. *J Pediatr Surg.* 2007;42:1251-1254.
2. Hadfield PJ, Lloyd-Faulconbridge RV, Almeyda J, et al. The changing indications for paediatric tracheostomy. *Int J Pediatr Otorhinolaryngol.* 2003;67:7-10.
3. Grundfast KM, Harley E. Vocal cord paralysis. *Otolaryngol Clin North Am.* 1989;22:569-597.
4. Wang RC. Three-dimensional analysis of cricoarytenoid joint motion. *Laryngoscope.* 1998;108:1-17.
5. de Gaudemar I, Roudaire M, Francois M, et al. Outcome of laryngeal paralysis in neonates: a long term retrospective study of 113 cases. *Int J Pediatr Otorhinolaryngol.* 1996;34:101-110.

6. Daya H, Hosni A, Bejar-Solar I, et al. Pediatric vocal fold paralysis: a long-term retrospective study. *Arch Otolaryngol Head Neck Surg.* 2000;126:21-25.

7. Cohen SR, Geller KA, Birns JW, et al. Laryngeal paralysis in children: a long-term retrospective study. *Ann Otol Rhinol Laryngol.* 1982;91:417-424.

8. Zbar RI, Smith RJ. Vocal fold paralysis in infants twelve months of age and younger. *Otolaryngol Head Neck Surg.* 1996;114:18-21.

9. Emery PJ, Fearon B. Vocal cord palsy in pediatric practice: a review of 71 cases. *Int J Pediatr Otorhinolaryngol.* 1984;8:147-154.

10. de Jong AL, Kuppersmith RB, Sulek M, et al. Vocal cord paralysis in infants and children. *Otolaryngol Clin North Am.* 2000;33:131-149.

11. Papasozomenos S, Roessmann U. Respiratory distress and Arnold-Chiari malformation. *Neurology.* 1981;31:97-100.

12. Lacy PD, Hartley BE, Rutter MJ, et al. Familial bilateral vocal cord paralysis and Charcot-Marie-Tooth disease type II-C. *Arch Otolaryngol Head Neck Surg.* 2001;127:322-324.

13. Boseley ME, Bloch I, Hartnick CJ. Charcot-Marie-Tooth Disease type 1 and pediatric true vocal fold paralysis. *Int J Pediatr Otorhinolaryngol.* 2006;70:345-347.

14. Dedo DD. Pediatric vocal cord paralysis. *Laryngoscope.* 1979;89:1378-1384.

15. Truong MT, Messner AH, Kerschner JE, et al. Pediatric vocal fold paralysis after cardiac surgery: rate of recovery and sequelae. *Otolaryngol Head Neck Surg.* 2007;137:780-784.

16. Steele NP, Myssiorek D. West Nile virus induced vocal fold paralysis. *Laryngoscope.* 2006;116:494-496.

17. Driscoll BP, Gracco C, Coelho C, et al. Laryngeal function in postpolio patients. *Laryngoscope.* 1995;105:35-41.

18. Clack ZA, Anand KJ, Fortenberry JD, et al. Bilateral vocal cord paralysis after meningitis due to Streptococcus pneumoniae. *South Med J.* 1998;91:660-662.

19. Parano E, Pavone L, Musumeci S, et al. Acute palsy of the recurrent laryngeal nerve complicating Epstein-Barr virus infection. *Neuropediatrics.* 1996;27:164-166.

20. Schroeter V, Belz GG, Blenk H. Paralysis of recurrent laryngeal nerve in Lyme disease. *Lancet.* 1988;2:1245.

21. Rafay MA. Tuberculous lymphadenopathy of superior mediastinum causing vocal cord paralysis. *Ann Thorac Surg.* 2000;70:2142-2143.

22. Amin MR, Koufman JA. Vagal neuropathy after upper respiratory infection: a viral etiology? *Am J Otolaryngol.* 2001;22:251-256.

23. Virgilis D, Weinberger JM, Fisher D, et al. Vocal cord paralysis secondary to impacted esophageal foreign bodies in young children. *Pediatrics.* 2001;107:E101.

24. Cohen SR. Pseudolaryngeal paralysis: a post-intubation complications. *Ann Otol Rhinol Laryngol.* 1981;90:483-488.

25. Burns BV, Shotton JC. Vocal fold palsy following vinca alkaloid treatment. *J Laryngol Otol.* 1998;112:485-487.

26. Cunningham MJ, Eavey RD, Shannon DC. Familial vocal cord dysfunction. *Pediatrics.* 1985;76:750-753.

27. Grundfast KM, Milmoe G. Congenital hereditary bilateral abductor vocal cord paralysis. *Ann Otol Rhinol Laryngol.* 1982;91:564-566.

28. Jacobs IN, Finkel RS. Laryngeal electromyography in the management of vocal cord mobility problems in children. *Laryngoscope.* 2002;112:1243-1248.

29. Swift AC, Rogers J. Vocal cord paralysis in children. *J Laryngol Otol.* 1987;101:169-171.

30. Tucker HM. Human laryngeal reinnervation. *Laryngoscope.* 1976;86:769-779.

31. Hartnick CJ, Brigger MT, Willging JP, et al. Surgery for pediatric vocal cord paralysis: a retrospective review. *Ann Otol Rhinol Laryngol.* 2003;112:1-6.

32. Suskind DL, Thompson DM, Gulati M, et al. Improved infant swallowing after gastroesophageal reflux disease treatment: a function of improved laryngeal sensation? *Laryngoscope.* 2006;116:1397-1403.

33. Bhattacharyya N, Kotz T, Shapiro J. Dysphagia and aspiration with unilateral vocal cord immobility: incidence, characterization, and

response to surgical treatment. *Ann Otol Rhinol Laryngol.* 2002;111:672-679.

34. Leder SB, Ross DA. Incidence of vocal fold immobility in patients with dysphagia. *Dysphagia.* 2005;20:163-167; discussion 168-169.

35. Friedman EM. Role of ultrasound in the assessment of vocal cord function in infants and children. *Ann Otol Rhinol Laryngol.* 1997;106:199-209.

36. Min YB, Finnegan EM, Hoffman HT, et al. A preliminary study of the prognostic role of electromyography in laryngeal paralysis. *Otolaryngol Head Neck Surg.* 1994;111:770-775.

37. Sittel C, Stennert E, Thumfart WF, et al. Prognostic value of laryngeal electromyography in vocal fold paralysis. *Arch Otolaryngol Head Neck Surg.* 2001;127:155-160.

38. Munin MC, Rosen CA, Zullo T. Utility of laryngeal electromyography in predicting recovery after vocal fold paralysis. *Arch Phys Med Rehabil.* 2003;84:1150-1153.

39. Berkowitz RG. Laryngeal electromyography findings in idiopathic congenital bilateral vocal cord paralysis. *Ann Otol Rhinol Laryngol.* 1996;105:207-212.

40. Wohl DL, Kilpatrick JK, Leshner RT, et al. Intraoperative pediatric laryngeal electromyography: experience and caveats with monopolar electrodes. *Ann Otol Rhinol Laryngol.* 2001;110:524-531.

41. Scott AR, Chong PS, Randolph GW, et al. Intraoperative laryngeal electromyography in children with vocal fold immobility: A simplified technique. *Int J Pediatr Otorhinolaryngol.* 2008;72:31-40.

42. O'Leary MA, Grillone GA. Injection laryngoplasty. *Otolaryngol Clin North Am.* 2006; 39:43-54.

43. Sipp JA, Kerschner JE, Braune N, et al. Vocal fold medialization in children: injection laryngoplasty, thyroplasty, or nerve reinnervation? *Arch Otolaryngol Head Neck Surg.* 2007;133:767-771.

44. Payr A. Plastik am Schildknorpel zur Behebung der Folgen einseitiger Stimmbandlahmung. *Dtsch Med Wochenschr.* 1915;43: 1265-1267.

45. Isshiki N, Morita H, Okamura H, et al. Thyroplasty as a new phonosurgical technique. *Acta Otolaryngol.* 1974;78:451-457.

46. Koufman JA. Laryngoplasty for vocal cord medialization: an alternative to Teflon. *Laryngoscope.* 1986;96:726-731.

47. McCulloch TM, Hoffman HT. Medialization laryngoplasty with expanded polytetrafluoroethylene. Surgical technique and preliminary results. *Ann Otol Rhinol Laryngol.* 1998;107:427-432.

48. Zeitels SM. New procedures for paralytic dysphonia: adduction arytenopexy, Gore-Tex medialization laryngoplasty, and cricothyroid subluxation. *Otolaryngol Clin North Am.* 2000;33:841-854.

49. Tucker HM. Combined laryngeal framework medialization and reinnervation for unilateral vocal fold paralysis. *Ann Otol Rhinol Laryngol.* 1990;99:778-781.

50. Link DT, Rutter MJ, Liu JH, et al. Pediatric type I thyroplasty: an evolving procedure. *Ann Otol Rhinol Laryngol.* 1999;108: 1105-1110.

51. Gardner GM, Altman JS, Balakrishnan G. Pediatric vocal fold medialization with Silastic implant: intraoperative airway management. *Int J Pediatr Otorhinolaryngol.* 2000;52: 37-44.

52. Paniello RC. Laryngeal reinnervation. *Otolaryngol Clin North Am.* 2004;37:161-681, vii-viii.

53. Su WF, Hsu YD, Chen HC, et al. Laryngeal reinnervation by ansa cervicalis nerve implantation for unilateral vocal cord paralysis in humans. *J Am Coll Surg.* 2007;204: 64-72.

54. Tucker HM. Long-term preservation of voice improvement following surgical medialization and reinnervation for unilateral vocal fold paralysis. *J Voice.* 1999;13:251-256.

55. Tucker HM. Long-term results of nerve-muscle pedicle reinnervation for laryngeal paralysis. *Ann Otol Rhinol Laryngol.* 1989; 98:674-676.

56. Bower CM, Choi SS, Cotton RT. Arytenoidectomy in children. *Ann Otol Rhinol Laryngol.* 1994;103:271-278.

57. Worley G, Bajaj Y, Cavalli L, et al. Laser arytenoidectomy in children with bilateral vocal fold immobility. *J Laryngol Otol.* 2007;121:25-27.

58. Woodman D. A modification to the extralaryngeal approach to arytenoidectomy for bilateral abductor paralysis. *Arch Otolaryngol Head Neck Surg.* 1946;43:63-65.

59. Kelly JD. Surgical treatment of bilateral paralysis of the abductor muscles. *Arch Otolaryngol Head Neck Surg.* 1941;33:293-304.

60. Orton HB. Extralaryngeal surgical approach for arytenoidectomy: bilateral abductor paralysis of the larynx. *Ann Otol Rhinol Laryngol.* 1944;53:302-307.

61. Priest RE, Ulvestad HS, Van De Water F, et al. Arytenoidectomy in children. *Ann Otol Rhinol Laryngol.* 1960;69:869-881.

62. Narcy P. Arytenoidopexy for laryngeal paralysis in children. *Int J Pediatr Otorhinolaryngol.* 1995;32(suppl):S101-S102.

63. Brigger MT, Hartnick CJ. Surgery for pediatric vocal cord paralysis: a meta-analysis. *Otolaryngol Head Neck Surg.* 2002;126: 349-355.

64. Inglis AF Jr, Perkins JA, Manning SC, et al. Endoscopic posterior cricoid split and rib grafting in 10 children. *Laryngoscope.* 2003; 113:2004-2009.

14

Pediatric Airway Reconstruction and the Voice

Karen B. Zur

INTRODUCTION

Pediatric airway reconstruction saw a surge in the early 1970s when Robin Cotton began applying surgical techniques that were developed in the adult population by Rethi and Feron, to manage children who suffered from laryngotracheal stenosis. His research and clinical work enabled technologically dependent children suffering from airway compromise due to acquired or congenital laryngotracheal pathology to lead a life without the need for a tracheostomy tube. Airway specialists throughout the United States and the world have adapted and expanded these techniques, allowing a significant rate of decannulation[1] and successful management of other airway disorders.

Now that the management of pediatric airway disorders has been mastered, attention is shifting toward the quality of life of these children. One of the main areas not previously addressed in a systematic fashion is the effect of airway disorders on a child's voice. Tracheostomy tube placement and airway reconstruction can lead to dysphonia, affecting a child's communication and quality of life. These voicing disturbances are due to multifactorial issues that are discussed at the end of this chapter.

Normally, the production of voice is related to the flow of air through the glottis, whose time-dependent shape is defined by the motion of the vocal folds and the translaryngeal pressure.[2] Airway lesions thus alter transglottic airflow patterns leading to either turbulent flow through the vocal folds or complete inability to cause vocal fold vibration due to a high-grade stenosis. Direct injury to the vocal folds may occur during intubation, use of the laser for management of myriad conditions affecting the airway, or open airway procedures (Fig 14-1).

The goal of this chapter is to introduce the reader to basic airway procedures and the voice-related issues following airway manipulation and reconstruction. A detailed description and definition of airway patholo-

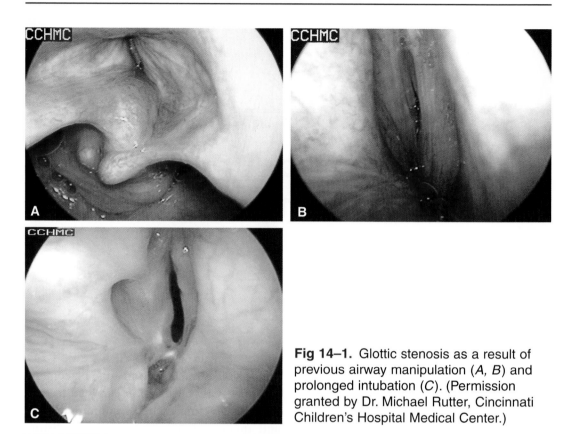

Fig 14–1. Glottic stenosis as a result of previous airway manipulation (*A, B*) and prolonged intubation (*C*). (Permission granted by Dr. Michael Rutter, Cincinnati Children's Hospital Medical Center.)

gies is beyond the scope of this chapter. The systematic, data-oriented paradigm of patient evaluation used by the author is discussed as well. This chapter focuses on the therapeutic interventions that are currently being used to rehabilitate these children.

OVERVIEW OF SURGICAL PROCEDURES TO IMPROVE AND/OR RECONSTRUCT THE AIRWAY

In cases of very mild subglottic or tracheal obstruction with no overt symptoms or complications, it is possible to closely observe the child. Interval endoscopies are performed to assess structural progression versus relative reduction of the obstruction. During the period of observation it is important to monitor underlying gastroesophageal reflux disease and eosinophilic esophagitis and to ensure optimal pulmonary status. In cases with more significant symptoms or obstruction, and following an adequate multidisciplinary evaluation, an appropriate intervention is chosen.

Tracheotomy

The indications for tracheotomy include: severe upper airway obstruction, long-term ventilation, and pulmonary toilet. When the tracheostomy is no longer medically necessary, the child will undergo a decannulation process to remove the tube. This will require another airway evaluation to ensure the airway caliber is adequate. Lesions that can be associated with chronic tracheostomies include suprastomal collapse and suprastomal granulation, and those should be managed prior to decannulation.

The greatest risk of an indwelling tracheostomy is death secondary to tube obstruction or an accidental dislodgement. Mortality related to the presence of a tracheostomy tube has been reported to approximate 0.5%.[3] It is therefore incumbent on the clinicians to educate the family and caretakers regarding proper care at home. Specific tracheotomy care protocols are often developed by many hospitals and medical centers.

Endoscopic Approaches to Repair of Glottic/Subglottic Stenosis

Certain conditions are amenable to endoscopic, "minimally invasive" approaches of repair. Discussion of the merits of various lasers (CO_2, KTP) versus "cold steel" is beyond the scope of this chapter. Base of tongue cysts/masses, glossoptosis (base of tongue collapse), recurrent respiratory papillomatosis (RRP), laryngomalacia, arytenoids prolapse, arytenoid subluxation leading to posterior glottic stenosis, small posterior glottic scar/web (Fig 14–2), bilateral vocal fold paralysis (Fig 14–3), small subglottic web, subglottic cysts and tracheal hemangiomas are but a few of airway lesions that may lead to stridor and airway compromise, and could potentially be managed transorally. All of these lesions can lead to dysphonia either due to the underlying

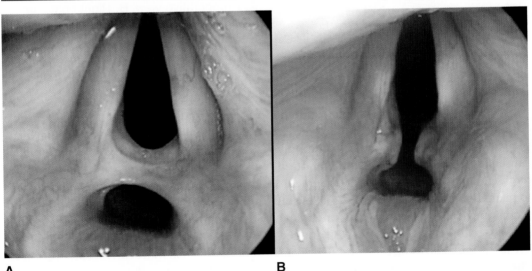

A   **B**

Fig 14–2. Endoscopic approach to manage a posterior glottic web. **A.** Preoperative view. **B.** Immediate postoperative view. This child had no sequelae from a voice or airway perspective.

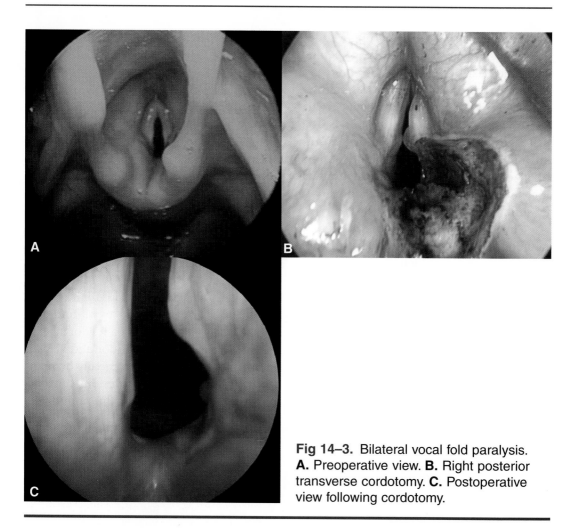

Fig 14–3. Bilateral vocal fold paralysis. **A.** Preoperative view. **B.** Right posterior transverse cordotomy. **C.** Postoperative view following cordotomy.

pathology or as a result of its management. For example, laryngotracheal recurrent respiratory papillomatosis, most commonly caused by HPV subtypes 6 and 11, often require numerous endoscopic debridements to maintain a safe airway (Fig 14–4). Several techniques have been utilized, including cold-dissection, laser techniques (CO_2, pulsed dye laser,[4] and KTP[5]) and the microdebrider.[6] The goal of management is to maintain a safe airway in the case of the obstructing papillomas, and to improve vocalization in milder situation by reducing the mass from the surface of the vocal fold. The goal of

restoring mucosal wave without causing irreparable damage to the underlying vocal folds and mucosa is the basic tenet of management, as direct vocal fold and anterior commissure injury can lead to chronic vocal fold scarring, webbing of the larynx, and stenosis. To date, basic science research has been focused on the management and prevention of vocal fold scarring. Mitomycin C, an antifibroblast and antitumor agent, has been used, with variable success, to prevent scarring in the larynx. More innovative tissue engineering technologies utilize injectates to preserve the viscoelastic properties of

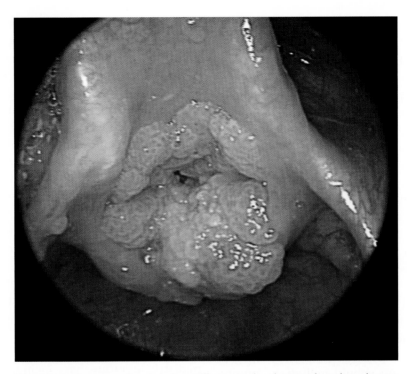

Fig 14–4. Laryngotracheal papillomatosis obstructing the airway.

the vocal folds. Prophylactic in vivo manipulation of the extracellular matrix with an injectable Carbylan-SX hydrogel appears to induce vocal fold tissue regeneration to yield optimal tissue composition and biomechanical properties favorable for phonation.[7] One hopes more clinical research and applications of these techniques will allow preservation of normal vocal fold morphology, while allowing proper management of the airway lesions, either endoscopically or via open surgical approaches.

Anterior Cricoid Split

Neonates who have been intubated for a prolonged period of time, who fail extubation due to minimal subglottic stenosis, and who meet strict eligibility criteria may benefit from performing a cricoid split to augment the airway.[8] This practice is falling out of favor in a population of neonates and infants who can avoid a tracheostomy tube placement. In this group, a thyroid ala graft is interposed between the cut ends of the cricoid cartilage (usually anteriorly) and the child remains intubated for a shorter duration than the cricoid split without the graft; this procedure is fondly referred to as the "mini-laryngotracheoplasty." Improved outcomes (88% success versus 83%) and shorter periods of intubation have made this procedure more favorable, whereas uncontrolled severe reflux, prematurity and low birth weight adversely affect the surgical results.[9]

Augmentation Procedures: Laryngotracheal Reconstruction (LTR)

Expansion procedures to aid in tracheostomy tube removal in the child with glottic/subglottic stenosis (Fig 14–5) include placement of anterior, posterior, or combined grafts to augment the cricoid and/or tracheal airway. Laryngotracheal reconstruction refers to an augmentation procedure with use of a graft(s). The aim of this surgical method is to re-establish airway continuity without the need for a tracheostomy tube and with preservation of laryngeal function for protection of the airway, swallowing, and voicing.[10] For this reason, the candidate for an LTR should have good pulmonary reserve, requiring no ventilatory support and be medically stable. The preoperative workup should include a comprehensive gastroenterological, pulmonary, and swallowing/aspiration evaluation.

Once the decision has been made to reconstruct, the surgical options include augmentation or resection. Resection is described in the next section. Another element that needs to be decided is whether or not the procedure should be single-staged or double-staged. A single-staged procedure means that at the conclusion of the surgery the tracheostomy tube will no longer be present, whereas a double-staged procedure implies that either a tracheostomy tube or a similar type of stent will be present at the end of the case (see next section).

The augmentation procedure involves placement of an autogenous cartilage graft between the split cricoid cartilage and/or split tracheal wall. Numerous graft materials have been reported in the literature over the years, but the most commonly used graft is the cartilaginous rib. Other sources of cartilage grafts, reported in both adult and pediatric literature, have included auricular cartilage, hyoid, thyroid ala, septal cartilage, and thyrotracheal autografts.[11-13] Regardless of the source of cartilage, studies have shown that autogenous cartilage used in the anterior and posterior pediatric larynx survives, grows and undergoes neovascularization.[14]

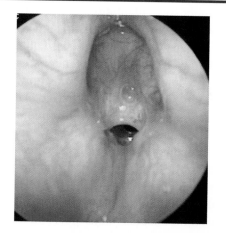

Fig 14–5. Laryngeal atresia. This patient underwent a tracheostomy tube placement at birth and is awaiting surgical reconstruction with a laryngotracheal reconstruction.

Resection Procedures: Partial Cricotracheal Resection

Patients with discrete levels of obstruction and those with high-grade stenoses (grade III-IV subglottic stenosis), often benefit from a graft-free resection procedure. Two resection procedures are used to manage either subglottic or tracheal stenosis; respectively, they are termed partial cricotracheal resection (CTR) or tracheal resection. This chapter focuses on the more complex CTR.

The CTR procedure involves: (1) resection of the anterior cricoid plate, remaining anterior to the cricothyroid joint; (2) resection of proximal tracheal stenosis, maintaining the first healthy tracheal ring intact; and (3) removing posterior cricoid scar in a submucosal plane, below the level of the cricoarytenoid joint. Once the scar is removed, the trachea is sutured to the posterior cricoid mucosa and to the anterior thyroid lamina (Fig 14–6). Chin to chest sutures are placed for 10 days to allow healing of the anastamosis without potential for head extension and tracheal separation in cases of patient agitation. The CTR, just like the LTR, can be performed in a single- or double-staged procedure, with similar indications for each as previously described.

AIRWAY RECONSTRUCTION AND THE VOICE

With the excellent decannulation rates discussed earlier in the chapter and the comfort of the pediatric airway surgeon in managing those cases, the focus of the multidisciplinary team caring for these children is now shifting toward improving their vocal quality of life. In his book *Odyssey of the Voice* Jean Abitbol states that " . . . feeling good about one's voice, just as feeling good about oneself, is essential for our communication with oneself and with others."[15] The ability

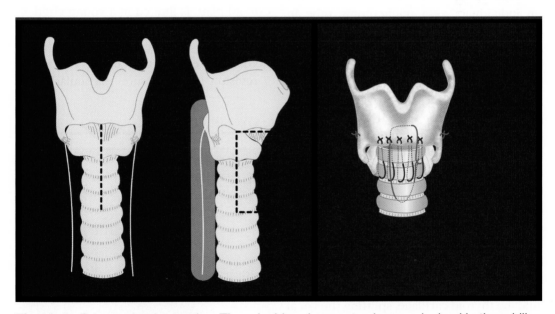

Fig 14–6. Cricotracheal resection. The cricoid and upper trachea are incised in the midline in a vertical fashion to allow exposure of the airway and to assess the stenotic lesion. At this point, the decision will be made whether an augmentation versus a resection procedure will be undertaken. For the partial CTR, the anterior cricoid plate and damaged tracheal rings are removed, anterior to the cricothyroid joint, with care to dissect in a subperichondrial plane, as to avoid the nearby recurrent laryngeal nerves. Once a circumferential dissection around the trachea is accomplished, sutures are placed between the trachea and inferior thyroid border, with two lateral detentioning sutures to secure the anastomosis. Hartley BE, Cotton RT. Pediatric Airway Stenosis: Laryngotracheal Reconstruction or Cricotracheal Resection? *Clin Otolaryngol Allied Sci.* 2000;25(5):342–349. Reprinted with permission.

to communicate effectively, effortlessly and with clarity is a secondary goal in the process of augmenting an airway. The focus of this section is on procedure-specific complications as they relate to the voice.

Chronic Tracheostomy

Dysphonia in children with tracheostomy tubes who can tolerate the placement of a Passy-Muir valve or cap, or in those children with a history of chronic subglottic stenosis who underwent surgical reconstruction, can be partly attributed to phonation patterns that involve the extensive use of supraglottic laryngeal structures.[16-19] When an individual has a tracheotomy tube in place, the direct airstream that can be utilized for vocal fold vibration is generated by inspiration through the tracheotomy tube. When the child is decannulated, he or she quite often continues the previously learned motor behavior for speech and breathing pattern. Reverse or inspiratory phonation is the compensatory speech characteristic used by children in this population.[21]

Glottic Insufficiency

Laryngofissure

A laryngofissure is created by incising the midline thyroid cartilage, splitting the vocal folds at the anterior commissure. Surgical procedures that require a laryngofissure such as those to manage laryngeal webs and high subglottic stenoses, can potentially lead to scarring and asymmetry at the level of the glottis. The laryngofissure is performed transcervically, often with the aid of an assistant surgeon who performs a simultaneous bronchoscopy to visualize the ante-

rior commissure. The author uses a No. 12 blade whose curvature and sharp tip allow direct placement of the knife at the commissure for lysis (Fig 14–7). During this maneuver, the vocal folds are at risk of direct injury and for asymmetric reapproximation of the vocal folds (Fig 14–8). This vertical asymmetry will lead to glottic insufficiency, wave irregularities, and potentially to breathy phonation. Furthermore, aggressive manipulation of the pre-epiglottic region could potentially lead to prolapse of the base (petiole) of the epiglottis (Fig 14–9).

The laryngofissure is often a component of the more extensive laryngotracheal surgery, providing an access to the posterior larynx when exposure of the posterior cricoid plate is limited in a young child, or when adjunct procedures are necessary at the level of the vocal process and arytenoids. In these circumstances, performing a revision laryngofissure, particularly in a

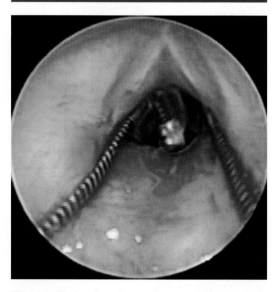

Fig 14–7. Lysis of anterior commissure utilizing simultaneous microlayngoscopy to assist in precise incision placement.

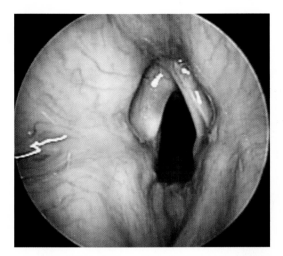

Fig 14–8. Asymmetric vocal fold height post-laryngotracheal reconstruction graft and a laryngofissure for management of a subglottic hemangioma.

young child, is unfavorable (Fig 14-10). Voice therapy techniques to minimize supraglottic compensation and to improve breath support and audibility should help in these cases. If voice therapy does not adequately augment the phonatory volume, augmentative or alternative communication devices should be considered. Another possible surgical option would be to plump a vocal fold with an injectate (such as Radiesse Gel, Cymetra, etc) to minimize the air escape through the glottis.

Glottic insufficiency can also result from prolonged intubation and a defect in the posterior glottis (Benjamin defect), preventing approximation of the arytenoids and vocal folds and leading to breathy dysphonia (Fig 14-11).

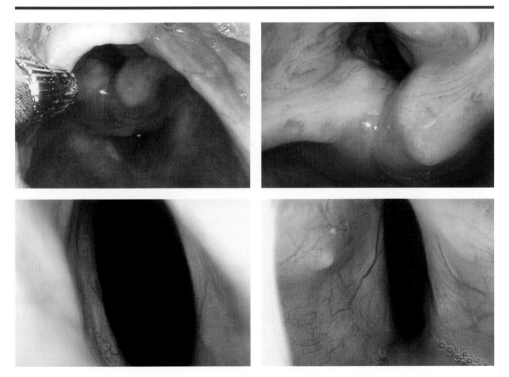

Fig 14–9. Intraoperative images of a patient long-term post-LTR with asymmetric vocal fold height, scarring, and petiole prolapse.

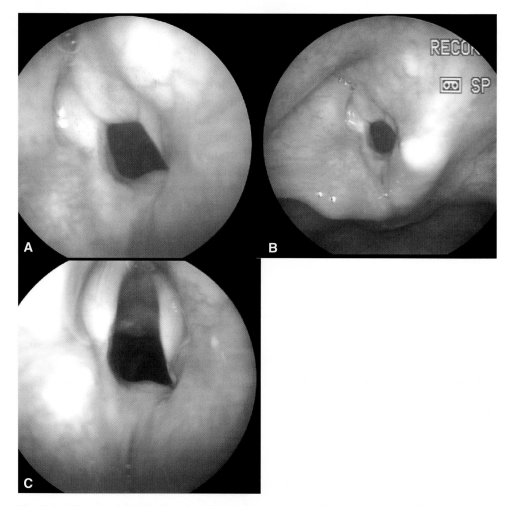

Fig 14–10. 14-year-old female, 30-week premature infant at birth with a history of prolonged intubation and resultant transglottic injury and grade 3 subglottic stenosis. She underwent a tracheostomy at 3 months of age and a subsequent LTR with anterior and posterior cartilaginous rib grafts at 2 years of age. Due to an anterior glottic stenosis at the commissure (*A,B*), she underwent a laryngofissure with a keel 2 years post-LTR. Five months later she was decannulated with a healthy airway (*C*) but a weak and breathy voice. Note the widened anterior commissure and mildly atrophic right vocal fold, slight asymmetric height approximation. On flexible transnasal stroboscopy she is noted to exhibit mild compression of ventricular folds and mild-moderate anterior-posterior compression with arytenoid prolapse. The vocal folds are mobile, but slightly atrophic.

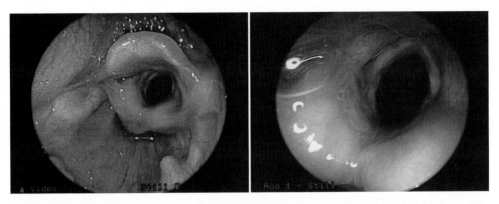

Fig 14–11. Intubation defect (Benjamin defect). One-week intubation history with associated breathy dyphonia due to a large posterior glottic chink.

Supraglottic Phonation

Posterior Cricoid Split

Surgical management of subglottic stenosis or posterior glottic stenosis may require a complete vertical division of the posterior plate to allow placement of a graft material or to allow fibrosis of a posterior cricoid split as described in the previous section. The posterior incision must be in the midline, to allow the proper placement of a posterior graft. This graft has to be of the proper vertical height to prevent postoperative posterior glottic/interarytenoid stenosis. Furthermore, the graft must not be too thick, in order to prevent postoperative dysphagia or extrusion (Fig 14–12).

A trend that has been noted by the author in over 200 dysphonic children evaluated following laryngotracheal reconstruction is anterior arytenoid prolapse with supraglottic compression. There are a couple of theories explaining the resultant prolapse. The first relates to destabilization of the arytenoid if the interarytenoid muscle is not cut during the posterior cricoid split.[20] Another issue related to placement of a posterior cricoid graft is the static distraction of the posterior glottis and the almost inevitable glottic insufficiency. To prevent air escape during phonation, a supraglottic sphincter is formed by the compensatory motion of the arytenoid cartilages onto the epiglottis. This is a child's natural way of adapting to the loss of volume generated at the level of the vocal folds, albeit creating a harsher tone with a deeper phonatory quality. In a recent study done ex vivo in excised larynges it was found that the false vocal folds and the epiglottis offer a positive contribution to the glottal resistance and sound intensity of the larynx. Also, vocal fold elongation and glottal medial compression caused an increase in glottal resistance. The pressure-flow relationships were approximately linear regardless of the structure.[21] It is the author's belief that early voice therapy techniques to minimize supraglottic compression can reduce these compensatory behaviors. It is imperative, however, to avoid placement of wider posterior grafts, to minimize overdistraction of this delicate region.

Supraglottic phonation in response to glottic insufficiency has also been shown

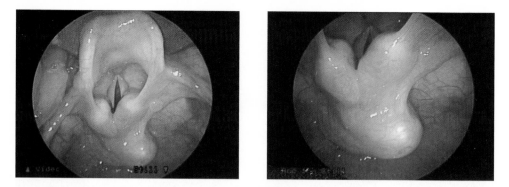

Fig 14–12. Images of a child who underwent a laryngotracheal reconstruction with a posterior cartilaginous rib graft. Both images depict a posterior cricoid bulge representing an extruded graft. It was subsequently removed and reimplanted with no long-term sequelae.

to promote formation of laryngoceles in a small group (n = 5) of children who previously underwent successful laryngotracheal reconstruction (Fig 14-13). Laryngocele formation represents the pathologic response of the larynx and supraglottis to increased intralaryngeal pressures. This is a well-recognized phenomenon in patients with laryngeal carcinoma, glass blowers, and those playing wind instruments.[22]

In a recent objective and subjective retrospective evaluation of postreconstruction dysphonia in a group of 12 patients it was shown that those children who used supraglottic structures for phonation were rated by experienced voice clinicians as demonstrating significantly more strain during voice production.[22] Hyperfunctional phonatory performance can adversely impact communication and social skills, as well as classroom performance. This was recently shown in a study utilizing the Pediatric Voice Handicap Index (pVHI), a proxy quality-of-life tool available for following dysphonia in children[23] (Appendix 14, pVHI). In this validation study, parents of 33 dysphonic children who underwent airway

reconstruction and had no voice therapy in the past, were asked to fill out a 23-item parental-proxy survey with a focus on the physical, emotional, and functional effects of their child's voice disorder. They were compared to a group of healthy controls without voicing issues. There was a statistically significant difference in the perception of a child's ability to integrate in school from an emotional and physical standpoint compared to a healthy child without a voice disorder.[23] The dysphonia group differed greatly from the control group on each subscale and on the total scores (Table 14-1).

Modulation and Pitch Range

Cricotracheal Resection (CTR)

The partial cricotracheal resection (CTR) involves the excision of the anterolateral cricoid plate and anastomosis of the distal tracheal ring to the proximal thyroid ala with suture lines placed in the posterior cricoid mucosa to attempt to reapproximate the trachealis to the more proximal cricoid

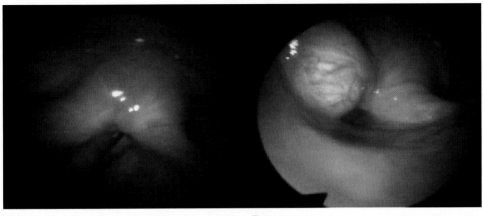

A   **B**

Fig 14–13. Glottic insufficiency with a chronic force of translaryngeal air and supraglottic compression may lead to laryngocele formation. **A.** View of the larynx at rest. **B.** With phonation, note the air-filled right aryepiglottic cyst and the muscle tension in the supraglottis. This is an 11-year-old female, 27-week premature infant at birth with a history of broncopulmonary dysplasia and prolonged intubation. She underwent a tracheostomy tube placement at the age of 4 months. She underwent a single staged laryngotracheal reconstruction with placement of anterior and posterior cartilaginous rib grafts following an unsuccessful tracheal resection and right laser arytenoidectomy the previous year. She has had an excellent airway, but experiences worsening dysphonia and loss of her soprano range.

Table 14–1. A Comparison of the Mean Scores Obtained for the Control Group and a Diverse Group of Dysphonic Airway Patients (*)

Scale	Control	Airway*
Functional	1.47	13.94
Physical	0.20	15.48
Emotional	0.18	12.15
TOTAL SCORE	1.84	41.58
Visual Analog Scale (VAS)		52.91

*The values reflect the pVHI subscales, total scores, and overall severity of the voice expressed by the child's parent (calculated from the visual analog scale, VAS). Reprinted from Zur KB, Cotton S, Kelchner L, Baker S, Weinrich B, Lee L. Pediatric Voice Handicap Index (pVHI): a new tool for evaluating pediatric dysphonia. *Int J Pediatr Otorhinolaryngol.* 2007;71(1): 77–82 with permission from Elsevier.

plate. This procedure is well suited for higher grade subglottic stenosis that has a healthy margin away from the vocal folds to allow for the proximal suture line.[24] Again, preservation of the vocal folds is imperative, and in the most complex of airway cases where there is an extension of the stenosis into the glottis, an extended CTR (eCTR) is often performed with judicious placement of a posterior cricoid graft.

It is intuitive that the CTR will lead to postoperative dysphonia due to obliteration of the cricothyroid membrane and removal of the cricothyroid muscle. Thus, patients are left with a deeper phonatory quality and loss of the higher pitch ranges. Furthermore, extensive scarring and manipulation of the prelaryngeal muscles during dissection, especially in revision laryngotracheal surgery, can render the patient dysphonic due to difficulties in modulating a sound.[25] Other potential complications may include arytenoid prolapse due to destabilization following manipulation of the lateral cricoarytenoid muscles, destabilization of the cricoarytenoid joint, and potential damage of the posterior cricoarytenoid ligament (if an extended CTR is performed with a posterior cricoid split).[26]

Additionally, vocal fold paralysis, albeit rare, may result if the dissection of the cricoid and trachea is not meticulous and the recurrent laryngeal nerve is injured. Other CTR-related complications that can lead to dysphonia include prolapse of the base (petiole) of the epiglottis leading to supraglottic phonation (Fig 14–14 and 14–15), and restenosis of the airway and webbing on the undersurface of the vocal folds leading to turbulent airflow through the glottis (Fig 14–16).

Given the potential complications following reconstruction, it is incumbent on the surgeon to recognize the potential pitfalls of the reconstructions and to deliberately attempt to preserve laryngeal function when possible. In general, successful decannulation is reported to be as high as 95% for CTR;[25-26] however, data concerning voice outcomes are less well defined.

SYSTEMATIC APPROACH TO EVALUATION OF PEDIATRIC DYSPHONIA

There is a wide spectrum of voice disorders and laryngeal dysfunction presented by individuals requiring LTR, and a systematic documentation of communication ability, laryngeal condition, voicing, and potential for voicing pre- and postreconstruction surgery is essential. Complicating this issue is the fact that many of the children who undergo reconstruction, have spent the formative years of their life (birth to 3 years) with a tracheostomy tube. This is a critical period for language development and often these children exhibit delays.[27] Meticulous record keeping should provide valuable data to surgeons and speech-language pathologists regarding medical, surgical, and behavioral interventions' timing and planning. Careful adaptation of evaluation protocols and a team approach including patient, caregivers, otolaryngologist, and speech-language pathologist is essential to address all key assessment and subsequent management issues.[28]

The initial evaluation of a child with chronic laryngotracheal stenosis should include overall assessment of the child's communication, potential for voicing (ie, can the child phonate with the tracheotomy tube covered, ability of the child to tolerate and phonate with a Passy-Muir valve), and use of any form of alternative communication (ie, sign language). In the prelinguistic child a formal preoperative voice assessment may be difficult; however, the presence and the quality of stridor, a cry, breathing, or babbling may be documented. An awake-transnasal fiberoptic laryngoscopy may reveal information regarding vocal fold mobility during breathing and/or crying.

As already alluded to, the focus of the parents of a young child with laryngotracheal stenosis is to establish an adequate airway, successful decannulation, safe swallowing, and some type of functional voicing. However, once an adequate airway is well established and as the child ages, vocal quality becomes increasingly important to the family. In order to provide effective guidance and treatment, the effect of the child's current vocal quality on peer interactions and ability to function appropriately in school and extracurricular activities should be evaluated. Inquiry into the specific accommodations the classroom teacher has

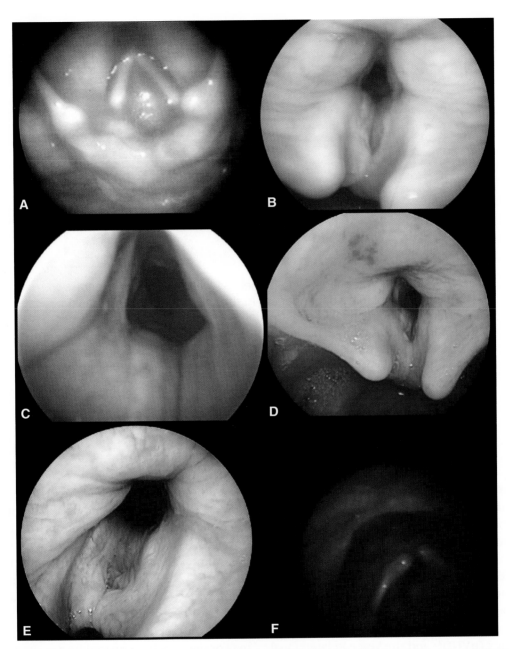

Fig 14–14. These images illustrate a potential pitfall from lack of voice therapy postcricotracheal resection. Note the progressive eversion of the false vocal folds with eventual loss of laryngeal architecture due to chronic supraglottic compensation. **A.** Preoperative view of a grade 4 subglottic stenosis **B.** Six months post-extended cricotracheal resection with laryngofissure and accidental injury to the right vocal fold **C.** Eighteen-months post-reconstruction **D.** Four-years post-reconstruction **E.** Ten-years postreconstruction. **F.** Ten-years postreconstruction, during flexible transnasal stroboscopy. The patient described in Figure 14–15 illustrates the benefit of front focus phonation with a lip buzz. Note an irregular neocord vibration at the onset. During the lip buzz maneuver, there is better regulation of the vibratory movement and a more crisp sound.

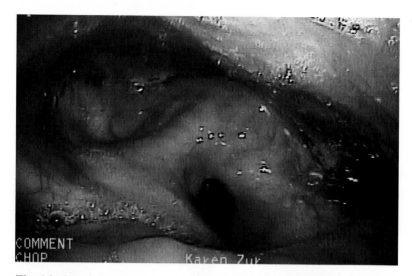

Fig 14–15. A teenager who presented with supraglottic stenosis and tracheostomy dependence. In the past, he underwent multiple laryngotracheal reconstructions with anterior and posterior cartilaginous grafts. This image is postsupraglottic reconstruction and petiole repositioning. He is decannulated and doing well. Transnasal stroboscopy reveals significant glottic insufficiency due to multiple prior reconstruction, supraglottic compression, and dysphonia.

made in order for the child to be heard and understood in class should also be made, as contact with the school's services can be made to help assist these children.[28]

Rating scales have recently been developed that can assist in determining these functional and social impact of voice impairment. Two such quality of life assessments include the Pediatric Voice Handicap Index (pVHI)[23] and the Voice-Related Quality of Life Index (V-RQOL).[29] Whichever tool is used to monitor the quality of life of a child, it is important to include it as part of the evaluation and management of these triumphant children as visualization of the larynx is not necessarily reflective of a child's vocal performance (Fig 14–17).

Although the potential exists for an increase of social, educational, and functional impairments for patients in the LTS population, as previously stated, it is not uncommon for caregivers and the child to view the vocal quality as a minor impairment when compared to previous airway concerns. Decannulation is the goal of airway reconstruction surgeries, and patients may or may not be prepared by the surgeon that the resulting vocal quality may not be normal. Further investigation of voice impairment scales in this population will assist in determining the impact of vocal quality, particularly throughout development into the adolescent years. Additionally, voice assessment teams will benefit from a better

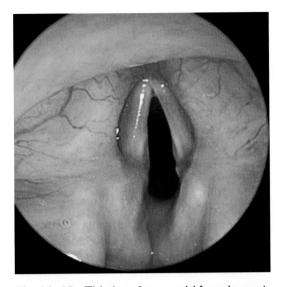

Fig 14–18. This is a 6-year-old female post-lye injection and interarytenoid scarring. She presented with inspiratory stridor and breathy phonation due to posterior glottic stenosis. She underwent a single-staged laryngotracheal reconstruction with a posterior cartilaginous rib graft. Voice therapy instituted several weeks postoperatively. She presents with a normal airway, no stridor on phonation, and no evidence of supraglottic compression 1 year postreconstruction.

possible and to restore a normalized childhood. Future research will allow the surgeon to pinpoint and avoid surgical maneuvers that increase the risk of voice disturbances postoperatively as well as incorporate tissue engineering to rehabilitee or prevent vocal fold scarring which is at times encountered during these procedures.

CONCLUSION

In conclusion, a comprehensive and multidisciplinary evaluation and management should provide valuable information to surgeons and voice therapists regarding medical, surgical, and behavioral intervention timing and planning. The evaluation should be precise and stringent, to allow consistent data collection among and within patients.

The field of medicine involves constant progress and innovation. With the maturation of laryngology as a subspecialty and with the advent of technologic innovation and interventions in the younger populations, it is incumbent on the pediatric specialist to nourish the field of pediatric laryngology to help carry these children to a healthy and integrated life.

on the effects of various surgical procedures on voicing. Currently, the available studies are limited and lack a combination of objective and subjective data to evaluate surgery-specific effects, utility of early voice therapy, benefits of various therapeutic maneuvers, and effectiveness of ancillary surgical interventions such as vocal fold injections to reduce glottic insufficiency.

The bottom line is providing a forum for management of dysphonic children following and during the perioperative reconstructive period to allow them to quickly integrate or reintegrate into their social setting and allow for as flawless a transition as

REFERENCES

1. Hartnick CJ, Hartley BE, Lacy PD, et al. Surgery for pediatric subglottic stenosis: disease-specific outcomes. *Ann Otol Rhinol Laryngol.* 2001;110(12):1109–1113.
2. Kucinschi BR, Scherer RC, Dewitt KJ, Ng TT. An experimental analysis of the pressures and flows within a driven mechanical model of phonation. *J Acoust Soc Am.* 2006; 119(5 pt 1):3011–3021.
3. Wetmore RF, Marsh RR, Thompson ME, et al. Pediatric tracheostomy: a changing

procedure? *Ann Otol Rhinol Laryngol.* 1999;108:695–699.

4. Valdez TA, McMillan K, Shapshay SM. A new laser treatment for vocal cord papilloma—585-nm pulsed dye. *Otolaryngol Head Neck Surg.* 2001;124(4):421–425.

5. Tasca RA, McCormick M, Clarke RW. British Association of Paediatric Otorhinolaryngology members experience with recurrent respiratory papillomatosis. *Int J Pediatr Otorhinolaryngol.* 2006;70(7):1183–1187.

6. Schraff S, Derkay CS, Burke B, Lawson L. American Society of Pediatric Otolaryngology members' experience with recurrent respiratory papillomatosis and the use of adjuvant therapy. *Arch Otolaryngol Head Neck Surg.* 2004;130(9):1039–1042.

7. Hansen JK, Thibeault SL, Walsh JF, Shu XZ, Prestwich GD. In vivo engineering of the vocal fold extracellular matrix with injectable hyaluronic acid hydrogels: early effects on tissue repair and biomechanics in a rabbit model. *Ann Otol Rhinol Laryngol.* 2005;114(9):662–670.

8. Cotton R. Management of subglottic stenosis. *Otolaryngol Clin North Am.* 2000;33: 111–130.

9. Forte V, Chang MB, Papsin BC. Thyroid ala cartilage reconstruction in neonatal subglottic stenosis as a replacement for the anterior cricoid split. *Int J Pediatr Otorhinolaryngol.* 2001;59(3):181–186.

10. Smith ME, March JH, Cotton RT, et al. Voice problems after pediatric laryngotracheal reconstruction: videolaryngostroboscopic, acoustic, and perceptual assessment. *Int J Pediatr Otorhinolaryngol.* 1993;25:173–181.

11. Cotton R. The problem of pediatric laryngotracheal stenosis: a clinical and experimental study on the efficacy of autogenous cartilaginous grafts placed between the vertically divided halves of the posterior lamina of the cricoid cartilage. *Laryngoscope* 1991;101:1–34.

12. Caputo V, Consiglio V. The use of patient's own auricular cartilage to repair deficiency of the tracheal wall. *J Thorac Cardiovasc Sur.* 1961;41:594–596.

13. Zur KB, Urken ML. Vascularized hemitracheal autograft for laryngotracheal reconstruction: a new surgical technique based on the thyroid gland as a vascular carrier. *Laryngoscope.* 2003;113:1494–1498.

14. Pashley N, Jaskunas J, Waldstein G. Laryngotracheoplasty with costochondral grafts—a clinical correlate of graft survival. *Laryngoscope.* 1984;94:1493–1496.

15. Abitbol J. *Odyssey of the Voice.* 1st ed. San Diego, Calif: Plural Publishing, 2006.

16. Weinrich B, Baker S, Kelchner L, et al. Examination of aerodynamic measures and strain by vibratory source. *Otolaryngol HNS.* 2007;136:455–458.

17. Clary RA, Pengilly A, Bailey M, et al. Analysis of voice outcomes in pediatric patients following surgical procedures for laryngotracheal stenosis. *Arch Otolaryngol Head Neck Surg.* 1996; 122:1189–1194.

18. MacArthur CJ, Kearns GH, Healy GB. Voice quality after laryngolotracheal reconstruction. *Arch Otolaryngol Head Neck Surg.* 1994;120:641–647.

19. Zalzal GH, Loomis SR, Fischer M. Laryngeal reconstruction in children: assessment of voice quality. *Arch Otolaryngol Head Neck Surg.* 1993;119:504–507.

20. Rutter MJ, Yellon RF, Cotton RT. Management and prevention of subglottis stenosis in infants and children. In: Bluestone CD, Stool SE, eds. *Pediatric Otolaryngology.* Vol. 2. 4th ed. Philadelphia, Pa: Saunders; 2003.

21. Alipour F, Jaiswal S, Finnegan E. Aerodynamic and acoustic effects of false vocal folds and epiglottis in excised larynx models. *Ann Otol Rhinol Laryngol.* 2007; 116(2):135–144.

22. Zur KB, Cotton RT, Willging JP, Rutter MJ. *Laryngocele Formation Following Pediatric Laryngotracheal Reconstruction.* Abstract and oral presentation, European Society of Pediatric Otolaryngology, June 2006.

23. Zur KB, Cotton S, Kelchner L, Baker S, Weinrich B, Lee L. Pediatric Voice Handicap Index (pVHI): a new tool for evaluating pediatric dysphonia. *Int J Pediatr Otorhinolaryngol.* 2007;71(1):77–82.

24. Rutter MJ, Hartley BE, Cotton RT. Cricotracheal resection in children. *Archives Otol Head Neck Surg.* 2001;127(3); 289–292.

25. Monnier P, Lang F, Savary M. Partial crico-tracheal resection for pediatric subglottic stenosis: a single institution's experience in 60 cases. *Eur Arch Otorhinolaryngol.* 2003;260:295-297.

26. Rutter MJ, Link DT, Hartley BE, et al. Arytenoid prolapse as a consequence of cricotracheal resection in children. *Ann Otol Rhinol Laryngol.* 2001;110:210-214.

27. Simon BM, Fowler SM, Handler SD. Communication development in young children with long-term tracheostomies: preliminary report. *Int J Pediatr Otorhinolaryngol.* 1983; 6(1): 37-50.

28. Baker S, Kelchner L, Weinrich B, et al. Pediatric laryngotracheal stenosis and airway reconstruction: a review of voice outcomes, assessment, and treatment issues. *J Voice.* 2006;20(4):631-641.

29. Hartnick CJ. Validation of a pediatric voice quality-of-life instrument. *Arch Otolaryngol HNS.* 2002;128:919-922.

APPENDIX 14

Pediatric Voice Handicap Index

Subject Number: _____   Date: _____

I would rate my/my child's talkativeness as the following (circle response)

1	2	3	4	5	6	7
Quiet Listener			Average Talker			Extremely Talkative

To be filled out by Staff:

F= _____
P= _____
E= _____
Total= _____

Talkativeness: _____

Instructions: These are statements that many people have used to describe their voices and the effects of their voices on their lives. Circle the response that indicates how frequently you have the same experience.

0=Never   1=Almost Never   2=Sometimes   3=Almost always   4=Always

Part I - F

1) My child's voice makes it difficult for people to hear him/her   0 1 2 3 4

2) People have difficulty understanding my child in a noisy room   0 1 2 3 4

3) At home, we have difficulty hearing my child when he/she calls through the house.   0 1 2 3 4

4) My child tends to avoid communicating because of his/her voice.   0 1 2 3 4

5) My child speaks with friends, neighbors, or relatives less often because of his/her voice.   0 1 2 3 4

6) People ask my child to repeat him/herself when speaking face-to-face.   0 1 2 3 4

7) My child's voice difficulties restrict personal, educational and social activities.   0 1 2 3 4

Part II – P

1) My child runs out of air when talking   0 1 2 3 4

2) The sound of my child's voice changes throughout the day   0 1 2 3 4

3) People ask, 'What's wrong with your child's voice?"   0 1 2 3 4

4) My child's voice sounds dry, raspy, and/or hoarse   0 1 2 3 4

5) The quality of my child's voice is unpredictable   0 1 2 3 4

6) My child uses a great deal of effort to speak (eg, straining)   0 1 2 3 4

7) My child's voice is worse in the evening   0 1 2 3 4

0=Never   1=Almost Never   2=Sometimes   3=Almost always   4=Always

8) My child's voice "gives out" when speaking   0 1 2 3 4

9) My child has to yell in order for others to hear him/her.   0 1 2 3 4

Part III – E

1) My child appears tense when talking to others because of his
    or her voice.   0 1 2 3 4

2) People seem irritated with my child's voice   0 1 2 3 4

3) I find other people don't understand my child's voice problem   0 1 2 3 4

4) My child is frustrated with his/her voice problem   0 1 2 3 4

5) My child is less outgoing because of his/her voice problem   0 1 2 3 4

6) My child is annoyed when people ask him/her to repeat   0 1 2 3 4

7) My child is embarrassed when people ask him/her to repeat   0 1 2 3 4

Overall Severity Rating of Voice
(Please place "X" mark anywhere along this line to indicate the severity of your child's voice; the verbal
descriptions serve as a guide)

_____

Normal   Severe

Reprinted from Zur KB, Cotton S, Kelchner L, Baker S, Weinrich B, Lee L. Pediatric Voice Handicap Index (pVHI):
a new tool for evaluating pediatric dysphonia. *Int J Pediatr Otorhinolaryngol.* 2007;71(1):77–82 with permission
from Elsevier.

Functional and Spasmodic Dysphonia's in Children

Marshall E. Smith
Nelson Roy
Cara Sauder

INTRODUCTION

The voice is an indicator of health, emotion, gender, and age. It forms part of one's individual identity and personality and is a primary means of communication and expression. In children this organ is developing in physical structure in concert with the rest of the speech mechanism. At this same time also proceeds the neurocognitive, behavioral growth and maturation of the child. As the larynx has highly developed neural connections it is not surprising that the voice is sensitive to neural input and control. This includes input derived from emotional centers in the brain. The larynx has been labeled "the valve of emotion."[1] It is highly responsive to emotional state and stress at all ages.

Studies of voice disorders in children have suggested that the majority of dysphonias are due to vocal abuse and misuse. The common manifestation of these is vocal nodules.[2,3] This disorder can be thought of as "functional" due to underlying dysfunction as the cause of tissue trauma that creates the nodules. That being said, there occasionally arises in children dysphonias for which no structural or physical pathologic change to the vocal folds can be identified. In this chapter, a functional voice disorder is defined as a voice disturbance which occurs in the absence of structural or neurologic laryngeal pathology. In adult voice clinics these disorders may account for up to 40% of cases.[4] In pediatric series, functional voice disorders occur less frequently. A series of 427 children referred to a tertiary pediatric voice disorders clinic reported that 7% of cases had a functional etiology.[2] In another recent series, only 4% of 136 children with voice disorder were labeled as functional or neurogenic.[3] In this review, the major manifestations of functional voice disorders in children are discussed. These include muscle tension dysphonia (MTD) and aphonia, and puberphonia or mutational falsetto.

Neurogenic dysphonias in children are due to a variety of causes, the most common of which is vocal fold paralysis. This chapter discusses other neurogenic movement disorders that affect the larynx. The major one is known as laryngeal dystonia or spasmodic dysphonia (SD). Other types of central neurologically based laryngeal disorders include essential vocal tremor and spastic dysarthrias, such as that associated with cerebral palsy. Laryngeal spasticity may affect the voice and airway in these patients.

FUNCTIONAL VOICE DISORDERS

MTD has gained common usage as a diagnostic label for functional dysphonias thought to be due to dysregulated or imbalanced laryngeal and paralaryngeal activity.[4] A variety of glottic and supraglottic patterns of laryngeal closure have been described.[5,6] Their diagnostic utility, however, has come into question because these closure patterns are not unique to MTD, and do not reliably distinguish them from normal speakers, or other voice disorders.[7]

The predominant auditory perceptual feature of MTD is a strained voice quality, disordered pitch (usually pitch elevation), and reduced loudness. These features may lead to diagnostic confusion with SD.[8] Periods of aphonia may also be present. These may be intermittent or persistent. Another feature that may be present in MTD is that periods of normal voice may occur in between the dysphonic intervals. On physical examination, exquisite tenderness to palpation in the thyrohyoid space, and narrowing of the thyrohyoid space are frequently encountered.

There have been a variety of explanations offered for MTD, including technical misuse due to excessive vocal demands, altered adaptation following upper respiratory infection, increased laryngeal tone due to local irritative conditions such as gastroesophageal reflux, compensation for underlying glottic insufficiency, and psychologic or personality traits that express excess laryngeal tension.[4]

The psychological traits of MTD patients have been studied in some depth. In the most extensive studies by Roy et al, personality profiles were obtained in large groups of patients with MTD, SD, vocal fold paralysis, vocal nodules, and normal controls.[9-11] MTD subjects scored high on dimensions of introversion, anxiety, depression, and emotionality. Vocal nodule patients scored similarly on anxiety and emotionality scales; however, instead of introversion (quiet, unsociable, passive, careful), they demonstrated extroversion (dominant, sociable, active). Patients with SD, vocal fold paralysis, and normal speakers demonstrated no distinguishing personality traits. MTD is described as muscularly inhibited voice production in the context of individuals with personality traits of introversion and neuroticism. In response to certain environmental cues or triggers elevated laryngeal tension creates incomplete or disordered vocal production in a structurally and neurologically intact larynx.[4]

Despite the above issues that involve the cause of MTD, successful treatment of MTD through behavioral management has been demonstrated in a number of reports.[5,12,13] This focuses on the proximate causes of the dysphonia and rebalancing the laryngeal mechanism to produce normal voice. The most effective technique in our experience is manual circumlaryngeal massage and laryngeal reposturing to lower the larynx.[5,12,14] This can yield remarkable improvement, with two-thirds of patients achieving normal voice return from a single treatment session. Successful treatment with behavioral therapy in nearly all patients is expected. Recalcitrant or resistant cases may respond after several sessions of therapy. In a case series of pediatric patients treated for "muscle tension dysphonia" recently published, seven of the eight children had vocal nodules with supraglottic hyperfunction seen on laryngoscopy.[15] One patient had aphonia without lesions. All patients improved with voice therapy. As an adjunct treatment for severe MTD, Dworkin et al reported the use of topical lidocaine spray to the larynx followed by voice therapy.[16] We have found this to be effective in pediatric patients (see case report below). We also used lidocaine block of the recurrent laryngeal nerve to facilitate phonation in a case of recalcitrant functional aphonia in an adolescent.[17] Sensory or motor perturbation of the laryngeal mechanism may relax excessive laryngeal muscle tension and help the patient gain confidence that they have the capacity to produce normal voice.

Case Report 1

A 14-year-old female had a 7-year history of voice loss, including both dysphonia and aphonia. She had been to several ENT physicians and speech pathologists but had not been able to regain her voice. On physical exam, the patient was mouthing words with articulation, but had no marked phonation and even had some difficulty whispering. She did not have a normal cough. A fiberoptic laryngoscopy revealed during phonation the vocal folds in a bowed posture and some abduction of the vocal fold observed during attempts at phonation, but normal vocal fold adduction during breath holding and Valsalva maneuver. The neck exam was remarkable for severe thyrohyoid region tenderness. As she was traveling

from a long distance, she worked with the speech pathologist for an extended therapy session on initiating glottal stops and vegetative glottal sounds. She returned 2 months later and underwent a laryngeal lidocaine wash given transcervically via the cricothyroid space. This was immediately followed by an extended therapy session, during which time she made considerable improvement. On follow-up examination 2 months later she demonstrated normal voice quality.

Case Report 2

A 9-year-old female was brought by her mother for a second opinion regarding complete voice loss of sudden onset when the child awoke 1 month earlier. She also complained of a sore throat and constant throat pain. She saw her primary care doctor and was treated with Augmentin® for 2 weeks. She saw a pediatric otolaryngologist who did a fiberoptic laryngoscopy and showed "no problems" and referred her to a speech pathologist. She also saw a school psychologist who reported that she had no psychological impairments. She had normal activity level and was active in tumbling and had no history of trauma to the neck. Her only notable health condition is that she was small for her age, below the fifth percentile for height and weight. On examination, the patient was noted to have aphonia with soft voice and slight whispering. Occasional phonatory sounds can be elicited with cough, throat clearing, and inhalatory phonation. Transnasal fiberoptic laryngoscopy showed the vocal folds positioned in a hyperadducted whispering posture with an open posterior chink, and mild true vocal fold edema was observed. The patient was treated with a course of prednisone without improvement. She underwent three weekly sessions of behavioral voice therapy using inhalation phonation, throat clear with phonation, glottal fry, throat focused /r/ phonation, and manual reposturing. These were also without progress. A transnasal fiberoptic laryngoscopy and lidocaine wash were then performed, with 4% lidocaine spray of the larynx and hypopharynx utilizing the curved spray atomizer (MAD 600, Wolfe-Tory, Inc, Salt Lake City, Utah). This provided excellent topical anesthesia of the vocal folds which were able to be palpated with the fiberscope and the subglottic larynx and trachea inspected through the vocal folds without any gagging or coughing. The speech pathologist then immediately worked with the patient on voice therapy techniques of inhalatory/exhalatory phonation and nasal voiced consonants with aggressive and persistent practice. After 30 minutes she was able to phonate and left the clinic speaking with a normal voice.

The voice of adolescence is characterized by pitch instability. This is true for both males and females but more so in males. In a study of children ages 10 to 17 without and with vocal complaints, acoustic measures of pitch stability on sustained vowel phonation were not found to statistically distinguish the normal from several disordered voice groups.[18] However, the group diagnosed with puberphonia had the most variability of frequency and amplitude. Puberphonia is a voice disorder of adolescent males. It has also been labeled mutational falsetto, adolescent male transitional dysphonia, incomplete mutation, and persistent falsetto. It can be seen in early adolescence, or can persist into late adolescence or adulthood. The voice does not successfully accomplish pitch change during puberty, between 12 and 14 years of age. The voice has been described as weak, thin, breathy, and hoarse in quality.[6,12] A recent

study in a large patient group with puberphonia measured the average speaking F_0 at 241 Hz.[19] It is frequently accompanied by downward pitch breaks into chest register. Coughing sound is also in chest register.[6] The voice of puberphonia may be described as a habituated use of falsetto register accompanied by pitch breaks rather than maintenance of the preadolescent voice. This pattern is commonly seen in MTD, so in our view, puberphonia is considered a variation of MTD seen in adolescent males. The larynx is generally positioned high in the neck, and excessive thyrohyoid tenderness and a narrow thyrohyoid space are found on palpation. Laryngeal lowering maneuvers, including head dorsiflexion, depression of the mandible, hyoid pushback and laryngeal pull-down, are combined with vocalization.[12] This may create a surprised patient and his mother when his normal deep chest register voice is produced for the first time.

The first-line treatment of puberphonia is behavioral voice therapy.[6,12] The same techniques of laryngeal lowering and reposturing combined with vocal cues that are used for MTD apply to the treatment of puberphonia. Ideally, this is conducted by a speech pathologist experienced in this approach. These techniques facilitate lowering of the larynx to engage the chest register and thyroarytenoid muscle activity. This lowers the pitch of the voice to the patient's normal male range. A recent study of 45 patients with puberphonia included 16 patients ages 11 to 15 years and 29 patients ages 16 to 40 years. All patients were treated successfully with behavioral therapy techniques with maintenance of improvement documented at 6 months.[19] For recalcitrant cases of puberphonia, novel approaches have been tried. These include a case report of the use of botulinum toxin to relax cricothyroid muscle function.[20]

Pitch lowering phonosurgical procedures including type III thyroplasty[21] and hyoid detachment/laryngeal lowering laryngoplasty[22] have also been described.

Case Report 3

An 18–year-old male complained of a 4-year history of voice problems. These coincided with onset of puberty. He was treated with speech therapy in schools for 1 year without improvement. He also was treated for allergies with fexofenadine, which did not affect his voice. On examination the voice demonstrated roughness, pitch breaks, and decreased loudness. An improvement in voice with engagement of the chest register was elicited with laryngeal reposturing maneuvers. Laryngostroboscopy demonstrated a normal laryngeal mechanism.

The patient was seen for a single session of voice therapy. Initially, laryngeal reposturing maneuvers were used to cue the patient to create chest register phonation during vegetative vocalizations and sustained vowels. Then the vocalizations were shaped into use with connected speech. The "new" voice was reinforced by having the patient read out loud, and by negative practice (temporarily reverting to the "old" voice and then back again). By the end of the therapy session he was able to consistently produced normal chest register phonation at normal male vocal pitch. He required no further therapy sessions.

The negative impact of these voice problems in children can be substantial. It may affect their ability to form and maintain social relationships with peers and adults, to communicate in school and home environments, and to enter the world of work. Although they are labeled "functional" because no underlying disease process

involving the organs of voice and speech is found, the significance of the problem should not be minimized. The organs of voice and speech are neurally controlled, and this neural control is profoundly influenced by central nervous system controls involving emotional state, personality, and stress response as described above. The impact of voice disorders in children on their social, emotional, and physical function is just beginning to be investigated (see Chapter 4 on pediatric voice quality of life measures). Providers caring for these children need to aggressively advocate for needed services, such as voice and speech therapy provided by experienced clinicians. Documentation by video and audio recordings, patient-based quality of life measures, and references from peer-reviewed publications may all be needed in making appeals to insurance providers to cover speech therapy services for these patients.

LARYNGEAL DYSTONIA

Dystonia is a neurologic disorder in which sustained muscle contractions cause twisting and repetitive movements or abnormal postures.[23] It occurs in several forms depending on how localized in the body are the symptoms. Focal dystonia affects an isolated part of the body. Examples include blepharospasm, writer's cramp, and laryngeal dystonia, also known as spasmodic dysphonia (SD). As more areas of the body are affected the manifestations are segmental (affecting adjoining parts of the body), multifocal, or generalized to the whole body. SD usually occurs as a focal dystonia. In the largest published series of over 900 patients, SD occurred as a focal condition in 64% of cases.[24] Others occurred with segmental or generalized symptoms, which is the usual presentation in children. Dystonia can occur as a primary disorder without underlying cause, or may be secondary to other causes such as neurologic disease, or exposure to drugs known to cause acquired dystonia (eg, phenothiazines). In Blitzer et al's series, 82.5% of their patients had primary dystonia, 17.5% had secondary dystonia. They also reported that 12% of their patients presenting with primary dystonia that included involvement of the larynx had symptom onset before age 20 years; 4% had symptom onset at or under 10 years of age. However, the initial symptoms did not usually involve the larynx.[23] In another prospective study of 168 patients, the youngest age of laryngeal symptom onset was 13 years.[25] Laryngeal dystonia has a high female preponderance, from 63 to 79%. Its onset has been associated with following an upper respiratory infection, and a history of childhood mumps or measles.[25] Females have a predominance of autoimmune diseases; however, an association of dystonia with specific autoimmune disease has not been made.

Although most dystonia patients are focal and primary, children usually present with more generalized symptoms.[23] Limb and axial symptoms are more commonly seen in children than cranial and cervical-based manifestations. They often have underlying neurologic conditions, including, but not limited to, Wilson's disease, Huntington's chorea, spinocerebellar ataxia, primary torsion dystonia, dopa-responsive dystonia (Segawa disease), and PANDAS. Primary torsion dystonia may present in adolescence in familial and nonfamilial forms. DYT gene mutation testing is recommended for these patients.[26] Dystonia presenting in childhood usually does not involve SD as a presenting feature.[27] However, cervical symptoms may occur and can include SD.[28,29] When there is no other identifiable etiology for the dystonia a trial of levo-dopa is recommended.

Some cases can be responsive to levo-dopa even in the absence of a positive genetic testing for dopa-responsive dystonias, for example, GTP-cyclohydrolase deficiency.[29]

Another movement disorder that may present in adolescence is essential tremor (ET). The age of onset has bimodal peaks in late adolescence/young adulthood and in older adulthood.[23] ET is the most common movement disorder. It is familial in at least 50 to 70% of cases. Transmission is autosomal dominant, with incomplete penetrance. In its classical form, a bilateral, largely symmetric postural or kinetic tremor involving hands and forearms is visible and persistent, with possible additional or isolated tremor in head but absence of abnormal posturing. Isolated tremor of the voice occurs in about 15% of cases. The effect on the voice can cause voice breaks similar to that of SD. Medications that are prescribed for ET, for example, propranolol and primidone, may not be helpful for voice tremor. For severe cases that create voice breaks and increased vocal effort, laryngeal botulinum toxin A injection can be effective.

SD manifests in several subtypes, including the adductor (vocal folds closing) or ADSD and abductor (vocal folds opening) or ABSD varieties. An irregular tremor, called dystonic tremor is present in about 25% of cases.[23] Rarely, it occurs during respiration, with symptoms of dyspnea. In the most common ADSD type, the speaker experiences intermittent overclosure of the vocal folds during speech. This creates debilitating voice breaks and an effortful, strain-strangled voice quality. A signature feature of dystonia is task specificity. This means that the symptoms are provoked by certain movements, postures, or tasks. Examples in SD include the observations that singing and whispering are less effortful and sound better than speaking. The same is often true for sustained vowel phonation versus connected speech. Task specificity in laryngeal dystonia implies that the frequency and severity of laryngeal spasms may vary with the specific voice or speech context.[30] Performance differences on speech tasks have been identified in ADSD patients comparing connected speech with sustained vowel phonation,[8] and sentences loaded with voiced versus voiceless consonants.[31,32] Patients with MTD generally do not display this task-dependent differential performance, for example, the voice sounds as poorly on sustained vowel phonation as on connected speech. When proposed in 1976, unilateral lidocaine block of the recurrent laryngeal nerve was described as a diagnostic test to identify candidacy for recurrent laryngeal nerve section for ADSD.[33] This positive effect was confirmed in a prospective study of ADSD patients using a combination of blinded listener, patient-based, and acoustic measures.[34] Unfortunately, in a subsequent prospective study the lidocaine block test was found not to distinguish MTD from ADSD patients with these measures.[35] Both groups responded positively to the lidocaine block, so it cannot be recommended as a method to separate the two disorders. At this time, the diagnosis of SD remains a clinical one, based on perceptual features as described above and examination for other manifestations of dystonia.

Treatment for SD may involve behavioral therapy, medications, injections, or surgery.[23] Behavioral therapy does not have a major role, but can help patients with mild symptoms compensate for the disorder or prolong the effect of botulinum toxin injections.[36] The current gold standard treatment of SD is laryngeal botulinum toxin injection.[37] For the ADSD form injections are placed into the laryngeal adductor muscles. ABSD is treated with injections in the posterior cricoarytenoid muscles.[38]

These are technically more difficult, and the response to injections is overall not as dramatic as the ADSD form. Patients with vocal tremor improve, but not to the degree that those without tremor do. Medications used to treat dystonia, for example, anticholinergics, clonazepam, may also ameliorate SD symptoms.[23] In surgical treatment of SD, unilateral RLN section is not generally performed now due to a high late relapse rate. A variation on this concept, the selective laryngeal adductor denervation-ansa reinnervation, (introduced in 1999), shows promising results.[39,40]

Case Report 4

A 22-year-old female complained of voice problems for the last 2 years. She described her voice as choppy and reports that the onset was gradual. She also noticed a shaking feeling in her body since age 14 and has noted a tremor in her head for at least the last 2 years. She complained of a chronically tense neck that sometimes causes the head to turn to the right, mildly shaking handwriting, and the occasional feeling of cramps in legs and feet. She had no family history of movement disorders. For her voice problem she saw an otolaryngologist who diagnosed her with reflux laryngitis and gave her some antireflux medicine. This did not help her voice at all and she discontinued the medication. On examination she had a notable strained-strangle quality to her voice with intermittent hypernasality and a fast irregular tremor audible both in running speech and sustained vowel phonation. She demonstrated a notable turning of the head to the right with side-to-side head tremor. Voice symptoms were more prominent when the head tremor was worse. Oral reading of task specific sentences revealed much more difficulty on voiced consonants and vowels than with those containing voiceless consonants. The voice was fluent and spasm-free in falsetto and whisper. On physical exam, marked tightness in the right sternocleidomastoid region was noted. A transnasal fiberoptic laryngoscopy was performed and this demonstrated notable tremor of the pharynx, larynx and palate during phonation attempts with interruption of vibration due to adductor spasms. Her Voice Handicap Index score was 108 (normal 0–5), and she rated her voice problem as severe. A diagnosis of adductor spasmodic dysphonia was made. The patient had a dystonic laryngeal tremor and segmental dystonia with torticollis. The SD was treated with laryngeal injections of botulinum toxin A with marked improvement in her voice. She was referred to a neurologist for treatment of torticollis with cervical muscle injections of botulinum toxin A.

OTHER NEUROLOGIC CONDITIONS AFFECTING THE LARYNX

Myriad neurologic disorders exist which can affect the voice and speech mechanism. This is expected, due to the extensive neural connections to the structures of the larynx and the rest of the speech articulatory system. Neurologic disorders of voice and speech are traditionally classified by site of lesion based on location. From peripheral to central, these include muscle, neuromuscular junction, lower motor neuron, upper motor neuron, extrapyramidal sytem, cortex, subcortex, and cerebellum.[41] A neurologic disorder that affects the neuromuscular junction is myasthenia gravis. In children, juvenile onset myasthenia gravis usually does not present with isolated voice weakness, but with other symptoms of fatigue, eyelid drooping, and difficulty swallowing or chewing. Dystonia is an example of a neurologic disorder localized to the extrapyramidal system. Other neurologic conditions that may affect the voice and speech of children, especially those with cerebral palsy, involve the upper motor neuron, cerebellar, and cortical and subcortical systems. Upper motor neuron lesions create spasticity which causes a strained, harsh, and hypernasal voice quality. The effects of speech and voice from cerebellar lesions are felt to be a breakdown in integration and alterations in motor programming (ataxia).[42] Causes of cerebellar lesions include cerebellar degeneration, infarcts, hemorrhage, or neoplasm. The characteristics of speech and voice in ataxic dysarthria included harsh voice, monopitch, monoloudness, and poor pitch or loudness control (bursts of loudness).[43] Lesions of the cortex and subcortical regions, such as those caused by stroke, head injury, or tumor, can produce apraxia of phonation, in conjunction with apraxia of respiration and articulation.[44] Apraxia is a loss of ability to program the coordinated movements of speech in the absence of other peripheral motor or sensory impairment. Phonatory characteristics can vary from mutism to trial-and-error nonspeech to whispered speech, with or without airflow.[45] Verbal and nonverbal vocalizations may be encountered in Gilles de la Tourette syndrome (TS). TS is a rare, chronic disorder of involuntary motor tics that begins in childhood and persists in adulthood.[46] It is seen predominantly in men, often runs in families, and may have an autosomal dominant mode of inheritance. The involuntary vocalizations in TS range from unintelligible nonverbal noises to verbal tics including coprolalia (repetition of obscene words), echolalia (repetition of the last syllable, word, or sentence spoken by others), or palilalia (repeating by the patient of the last word or sentence in a phrase). Laryngeal botulinum toxin injection has been used to reduce vocal volume and the social embarrassment of vocal tics.[47,48]

Some neurologic conditions may impair the abductory function of the vocal folds and obstruct the airway. The most common examples are bilateral vocal fold paralysis and cerebral palsy. The pediatric airway can also be treated with botulinum toxin A to the vocal folds. Children with cerebral palsy can develop laryngospasm. Bilateral vocal fold paralysis patients may develop laryngeal synkinesis, whereby the laryngeal adductor muscles activate during inspiration. These conditions may benefit from vocal fold botulinum toxin injection to improve the airway through relaxation of the thyroarytenoid muscles.[49,50]

REFERENCES

1. Roy N, McGrory JJ, Tasko SM, Bless DM, Heisey D, Ford CN. Psychological correlates of functional dysphonia: an investigation using the Minnesota Multiphasic Personality Inventory. *J Voice.* 1997;11:443–451.
2. Campbell TF, Dollaghan CA, Yaruss JS. Disorders of language, phonology, fluency, and voice in children: indicators for referral. In: Bluestone CD, Stool SE, et al, eds. *Pediatric Otolaryngology.* 4th ed. Philadelphia, Pa: Saunders; 2003:1773–1787.
3. Wuyts FL, Heylen L, Mertens F, et al. Effects of age, sex, and disorder on voice range profile characteristics of 230 children. *Ann Otol Rhinol Laryngol.* 2003;112:540–548.
4. Roy N. Functional dysphonia. *Curr Opin Otolaryngol Head Neck Surg.* 2003;11:144–148.
5. Roy N, Ford CN, Bless DM. Muscle tension dysphonia and spasmodic dysphonia: the role of manual laryngeal tension reduction in diagnosis and treatment. *Ann Otol Rhinol Laryngol.* 1996;105:851–856.
6. Morrison MD, Rammage LA. *The Management of Voice Disorders.* San Diego, Calif: Singular Publishing Group; 1994.
7. Sama A, Carding PN, Price S, et al. The clinical features of functional dysphonia. *Laryngoscope.* 2001;111:458–463.
8. Roy N, Gouse M, Mauszycki SC, Merrill RM, Smith ME. Task specificity in adductor spasmodic dysphonia versus muscle tension dysphonia. *Laryngoscope.* 2005;115:311–316.
9. Roy N, Bless DM. Toward a theory of the dispositional bases of functional dysphonia and vocal nodules: exploring the role of personality and emotional adjustment. In: Kent RD, Bass MJ, eds. *Voice Quality Measurement.* San Diego, Calif: Singular Publishing Group; 2000:461–480.
10. Roy Bless DM, Heisey D. Personality and voice disorders: a superfactor trait analysis. *J Speech Lang Hear Res.* 2000;43:749–768.
11. Roy N, Bless DM, Heisey D. Personality and voice disorders: a multitrait-multidisorder analysis. *J Voice.* 2000;14:521–548.
12. Aronson AE. *Clinical Voice Disorders: An Interdisciplinary Approach* 3rd ed. New York, NY: Thieme-Stratton; 1990.
13. Ramig LO, Verdolini K. Treatment efficacy: voice disorders. *J Speech Lang Hear Res.* 1998;41:S101–S116.
14. Roy N, Leeper HA. Effects of the manual laryngeal musculoskeletal tension reduction technique as a treatment for functional voice disorders: perceptual and acoustic measures. *J Voice.* 1993;7:242–249.
15. Lee EK, Son YI. Muscle tension dysphonia in children: voice characteristics and outcome of voice therapy. *Int J Pediatr Otorhinolaryngol.* 2005;69:911–917.
16. Dworkin JP, Meleca RJ, Simpson ML, et al. Use of topical lidocaine in the treatment of muscle tension dysphonia. *J Voice.* 2000;14:567–574.
17. Smith ME, Darby KP, Kirchner K, Blager FB. Simultaneous functional laryngeal stridor and functional aphonia in an adolescent. *Am J Otolaryngol.* 1993;5:366–369.

18. Boltezar IH, Burger ZR, Zargi M. Instability of voice in adolescence: patholgic condition or normal developmental variation? *J Pediatr.* 1997;130:185–190.

19. Kagli M, Sati I, Acar A, et al. Mutational falsetto: intervention outcomes in 45 patients. *J Laryngol Otol* . In press.

20. Woodson GE, Murry T. Botulinum toxin in the treatment of recalcitrant mutational dysphonia. *J Voice.* 1994;8:347–351.

21. Li GD, Mu L, Yang S. Acoustic evaluation of Isshiki type III thyroplasty for treatment of mutational voice disorders. *J Laryngol Otol.* 1999;113:31–34.

22. Pau H, Murty GE. First case of surgically corrected puberphonia. *J Laryngol Otol.* 2001; 115:60–61.

23. Brin MF, Fahn S, Blitzer A, Ramig LO, Stewart C. Movement disorders of the larynx. In: Blitzer A, Brin MF, Sasaki CT, Fahn S, Harris KS, eds. *Neurologic Disorders of the Larynx.* New York, NY: Thieme; 1992: 248–278.

24. Blitzer A, Brin MF, Stewart CF. Botulinum toxin management of spasmodic dysphonia (laryngeal dystonia): a 12-year experience in more than 900 patients. *Laryngoscope.* 1998;108(10):1435–1441.

25. Schweinfurth JM, Billante M, Courey MS. Risk factors and demographics in patients with spasmodic dysphonia. *Laryngoscope.* 2002;112:220–223.

26. Fasano A, Nardocci N, Elia AE, Zorzi G, Bentivoglio AR, Albanese A. Non-DYT1 early-onset primary torsion dystonia: comparison with DYT1 phenotype and review of the literature. *Mov Disord.* 2006;21(9):1411–1418.

27. O'Riordan S, Raymond D, Lynch T, Saunders-Pullman R, Bressman SB, Daly L, Hutchinson M. Age at onset as a factor in determining the phenotype of primary torsion dystonia. *Neurology.* 2004;63(8):1423–1426.

28. Boseley ME, Gherson S, Hartnick CJ. Spasmodic dysphonia in an adolescent patient with an autoimmune neurologic disorder. *Am J Otolaryngol.* 2007;28:140–142.

29. Schneider SA, Mohire MD, Trender-Gerhard I, et al. Familial dopa-responsive cervical dystonia. *Neurology.* 2006;66:599–601.

30. Bloch CS, Hirano M, Gould WJ. Symptom improvement of spastic dysphonia in response to phonatory tasks. *Ann Otol Rhinol Laryngol.* 1985;94:51–54.

31. Erickson M. Effects of voicing and syntactic complexity on sign expression in adductor spasmodic dysphonia. *Amer J Speech Lang Pathol.* 2003;12:416–424.

32. Roy N, Mauszycki SC, Merrill RM, Gouse M, Smith M. Toward improved differential diagnosis of adductor spasmodic dysphonia and muscle tension dysphonia. *Folia Phoniatr Logop.* 2007;59:83–90.

33. Dedo HH. Recurrent laryngeal nerve section for spastic dysphonia. *Ann Otol Rhinol Laryngol.* 1976;85:451–459.

34. Smith ME, Roy N, Wilson C. Lidocaine block of the recurrent laryngeal nerve in adductor spasmodic dysphonia: a multi-dimensional assessment. *Laryngoscope.* 2006;116:591–595.

35. Roy N, Smith ME, Allen B, Merrill RM. Adductor spasmodic dysphonia versus muscle tension dysphonia: examining the diagnostic value of recurrent laryngeal nerve lidocaine block. *Ann Otol Rhinol Laryngol.* 2007;116:161–168.

36. Murry T, Woodson GE. Combined-modality treatment of adductor spasmodic dysphonia with botulinum toxin and voice therapy. *J Voice.* 1995;9:460–465.

37. Sulica L. Contemporary management of spasmodic dysphonia. *Curr Opin Otolaryngol Head Neck Surg.* 2004;12:543–548.

38. Woodson G, Hochstetler H, Murry T. Botulinum toxin therapy for abductor spasmodic dysphonia. *J Voice.* 2006;20:137–143.

39. Berke GS, Blackwell KE, Gerratt BR, Verneil A, Jackson KS, Sercarz JA. Selective laryngeal adductor denervation-reinnervation: a new surgical treatment for adductor spasmodic dysphonia. *Ann Otol Rhinol Laryngol.* 1999;108:227–231.

40. Chhetri DK, Mendelsohn AH, Blumin JH, Berke GS. Long-term follow-up results of selective laryngeal adductor denervation-reinnervation surgery for adductor spasmodic dysphonia. *Laryngoscope.* 2006;116: 635–642.

41. Smith ME, Ramig LO. Neurological disorders and the voice. In: Rubin JS, Sataloff R, Korovin G, eds. *Diagnosis and Treatment of Voice Disorders.* 2nd ed. New York, NY: Thomson/Delmar Learning; 2002: 409-433.

42. Kent RD, Netsell R, Abbs JH: Acoustic characteristics of dysarthria associated with cerebellar disease. *J Speech Hear Res.* 1979; 22:627-648.

43. Zwirner P, Murry T, Woodson GE: Phonatory function in neurologically impaired patients. *J Commun Disord.* 1991;24:287-300.

44. Aronson AE. *Clinical Voice Disorders.* 3rd ed, New York, NY: Thieme; 1990.

45. Duffy J. Apraxia of speech. In: Duffy J. *Motor Speech Disorders: Substrates, Differential Diagnosis, and Management.* St. Louis, Mo: Mosby; 1995:259-281.

46. Tolosa E, Peña J: Involuntary vocalizations in movement disorders. *Adv Neurol.* 1988;49: 343-363.

47. Salloway S, Stewart CF, Israeli L, et al. Botulinum toxin for refractory vocal tics. *Mov Disord.* 1996;11:746-748.

48. Porta M, Maggioni G, Ottaviani F, Schindler A. Treatment of phonic tics in patients with Tourette's syndrome using botulinum toxin type A. *Neurol Sci.* 2004;24:420-423.

49. Worley G, Witsell DL, Hulka GF. Laryngeal dystonia causing inspiratory stridor in children with cerebral palsy. *Laryngoscope.* 2003;113:2192-2195.

50. Smith ME, Park AH, Muntz HR, Gray SD. Airway augmentation and maintenance through laryngeal chemodenervation in children with impaired vocal fold mobility. *Arch Otolaryngol Head Neck Surg.* 2007;133:610-612.

Diagnosis and Treatment of Velopharyngeal Insufficiency

Matthew T. Brigger
Jean E. Ashland
Christopher J. Hartnick

CLINICAL CASE

A 4-year-old boy presented for evaluation of his "abnormal voice." His mother reports that since he has been able to speak he has never made clear "s" and "p" sounds. She reports that to most people he is unintelligible. She is seeking options for therapy, but currently lives on a Caribbean island with minimal access to speech services or surgical care. The child has no other medical problems, feeds well, and has no previous surgical history. His examination shows a healthy energetic boy with no evidence of craniofacial dysmorphisms. However, he demonstrates markedly hypernasal speech. Fiberoptic examination demonstrates a short palate with decent lateral wall motion. Nasometry is consistent with marked nasal air escape. Given his anatomic deficit, surgical management was offered. In discussing the potential risks and benefits of each surgical option with his mother, she pro-

vided additional history that suggested he might have some degree of sleep apnea. She gave support to the notion that, were he to develop worse sleep apnea postoperatively, there would be no access on the island to anyone with expertise in diagnosing and managing such a condition. Given the history, a sphincter pharyngoplasty was offered in place of a posterior pharyngeal flap. The child underwent surgery uneventfully and noticed immediate improvement. Six months later his results were maintained.

INTRODUCTION

The complex neuromuscular functions that regulate human speech are not limited to the larynx. The sphincteric interaction of the palate (velum) within the pharynx is critical to the production of intelligible speech. Velopharyngeal insufficiency (VPI), or the inability to effectively seal the nasopharynx, results in loss of resonant control of speech and in some cases, optimal intraoral pressure to achieve orally directed speech sounds. Given that the nasopharynx is effectively closed during the vast majority of speech, this can significantly impact speech intelligibility. A lack of speech intelligibility has an obvious detrimental effect to affected children, but even mild cases of VPI can alter a child's effective communication and their well-being as speech provides a bridge to the people around us. The etiology of VPI varies from residual speech patterns after cleft palate repair to congenital anomalies of the soft palate (eg, shortness, submucous cleft) as well as weakness or motor planning difficulties.[1] Subsequently, the approaches to assessment and intervention are variable and often need to be tailored to the individual child.

SEMANTICS

Terminology used within the VPI literature is limited by redundancy and inconsistencies. In addition to velopharyngeal insufficiency, commonly used terms include velopharyngeal dysfunction, velopharyngeal inadequacy, and velopharyngeal incompetence. These terms are often used interchangeably. When specific terminology is used, variations of the classification introduced by Trost in 1981 seem to be the most common.[2] In the classification, an all encompassing term velopharyngeal inadequacy is used to describe velopharyngeal mislearning (faulty learning of articulation patterns), velopharyngeal incompetence (neurologic dysfunction leading to impaired motor control of the palate), and velopharyngeal insufficiency (an anatomic deficiency of insufficient tissue for closure). A similar, widely used all encompassing term is velopharyngeal dys-

function (VPD).[3] For the purposes of this chapter, VPI is used to connote velopharyngeal inadequacy.

PERTINENT ANATOMY

A brief review of anatomy is requisite to understanding the problem of VPI and the potential implications regarding evaluation and treatment. In general terms, the velopharyngeal port is a sphincter that regulates airflow through the nasopharynx. The degree of regulation manifests in the production (or lack thereof) of nasal resonance. In simple terms, six muscles constitute the sphincter. These include the levator veli palatini, tensor veli palatini, palatoglossus, palatopharyngeus, muscular uvula, and superior pharyngeal constrictor. All except for the superior constrictor comprise the soft palate, also known as the velum. Anatomically, the soft palate is located at the posterior aspect of the maxilla protruding from the hard palate. The Latin term velum refers to a "ship's sail" and connotes the flat sheet-like shape of the soft palate as it protrudes posteriorly. By separating the oropharynx from the nasopharynx, the palate has both an oral and nasal surface.

Regarding the musculature, motor control is primarily mediated through branches of cranial nerve X except for the tensor veli palatini which is innervated by a motor branch of cranial nerve V. The paired levator palatini serve as the primary muscle mass of the soft palate and form a sling suspended from the skull base.[4] The muscle serves to elevate the palate in a posterior direction. This motion is counteracted by the action of the palatoglossus (anterior tonsillar pillar) and the palatopharyngeus (posterior tonsillar pillar). Although the levator veli palatini provides the muscular mass of the velum, the tensor veli palatini contributes the majority of the fibrous component referred to as the palatal aponeurosis.[4] The primary action of the tensor veli palatini is to facilitate middle ear aeration and overall has a minimal effect on velopharyngeal closure.[5] The muscular uvula tenses the palate as well as providing a bulge on the posterior nasal surface of the palate which has been postulated to be instrumental in tight velopharyngeal closure.[6] The superior pharyngeal constrictor serves to provide lateral wall motion of the nasopharynx to close the velopharyngeal port.[7] Additionally, it may contribute to the presence of Passavant's ridge, a transverse mucosal bulge along the posterior pharyngeal wall noted in 20% of the population.[8]

From a functional standpoint, an interesting distinction is made between the physiology involved in closing the nasopharynx during swallowing versus speech exercises. A common situation is seen when children have evidence of severe VPI with speech, but exhibit no nasal regurgitation during swallowing. Shprintzen and colleagues classified differences in pneumatic (speech, blowing, and whistling) and nonpneumatic (gagging and swallowing) closure mechanisms based on videofluoroscopic findings.[7] Furthermore, an electromyographic (EMG) study of levator function during speech, blowing, and swallowing suggests that different muscle types are activated during swallowing exercises as compared to speech and blowing exercises.[9] By determining the mean power frequencies of EMG signals, Nohara et al. concluded that pneumatic activities tend to activate slow-twitch motor units while swallowing tends to trigger fast twitch motor units.[9] This work is corroborated by the hypothesis that the human pharyngeal constrictors possess a subspecialized slow twitch inner layer of muscle fibers that appears to be related to speech

and respiration.[10] Ultimately the complex neuromuscular interaction and subspecialization of muscle fibers highlights the importance of approaching VPI as more than a simple anatomic deficit and realizing that the manifestations of VPI can result from a variety of insults.

Closure Patterns

The relatively simplistic discussion of the musculature involved in velopharyngeal closure described above fails to reveal the high degree of coordination, complexity, and variation involved. The sum motion is one in which the palate elevates posteriorly and contacts the pharyngeal wall circumferentially. On a lateral view, the palate appears to flex like a knee due to the bulge of the uvula maximizing contact with the posterior pharyngeal wall (Fig 16–1).[11] Perhaps a

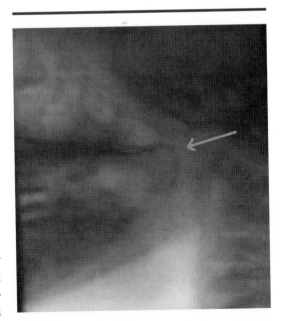

Fig 16–1. Lateral fluoroscopic view demonstrating "kneelike" contact between palate and posterior pharyngeal wall.

better way to look at velopharyngeal anatomy is through closure patterns. In 1973, Skolnick and associates used videofluoroscopy to delineate four patterns of velopharyngeal closure.[12] The most commonly observed pattern is the situation in which the posterior surface of the velum comes into broad apposition with the posterior pharyngeal wall in the absence of lateral pharyngeal wall motion. Two circular patterns of closure are described. The first pattern involves a combination of lateral wall motion and posterior velar movement to achieve velopharyngeal closure. A secondary circular pattern with posterior pharyngeal motion (Passavant's ridge) is described. However, this motion pattern must be interpreted with caution as Passavant's ridge does not always correspond to the level of closure. The least common closure pattern is referred to as sagittal and demonstrates minimal velar movement combined with medial apposition of the lateral pharyngeal walls. An

assessment of closure patterns is instrumental in characterizing the nature and location of the velopharyngeal air escape. Such knowledge is critical in selecting operative procedures to effectively seal the gap.

Normal Versus Abnormal Speech

Etiology and Pathophysiology

VPI is most commonly seen in children with associated craniofacial developmental anomalies of which cleft palate is the most common. Despite successful palatoplasty, post repair prevalence of VPI has been reported to be 20 to 50%.[11,13] A special case is the submucosal (occult) cleft palate. In this situation, no overt cleft is seen, but a failure of the midline fusion of the velar muscles is present often manifesting as a bifid uvula, hard palate notch, or a bluish line of a visible diastasis (Fig 16-2). The

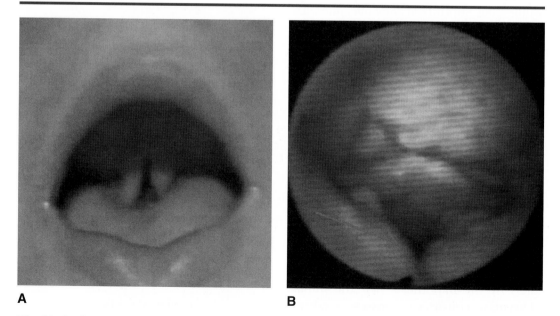

A   **B**

Fig 16–2. Submucous cleft with bifid uvula. **A.** Intraoral view. **B.** Intranasal view, note midline groove.

majority of these children will have no speech deficits during their lifetime.[14] However, a subset will present with VPI often after adenotonsillar surgery. In a review of 126 children with VPI after adenoidectomy, 26% were noted to have a previously unidentified submucosal cleft palate or bifid uvula.[15] In a different study, 55% of children with VPI in the absence of an overt bony cleft were noted to have a submucous cleft on endoscopic examination.[16]

Associated Syndromes

Over 200 syndromes have been described where cleft palate is a reported manifestation. Any such syndrome can be associated with VPI. Of special note is velocardiofacial syndrome which typically does not manifest an overt palatal cleft. The syndrome was first described in 1977 by Shprintzen and colleagues.[17] The syndrome has a wide spectrum of phenotypes including congenital cardiac anomalies, VPI, and characteristic facial dysmorphisms.[18] The prevalence in the United States is estimated to be 1:2000.[18] The difficulty lies in the wide variability of presentations and propensity to be underdiagnosed. Proper diagnosis is essential in that patients with VCFS must be screened for potentially lethal cardiac anomalies. From a surgical standpoint, there have been a number of reports of carotid artery medialization which may possibly represent hazardous surgical anatomy (Fig 16–3).[19,20] Additionally, surgical outcomes for VPI have been reported to be inferior to the results achieved in children without VCFS.[21]

Postadenoidectomy

VPI manifesting after adenoidectomy is relatively rare and generally of short duration, with most cases resolving within 6 weeks. Given the bulk of adenoid tissue, many children produce velopharyngeal closure by

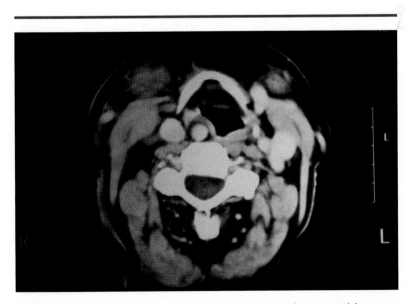

Fig 16–3. Computed tomography demonstrating carotid artery medialization.

approximating the velum to their adenoid pad. In most children, removal of the adenoid pad is of no consequence because their velum has adequate length to reach the posterior pharyngeal wall. However, in select children, the new dynamics of velopharyngeal closure do not allow adequate apposition. Permanent VPI after adenoidectomy requiring intervention is reported to occur in approximately 1:1500 adenoidectomies.[22,23] In retrospect, many children have suggestions of marginal velopharyngeal competence including physical stigmata of a submucosal cleft, preoperative hypernasality or regurgitation (Table 16-1). In a review of 23 children with VPI after adenoidectomy, 14 children were found to carry the VCFS genotype.[24] In situations where an adenoidectomy appears to be indicated in a child with features concerning for marginal velopharyngeal competence, a superior pole adenoidectomy can be performed in which the inferior aspect of the adenoid pad is maintained to prevent the development of VPI.

Other Causes

VPI has been noted in a variety of other settings. Any surgery that involves orthognathic maxillary advancement (often performed in children with craniofacial abnormalities) by definition puts a child at risk for developing VPI. Hypertrophied tonsils have been associated with clinical VPI and resolution has been documented after tonsillectomy.[25] Additionally, neuromuscular disorders resulting in poor control of pharyngeal musculature can result in hypernasality and dysarthria.

DIAGNOSTIC EVALUATION

As delineated above, VPI represents a complex problem with a variety of manifestations. The degree of complexity mandates a multidisciplinary approach to the diagnosis and treatment of affected children. Often these children are best served in the setting of a tertiary care referral center with coordinated access to speech pathologists, surgeons, dentists, audiologists, and social workers.

History

Evaluation of a child with suspected VPI starts by simply listening with a keen ear. Although children are often referred for grossly abnormal speech, a great deal can be learned by listening to the child speak. Using standard phrases weighted with sibilants and plosives will help to uncover the extent of VPI. A comprehensive history is imperative for all children. Particular emphasis on any developmental anomalies, past medical history and past surgical history may yield clues to syndromic associations or other problems that can be seen in the setting of VPI. Eliciting any history of hearing loss or other anomalies that potentially increase the child's communication difficulties is essential. A developmental and psychological history is useful in determining the extent of disability imparted by the communication difficulties.

Table 16–1. Physical Examination Findings for a Submucosal Cleft Palate

Prevention of Postadenoidectomy VPI: Recognize the Signs of a Submucosal Cleft
bifid uvula
hard palate notch
bluish line of a visible diastasis

Physical Examination

A comprehensive physical examination is requisite in all children with VPI. All children must be assessed for the presence of syndromic stigmata, craniofacial dysmorphisms and the presence of cardiac abnormalities. A thorough head and neck examination includes an assessment of the middle ear status. An oral exam is performed to identify the presence of a cleft and status of repair. As described below, flexible nasopharyngoscopy has proven to be a well tolerated and invaluable tool in examining and formulating a treatment plan for these children.

A further note on orofacial examination is necessary at this point. The complete evaluation consists of close intraoral examination with attention to oromotor skills, the occlusal and dental status as well as direct visualization and palpation of the velum. Facial examination during speech in relation to characteristic grimaces and gestures are often noted.

Perceptual Evaluation

Several perceptual evaluation scales have been developed and validated. One of the most commonly used is that of McWilliams and Phillips which is sometimes referred to as the Pittsburgh Weighted Speech Scale.[26] This weighted scale rates five components of speech including nasal emission, facial grimace, nasality, phonation, and articulation (Fig 16–4). Points are assigned for each subgroup and summed to give an overall score that can be used to track outcomes.

Nasometry

Nasometry is based on the measurement of nasal acoustic energy within speech.[27]

A headset with two directional microphones (nasal and oral) is connected through a converter to a computer. The child being evaluated wears the headset and voices standardized passages. A nasalence score relating the nasal acoustic energy as related to the total acoustic energy is displayed graphically on the computer screen and a nasalence score is generated. The score is then compared to normative data, such as with the MacKay-Kummer Simplified Nasometric Assessment Procedures (SNAP) test.[28] Additionally, nasometry can be useful in therapy in the form of biofeedback as discussed below.

Assessment of Velopharyngeal Closure

Flexible Nasapharyngoscopy

Flexible nasopharyngoscopy has become indispensable in the evaluation of children with VPI. The development of high-quality small-caliber flexible endoscopes permits excellent visualization in most children. The flexible endoscope is passed transnasally to a position in the posterior nasal cavity allowing a complete view of the velum and nasopharynx. Children of all ages can be evaluated anatomically; however, it is generally around age six that children can cooperate and perform comprehensive volitional vocalizing tasks for a complete evaluation. Flexible nasopharyngoscopy provides an excellent view of the nasal surface of the palate and may provide the only sign of a submucous cleft palate as described above. Additionally, flexible nasopharyngoscopy allows an examination of the larynx, which may uncover additional pathologies associated with compensatory measures, such as vocal nodules, that may have developed in response to the VPI.

WEIGHTED SPEECH SCORE: VPI SCALE

R	L		ARTICULATION
		0	Normal
		0	Articulation errors
		0	Articulation errors related to dentition
		0	Compensatory errors in the presence of a competent mechanism
		0	Phonological errors
		2	Slightly reduced intraoral pressure
		3	Significantly reduced intraoral pressure
		4	Compensatory errors with reduced intraoral air pressure, eg. Glottal stops, pharyngeal fricatives, pharyngeal stops, nasal snorts, implosions, etc.
		Total	

R	L		NASAL EMISSION
		0	Not present
		0	Nasal emission as an articulation error
		1	Inconsistent audible nasal emission
		1	Inconsistent inaudible nasal emission
		2	Nasal turbulence
		2	Consistent inaudible nasal airflow
		3	Consistent audible nasal emission
		Total	

	QUALITY: LARYNGEAL RESONANCE
0	Normal
1	Mild hoarseness and/or breathiness
1	Moderate hoarseness and/or breathiness
1	Reduced loudness
1	Severe hoarseness and/or breathiness
0	Other(tonsillar, pharyngeal, harsh):

	QUALITY: NASAL RESONANCE
0	Hyponasal
0	Nasality as a function of articulation (phoneme specific)
0	Assimilated nasality
1	Inconsistent nasality
1	Slight
1	Mild
2	Cul de sac or mild to moderate
3	Moderate
4	Severe
Total	

	FACIAL GRIMACE
0	Absent or Mild
1	Moderate or Severe
Total	

TOTAL SCORE	
0-1	Competent valving mechanism
2	Inconsistently competent
3-6	Borderline valving mechanism
7+	Incompetent valving mechanism

Fig 16–4. Perceptual weighted speech score used at Massachusetts General Hospital. Adapted from McWilliams and Phillips.[26]

Multiview Fluoroscopy

Multiview fluoroscopy was for many years the primary means of assessing velopharyngeal closure. Three views are traditionally used after instilling a small amount of high-density barium into the child's nose to coat the nasopharynx. The anteriorposterior view allows assessment of lateral pharyngeal wall motion (Fig 16–5). The lateral view allows visualization of palatal motion and the posterior pharyngeal wall (see Fig 16-1). The closure pattern of the sphincter is viewed directly in the base view (Fig 16–6). Videofluoroscopy allows excellent visualization of the shape of the velum and angle of elevation in lateral view and may serve as a better tolerated alternative for children who are noncompliant with nasendoscopy The requirement of ionizing radiation in addition to potential difficulties in standard positioning with resultant child compliance issues are potential limitations of the study. An important concept is that often videofluoroscopy and nasopharyngoscopy provide complementary information.

Grading and Standardization of Velopharyngeal Closure Measurements

In 1990, an international working group of clinicians and researchers headed by Karen Golding-Kushner reported a standardized grading scale for reporting findings on nasopharyngoscopy and multiview fluoroscopy.[29] The scale serves to outline both quantitative and qualitative scoring to accurately describe and grade the anatomic defects associated with VPI.

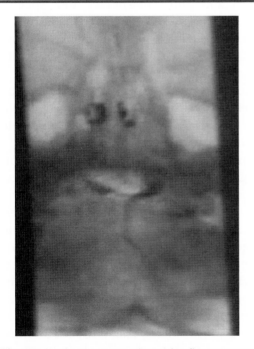

Fig 16–5. Anteroposterior videofluoroscopy demonstrating visualization of lateral wall motion.

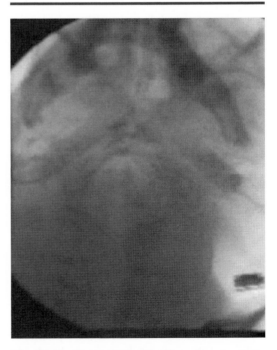

Fig 16–6. Base view videofluoroscopy demonstrating closure pattern.

Nasopharyngoscopy, Multiview Fluoroscopy, or Both?

Over time, much has been written about the merits and disadvantages of both nasopharyngoscopy and multiview fluoroscopy. Both are used to accurately assess velopharyngeal anatomy to assist in developing a treatment plan, particularly surgical methods. Nasopharyngoscopy allows an excellent view of velopharyngeal closure patterns, but can be limited by optical distortion and tolerance by the child undergoing the exam. Multiview fluoroscopy allows an excellent view of lateral wall motion as well as closure patterns. As stated above, the closure patterns of the velopharynx were initially described based on fluoroscopic studies. Difficulties arise in interpreting anatomic findings in the presence of multiple shadows. Additionally, postsurgical examination particularly in the setting of a pharyngeal flap is quite difficult with fluoroscopy, but is easily visualized directly with nasopharyngoscopy. A recent review suggests that both modalities provide complementary data, but that nasopharyngoscopy may provide a higher correlation with VPI severity.[30] Currently, our practice is to perform flexible nasopharyngoscopy on all children to visualize anatomy and assist in surgical planning and proceed to multiview fluoroscopy in children where additional information may prove useful, particularly in children under six years of age who have limited cooperation for a functional endoscopic assessment.

TREATMENT: BASIC TENETS

Prior to surgical repair of a cleft palate or primary VPI, a speech-language pathologist with specialized training can help guide parents to elicit sound play with their infant,

expand consonant repertoires, and to minimize patterns of glottal stops.

As language and speech emerge for the toddler and preschool age child, it is important to discern if speech errors are developmental, obligatory, or compensatory. When children with cleft or noncleft velopharyngeal problems display articulation errors and resonance abnormalities, the developmentally appropriate articulation issues are addressed first. It is important to remediate these developmental speech errors as well as establish accurate placement of the articulators and manner of production (eg, fricative versus stop consonants), even when the anatomy prohibits the ability to achieve an orally produced sound. This is especially true for children under four years of age with a cleft palate who are often too young for consideration of a secondary surgery.

Behavioral therapy with a speech-language pathologist can be helpful in mild VPI and phoneme-specific VPI. Speech/resonance therapy is not indicated when: (a) nasal emissions are present in all nonnasal consonants with subsequent hypernasality related to a short or poor moving palate or excessively deep pharynx, (b) nasal air loss related to a palatal fistula, or (c) articulation errors related to severe dental malocclusions that require physical management.[31,32] Speech/resonance therapy cannot work against atypical anatomy and if attempted may cause undue frustration to the child.

Perhaps the primary concern for every child, parent, and VPI surgeon is to avoid operating when a child has a functional speech abnormality that can be masking as what appears to be VPI secondary to anatomic deficit. A thorough evaluation by a speech and language pathologist is often necessary to accurately diagnose such disorders preoperatively. As described below, comprehensive therapy often involves much more than simply filling the anatomic defect.

Speech Therapy: Resonance Therapy

Resonance therapy is helpful in certain conditions: mild velopharyngeal dysfunction that results in inconsistent nasal air emissions related to articulation errors and in the postoperative period.[33,34] Short-term speech therapy preoperatively is helpful to establish accurate patterns so that the child can experience maximum success following surgery. Also, speech therapy may be considered for young children with a repaired cleft palate who are too young for secondary surgery but who have either difficulties with accurate articulation placement or have compensatory strategies considered as speech errors, such as glottal stops.[34] Treatment approaches generally include establishing auditory discrimination of nasal and nonnasal speech productions, maximizing oral airflow for nonnasal speech sounds, facilitating accurate articulation placement, production, and manner; and diminishing deviant compensatory speech patterns, such as glottal stops. Approaches may include articulation strategies to foster oral airflow, such as a prolonged plosive sound "t" to glide into a sibilant "s," whispered speech with initial sounds "h" or "w" paired with low front vowels (eg, "haha" or "wah wah").[32,35] Low resistance blowing toys can be helpful for the concept of oral airflow, but should not be used to "strengthen" the palate muscle as research does not support that an "exercise model" results in improved palate motion.[36,37] Other approaches that may help with improved resonance balance include: vowel prolongation, increased mouth opening, and increased vocal loudness. In addition, visual and auditory feedback in therapy can offer additional modalities to help the child see or hear the degree of nasal air escape. Feedback can be seen via fogging on a nasal mirror, use of a SeeScape® device which uses a nasal tip to capture nasal airflow and provides the visual correlation of an object moving up a tube to reflect degree of flow, the new Oral & Nasal Listener® device with connected dual stethoscopes to provide auditory feedback, or a computer program using a nasometer to display nasal airflow in graphic form.[35,38]

Of note, resonance therapy will not be helpful for moderate to severe VPI when the physical ability of the palate to achieve closure during speech is not possible. This would include unintelligible speech related to hypernasality and velopharyngeal incompetence, inability to achieve nonnasal consonants because of nasal air leakage and poor intraoral pressure.[39]

Obturators and Prostheses

In some children, the use of a dental appliance to serve as a palatal lift or nasopharyngeal obturator may serve as a useful therapy alternative. Palatal lifts serve to elevate the neurogenic palate that has reduced motion or decreased accurate timing of soft palate elevation to achieve VP closure. Generally such children will have adequate velar length, but poor muscle tone. In contrast, speech bulbs or obturators are fashioned to fill the open space or gap between the soft palate and posterior pharyngeal wall in cases of insufficient palatal length (Fig 16-7). The lateral and posterior walls of the pharynx can then close against the obturator.[40] Ideally, a speech appliance (either lift or bulb) provides the closure between the soft palate and pharyngeal wall to remediate nasal emissions and/or hypernasality associated with VPI.[41,42] In general, prosthetic management of VPI is not generally a first-line approach due to compliance issues and the need for adequate stable dentition.[40] However, such devices can be useful when secondary surgical

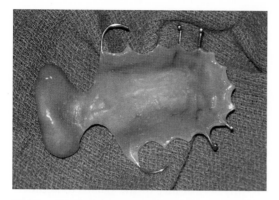

Fig 16–7. Velopharyngeal obturator (photo courtesy of Dr. Matthew Jackson).

management, such as a pharyngeal flap, is contraindicated as in the case of a child with potential surgical comorbidities such as severe obstructive sleep apnea or cardiac anomalies. The devices can often serve as a temporary approach until surgery can be completed, or to offer insight if surgery will be beneficial.[43]

A team approach for speech appliance selection and fitting is useful. In general, the team should consist of a speech language pathologist, dental specialist, and orthodontist or prosthodontist to maximize successful outcomes.[43] Some studies have documented improved VP muscle function following use of speech appliances in electromyography measures, such as increased activiation signal of the levator veli palatini muscle.[41]

Careful selection of patients is requisite for success. Potential candidates include children with wide clefts in whom a lack of available tissue may compromise potential repair techniques, children with significant neuromuscular deficits of the soft palate or when surgery is contraindicated or delayed for any reason.[44] In general, the limitations of such devices are realized through noncompliance. Extensive dental caries precludes the use of such devices as well.[44]

Surgical Treatment

Surgical treatment is the cornerstone of effective therapy for the anatomic defect associated with VPI. A variety of techniques have been developed over time to address the various configurations of closure patterns and degree of difficulties experienced by individual children. Most surgeons accept that a basic tenet of VPI surgery is that procedures must be tailored to the specific difficulty and anatomic deficiency present in each child.

The timing of such procedures depends on a variety of factors including age at diagnosis, etiology of VPI, access to trained therapists and neurocognitive development. In general, as discussed above, adequate diagnosis of VPI often does not occur until the child is approximately 3 to 4 years of age. Once diagnosed, most surgical procedures can be safely performed in children as young as 3 years old. A special note regarding selection of procedure type is the presence of baseline obstructive sleep apnea. As procedures designed to address VPI constrict the nasopharyngeal airway by definition, the theoretical possibility of exacerbating or introducing obstructive sleep apnea must be considered.

Posterior Pharyngeal Flap

Efforts to lessen the nasal emission of VPI were first described by Passavant in 1865 when he reported adhesion of the soft palate to the posterior pharyngeal wall.[45] This was subsequently followed in 1875 when Schoenborn described the inferiorly based posterior pharyngeal flap followed by his introduction of a superior based flap 10 years later.[46] The procedure has subsequently undergone numerous modifications since that time, but the principle remains the same. The goal of a posterior pharyngeal flap is to effectively obturate the nasopharynx with a biologic obturator. The procedure involves creating a flap of tissue from the posterior pharyngeal wall that is raised from an inferior point superiorly where it remains attached to the posterior pharynx. The elevated inferior aspect is subsequently secured to the nasal surface of the soft palate. This can be accomplished either with or without splitting the soft palate. Once completed, the central region of the nasopharynx is obturated by the tissue, whereas lateral ports for air escape remain open to allow an attenuated degree of nasal transmission (Fig 16–8).

The development of the procedure over time has placed attention to the proper construction of the lateral ports. A prevailing concept is that children with some degree of lateral wall motion may benefit most from a pharyngeal flap as the existing lateral wall motion may be used to control the release of air through the ports.[47]

Sphincter Pharyngoplasty

In distinction to the static obturator created by a pharyngeal flap, the sphincter pharyngoplasty operation was developed in an effort to recreate a dynamic sphincter. First introduced in 1950 by Hynes with further modifications by Orticochea, Jackson, and others, the sphincter pharyngoplasty involves elevating two lateral superiorly based flaps from the region of the posterior tonsillar pillars.[48-50] A transverse incision is made in the posterior pharyngeal wall mucosa, and the flaps are rotated 90 degrees and subsequently inset into the transverse incision potentially placing dynamic muscle (palatophayngeus) into an orientation to create a dynamic sphincteric effect (Fig 16–9). A study comparing pre and postoperative operative videofluoroscopy suggested that there is some degree of dynamism after sphincter pharyngoplasty, but that it is difficult to quantify.[51] Ultimately, sphincter pharyngoplasty is generally pursued in the setting of a child with adynamic lateral pharyngeal walls.

Posterior Wall Augmentation

In some children with a mild to moderate degree of VPI and a clearly evident small velopharyngeal gap, posterior pharyngeal wall augmentation may provide significant speech improvement. The concept involves placing the augmentation material in a location that allows adequate velopharyngeal closure by displacing the posterior pharyngeal wall anteriorly to allow contact with the soft palate. A variety of materials have been advocated including cartilage, fat, fascia, paraffin, silicone, acellular dermis, polytetrafluoroethylene, and calcium hydroxylapatite (CaHA).[4,52-56] Placement methods have included direct incision over the pharyngeal mucosa, transcervical approaches, and injection. Teflon is associated with an unclear safety profile and migration leading to a sharp decrease in its use in recent years.[4] Recently, our center has had a favorable experience with CaHA which serves as a stable, easily placed injectable augmentation

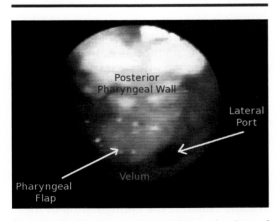

Fig 16–8. Postoperative endoscopic view of a superior based pharyngeal flap.

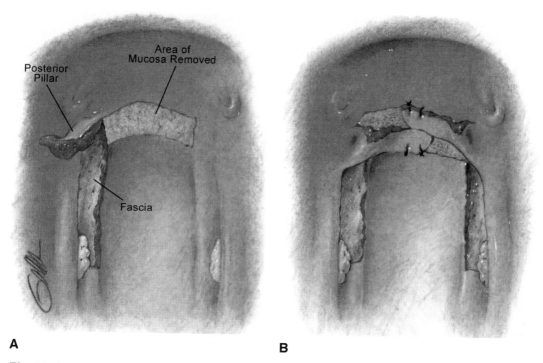

A   **B**

Fig 16–9. A. Transverse mucosal incision and elevation of superiorly based lateral flaps. **B.** Flaps rotated 90 degrees and inset on posterior pharyngeal wall.

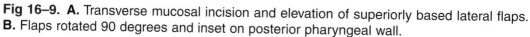

agent (Fig 16–10).[56] To date, we have used CaHA augmentation in 12 patients. Eight children demonstrated success defined as normalized nasometry and improved perceptual scores at 3 months. Four children have been followed for over 24 months and have demonstrated sustained success. Three of the 4 failures occurred very early in our experience and it became evident that the technique is both operator and patient dependent. From a technique standpoint, a mimimum of 2 to 3 mL of CaHA must be injected. This is performed under direct visualization using a 120-degree endoscope with a soft palate retractor. Of note, we have had no cases of CaHA migration. In our experience, older children with mild to moderate VPI with a clear anatomic deficit seem to benefit most from the procedure.

An alternative method of posterior wall augmentation is elevating a superiorly based posterior pharyngeal wall flap and rolling it onto itself instead of attaching it to the soft palate as in typical pharyngeal flap surgery. This creates a mound of tissue that ultimately scars and provides for a contact point in the soft palate. Patient selection is critical as this method is only appropriate in children with small gaps. A particular advantage with injection methods is the ability to precisely locate the area of deficiency and to endoscopically target only the area that requires treatment.

Palatoplasty Methods

In some children, the configuration of their palate or previous surgeries may make palato-

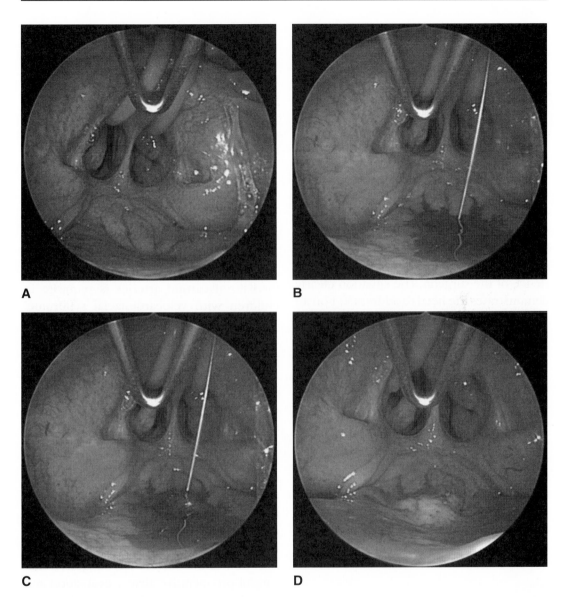

A

B

C

D

Fig 16–10. Posterior pharyngeal wall augmentation with injectable calcium hydroxylapatite viewed with 120-degree endoscope placed transorally viewing superiorly into nasopharynx. **A.** Prior to injection. **B.** Needle in place. **C.** During injection. **D.** Post injection.

plasty techniques more useful. In particular, children with submucous cleft palate or congenitally short palate and associated VPI may benefit from a palatal lengthening procedure such as a Furlow palatoplasty or V-Y push-back palatoplasty. Both of these methods serve to effectively lengthen the soft palate. The Furlow method involves using opposing Z-plasties whereas the V-Y method uses soft tissue elevated from the hard palate.

Special Case: Unilateral Deficits

Special consideration must be given in the setting of VPI in children with unilateral deficits as is commonly seen with hemifacial microsomia or unilateral neurologic injury.[57] In these children, the anatomic defect results in a unilateral escape of air on the affected side. Surgical therapy can be accomplished with unilateral sphincter pharynoplasty techniques, offset superior based pharyngeal flaps or possibly directed posterior wall augmentation.[57,58] The decision on the best procedure is dictated by the child's anatomy, underlying features and the experience of the surgeon. The situation clearly demonstrates the need to address VPI on an individual case by case basis.

Tonsillectomy

A rarely described, but clinically important cause of VPI is obstructed velar closure secondary to hypertrophic tonsils. Tonsillectomy can be curative in such children.[25] In such children examination will demonstrate significant tonsillar hypertrophy, but confirmation requires an endoscopic or fluoroscopic examination to determine the presence of the velopharyngeal gap and to visualize the role that the tonsils play in contributing to the overall gap dimensions.

Surgical Outcomes

Each of the described methods has been shown to be effective in representative case series. Definitions of success vary and the heterogeneity of the problem leads to preoperative characteristics that are not uniform in studies addressing surgical outcomes. In general, success rates described as resolution of VPI vary from 62 to 98% with most accounts being in the realm of 75% resolution.[58-67] Of note, several studies have looked to differentiate success rates between pharyngeal flaps and sphincter pharyngoplasty. Unfortunately, the relative rarity of the problem coupled with different techniques among different surgeons clouds the literature. An underpowered multicenter trial in 2005 suggested that outcomes were similar.[68]

Perhaps a greater concern might be the risk of complications between the various procedures. Moderate to severe bleeding seen after both pharyngeal flap surgery and sphincter pharyngoplasty is generally rare, but may occasionally require transfusion. As described above, prudence in detecting medialized carotid arteries is requisite in children with velocardiofacial syndrome. Complications associated with posterior wall augmentation procedures are related to the material used. Extrusion, infection, resorption and migration are all possibilities and occur at varying rates. Our material of choice, calcium hydroxylapatite, has not demonstrated any such complications to date.[56]

The development of obstructive sleep apnea is likely one of the most worrisome complications associated with the surgical management of VPI. Obstructive sleep apnea is almost exclusively seen in pharyngeal flap surgery and several postoperative deaths have been reported.[69,70] Recent attention to the subject has suggested that careful preoperative airway evaluation and consideration of preoperative tonsillectomy may be useful in preventing untoward outcomes.[60]

When considering patient selection for various procedures, a certain degree of tailoring is necessary. A combination of the child's anatomy, neurocognitive development, social situation, and access to therapy coupled with the surgeon's experience are all factors in selecting the appropriate procedure for each child.

FUTURE DIRECTIONS

The management of velopharyngeal insufficiency continues to be an evolving field. Recent advances in evaluation include the widespread use and acceptance of nasal endoscopy. Of recent note, the utility of magnetic resonance imaging (MRI) as an evaluation tool has emerged as stronger magnets and imaging algorithms have allowed the development of cine MRI sequences which provide high-resolution detailed velopharyngeal movement visualized without ionizing radiation.[71] Further developments in surgical technique including the novel materials for posterior wall augmentation as well as alternative procedures such as cerclage pharyngoplasty and creation of a palatopharyngeal sling have been described and represent exciting advances in the field.[56,72,73]

CONCLUSIONS

Overall, the evaluation and management of VPI remains both challenging and rewarding. The heterogeneity of the problem leads to a wide variety of manifestations and therapies. The care of these children requires an individualized approach to each patient in a multidisciplinary fashion. Fortunately, given the opportunity, most children can ultimately achieve intelligible speech and experience minimal vocal disability over the long term.

REFERENCES

1. Johns DF, Rohrich RJ, Awada M. Velopharyngeal incompetence: a guide for clinical evaluation. *Plast Reconstr Surg.* 2003;112:1890–1897; quiz 1898, 1982.
2. Trost JE. Articulatory additions to the classical description of the speech of persons with cleft palate. *Cleft Palate J.* 1981;18:193–203.
3. Kummer AW. Velopharyngeal dysfunction (VPD) and resonance disorders. In: *Cleft Palate and Craniofacial Anomalies: The Effects on Speech and Resonance.* San Diego, CA: Singular; 2001:145–176.
4. Willging JP, Cotton RT. Velopharyngeal insufficiency. In Bluestone CD, Stool SE, Alper CM, eds. *Pediatric Otolaryngology.* 4th ed. Philadelphia, PA: Saunders; 2003:1789–1799.
5. Kamerer DB, Rood SR. The tensor tympani, stapedius, and tensor veli palatini muscles—an electromyographic study. *Otolaryngology.* 1978;86:416–421.
6. Azzam NA, Kuehn DP. The morphology of musculus uvulae. *Cleft Palate J.* 1977;14:78–87.
7. Shprintzen RJ, McCall GN, Skolnick ML, et al. Selective movement of the lateral aspects of the pharyngeal walls during velopharyngeal closure for speech, blowing, and whistling in normals. *Cleft Palate J.* 1975;12:51–58.
8. Dickson DR, Dickson WM. Velopharyngeal anatomy. *J Speech Hear Res.* 1972;15:372–381.
9. Nohara K, Kotani Y, Ojima M, et al. Power spectra analysis of levator veli palatini muscle electromyogram during velopharyngeal closure for swallowing, speech, and blowing. *Dysphagia.* 2007;22:135–139.
10. Mu L, Sanders I. Neuromuscular specializations within human pharyngeal constrictor muscles. *Ann Otol Rhinol Laryngol.* 2007;116:604–617.
11. Kummer AW. Anatomy and Physiology: The orofacial structures and velopharyngeal valve. In: *Cleft Palate and Craniofacial Anomalies: The Effects on Speech and Resonance.* San Diego, CA: Singular; 2001:3–32.
12. Skolnick ML, Mc CG, Barnes M. The sphincteric mechanism of velopharyngeal closure. *Cleft Palate J.* 1973;10:286–305.
13. Morris HL. Velopharyngeal competence and primary cleft palate surgery, 1960–1971: a critical review. *Cleft Palate J.* 1973;10:62–71.

14. McWilliams BJ. Submucous clefts of the palate: how likely are they to be symptomatic? *Cleft Palate Craniofac J.* 1991;28: 247–249; discussion 250–251.

15. Witzel MA, Rich RH, Margar-Bacal F, et al. Velopharyngeal insufficiency after adenoidectomy: an 8-year review. *Int J Pediatr Otorhinolaryngol.* 1986;11:15–20.

16. Trier WC. Velopharyngeal incompetency in the absence of overt cleft palate: anatomic and surgical considerations. *Cleft Palate J.* 1983;20:209–217.

17. Shprintzen RJ, Goldberg RB, Lewin ML, et al. A new syndrome involving cleft palate, cardiac anomalies, typical facies, and learning disabilities: velo-cardio-facial syndrome. *Cleft Palate J.* 1978;15:56–62.

18. Robin NH, Shprintzen RJ. Defining the clinical spectrum of deletion 22q11.2. *J Pediatr.* 2005;147:90–96.

19. MacKenzie-Stepner K, Witzel MA, Stringer DA, et al. Abnormal carotid arteries in the velocardiofacial syndrome: a report of three cases. *Plast Reconstr Surg.* 1987;80: 347–351.

20. D'Antonio LD, Marsh JL. Abnormal carotid arteries in the velocardiofacial syndrome. *Plast Reconstr Surg.* 1987;80:471–472.

21. Butts SC, Tatum SA 3rd, Mortelliti AJ, et al. Velo-cardio-facial syndrome: the pediatric otolaryngologist's perspective. *Curr Opin Otolaryngol Head Neck Surg.* 2005;13: 371–375.

22. Gibb AG. Hypernasality (rhinolalia aperta) following tonsil and adenoid removal. *J Laryngol Otol.* 1958;72:433–451.

23. Skolnick ML. Velopharyngeal function in cleft palate. *Clin Plast Surg.* 1975;2:285–297.

24. Perkins JA, Lewis CW, Gruss JS, et al. Furlow palatoplasty for management of velopharyngeal insufficiency: a prospective study of 148 consecutive patients. *Plast Reconstr Surg.* 2005;116:72–80; discussion 81–84.

25. Kummer AW, Billmire DA, Myer CM 3rd. Hypertrophic tonsils: the effect on resonance and velopharyngeal closure. *Plast Reconstr Surg.* 1993;91:608–611.

26. McWilliams BJ, Phillips BJ. In: *Velopharyngeal Incompetence: Audio Seminars in Speech Pathology.* Philadelphia, PA: WB Saunders; 1979.

27. Kummer AW. Nasometry. In: *Cleft Palate and Craniofacial Anomalies: The Effects on Speech and Resonance.* San Diego, CA: Singular; 2001; 311–330.

28. MacKay I, Kummer A. Simplified nasometric assessment procedures. *The MacKay-Kummer SNAP Test.* Lincoln, NJ: Kay Elemtrics Corporation; 1994.

29. Golding-Kushner KJ, Argamaso RV, Cotton RT, et al. Standardization for the reporting of nasopharyngoscopy and multiview videofluoroscopy: a report from an International Working Group. *Cleft Palate J.* 1990;27: 337–247; discussion 47–48.

30. Lam DJ, Starr JR, Perkins JA, et al. A comparison of nasendoscopy and multiview videofluoroscopy in assessing velopharyngeal insufficiency. *Otolaryngol Head Neck Surg.* 2006;134:394–402.

31. Peterson-Falzone S, Trost-Cardamone J, Karnell M, et al. Articulation therapy for school-age children. In: *The Clinician's Guide to Treating Cleft Palate Speech.* St. Louis, MO: Mosby; 2005:124–160.

32. Golding-Kushner KJ. Therapy techniques for cleft palate speech and related disorders. In Golding-Kushner KJ, ed. *Therapy Techniques for Cleft Palate Speech and Related Disorders.* San Diego, CA: Singular; 2001.

33. Smith BE, Kuehn DP. Speech evaluation of velopharyngeal dysfunction. *J Craniofac Surg.* 2007;18:251–261; quiz 266–267.

34. Rudnick EF, Sie KC. Velopharyngeal insufficiency: current concepts in diagnosis and management. *Curr Opin Otolaryngol Head Neck Surg.* 2008;16:530–535.

35. Kummer AW. *Cleft Palate and Craniofacial Anomalies: Effects on Speech and Resonance.* 2nd ed. San Diego, CA: Singular/ Thomas Learning; 2008.

36. Ruscello D. Considerations for behavioral treatment of velopharyngeal closure for speech. In Bzoch KR, ed. *Communicative Disorders Related to Cleft Lip and Palate.* Austin, TX: Pro-Ed; 2004:763–796.

37. Kummer AW, Marty-Grames L, Jones DL, et al. Response to "Velopharyngeal dysfunction:

speech characteristics, variable etiologies, evaluation techniques, and differential treatments" by Dworkin, Marunick, and Krouse, October 2004. *Lang Speech Hear Serv Sch.* 2006;37:236-238; author reply 239-243.

38. Retrieved 11/22/08 from http://www.super duperinc.com/products/view.aspx?pid= ONL22 .

39. Retrieved 11/22/2008 from http://www .choa.org/default.aspx?id=762 .

40. Willging JP. Velopharyngeal insufficiency. *Curr Opin Otolaryngol Head Neck Surg.* 2003;11:452-455.

41. Tachimura T, Nohara K, Wada T. Effect of placement of a speech appliance on levator veli palatini muscle activity during speech. *Cleft Palate Craniofac J.* 2000;37:478-482.

42. Dworkin JP, Marunick MT, Krouse JH. Velopharyngeal dysfunction: speech characteristics, variable etiologies, evaluation techniques, and differential treatments. *Lang Speech Hear Serv Sch.* 2004;35:333-352.

43. Sell D, Mars M, Worrell E. Process and outcome study of multidisciplinary prosthetic treatment for velopharyngeal dysfunction. *Int J Lang Commun Disord.* 2006;41:495-511.

44. Kumar S, Hedge V. Prosthodontics in velopharyngeal insufficiency. *J Ind Prosthodont Soc.* 2007;7:12-16.

45. Passavant G. Ueber die Beseitigung der naselnden Sprache bei angeborenen Spalten des harten und weichen Gaumens. *Arch Klin Chir.* 1865;6:333-349.

46. Schoenborn D. Vorstellung eines Falles staphyloplastik. *Verhandlungen der Deutschen Gesellschaft fur Chirurgie.* 1886;15:57.

47. Cotton RT, Quattromani F. Lateral defects in velopharyngeal insufficiency. Diagnosis and treatment. *Arch Otolaryngol.* 1977;103: 90-93.

48. Hynes W. Pharyngoplasty by muscle transplantation. *Br J Plast Surg.* 1950;3:128-135.

49. Orticochea M. Construction of a dynamic muscle sphincter in cleft palates. *Plast Reconstr Surg.* 1968;41:323-327.

50. Jackson IT. Sphincter pharyngoplasty. *Clin Plast Surg.* 1985;12:711-717.

51. Witt PD, Marsh JL, Arlis H, et al. Quantification of dynamic velopharyngeal port excursion

following sphincter pharyngoplasty. *Plast Reconstr Surg.* 1998;101:1205-1211.

52. Lando RL. [Transplant of cadaveric cartilage into the posterior pharyngeal wall in treatment of cleft palate.] *Stomatologiia (Mosk).* 1950;4:38-39.

53. Hagerty RF, Hill MJ. Cartilage pharyngoplasty in cleft palate patients. *Surg Gynecol Obstet.* 1961;112:350-356.

54. Bluestone CD, Musgrave RH, McWilliams BJ, et al. Teflon injection pharyngoplasty. *Cleft Palate J.* 1968;5:19-22.

55. Blocksma R. Correction of velopharyngeal insufficiency by Silastic pharyngeal implant. *Plast Reconstr Surg.* 1963;31:268-274.

56. Sipp JA, Ashland J, Hartnick CJ. Injection pharyngoplasty with calcium hydroxyapatite for treatment of velopalatal insufficiency. *Arch Otolaryngol Head Neck Surg.* 2008; 134:268-271.

57. Funayama E, Igawa HH, Nishizawa N, et al. Velopharyngeal insufficiency in hemifacial microsomia: analysis of correlated factors. *Otolaryngol Head Neck Surg.* 2007;136: 33-37.

58. Argamaso RV, Levandowski GJ, Golding-Kushner KJ, et al. Treatment of asymmetric velopharyngeal insufficiency with skewed pharyngeal flap. *Cleft Palate Craniofac J.* 1994;31:287-294.

59. Armour A, Fischbach S, Klaiman P, et al. Does velopharyngeal closure pattern affect the success of pharyngeal flap pharyngoplasty? *Plast Reconstr Surg.* 2005;115:45-52; discussion 53.

60. Chegar BE, Shprintzen RJ, Curtis MS, et al. Pharyngeal flap and obstructive apnea: maximizing speech outcome while limiting complications. *Arch Facial Plast Surg.* 2007;9:252-259.

61. de Serres LM, Deleyiannis FW, Eblen LE, et al. Results with sphincter pharyngoplasty and pharyngeal flap. *Int J Pediatr Otorhinolaryngol.* 1999;48:17-25.

62. Lendrum J, Dhar BK. The Orticochea dynamic pharyngoplasty. *Br J Plast Surg.* 1984;37:160-168.

63. Meek MF, Coert JH, Hofer SO, et al. Short-term and long-term results of speech

improvement after surgery for velopharyngeal insufficiency with pharyngeal flaps in patients younger and older than 6 years old: 10-year experience. *Ann Plast Surg.* 2003; 50:13–17.

64. Pryor LS, Lehman J, Parker MG, et al. Outcomes in pharyngoplasty: a 10-year experience. *Cleft Palate Craniofac J.* 2006;43: 222–225.

65. Seagle MB, Mazaheri MK, Dixon-Wood VL, et al. Evaluation and treatment of velopharyngeal insufficiency: the University of Florida experience. *Ann Plast Surg.* 2002; 48:464–470.

66. Sie KC, Chen EY. Management of velopharyngeal insufficiency: development of a protocol and modifications of sphincter pharyngoplasty. *Fac Plast Surg.* 2007;23: 128–139.

67. Sie KC, Tampakopoulou DA, de Serres LM, et al. Sphincter pharyngoplasty: speech outcome and complications. *Laryngoscope.* 1998;108:1211–1217.

68. Abyholm F, D'Antonio L, Davidson Ward SL, et al. Pharyngeal flap and sphincterplasty for velopharyngeal insufficiency have equal outcome at 1 year postoperatively: results of a randomized trial. *Cleft Palate Craniofac J.* 2005;42:501–511.

69. Sloan GM. Posterior pharyngeal flap and sphincter pharyngoplasty: the state of the art. *Cleft Palate Craniofac J.* 2000;37: 112–122.

70. Kravath RE, Pollak CP, Borowiecki B, et al. Obstructive sleep apnea and death associated with surgical correction of velopharyngeal incompetence. *J Pediatr.* 1980;96:645–648.

71. Sato-Wakabayashi M, Inoue-Arai MS, Ono T, et al. Combined fMRI and MRI movie in the evaluation of articulation in subjects with and without cleft lip and palate. *Cleft Palate Craniofac J.* 2008;45:309–314.

72. Ragab A. Cerclage sphincter pharyngoplasty: a new technique for velopharyngeal insufficiency. *Int J Pediatr Otorhinolaryngol.* 2007;71:793–800.

73. Abdel-Aziz M. Palatopharyngeal sling: a new technique in treatment of velopharyngeal insufficiency. *Int J Pediatr Otorhinolaryngol.* 2008;72:173–177.

Paradoxic Vocal Fold Motion

Venu Divi
Mary J. Hawkshaw
Robert T. Sataloff

INTRODUCTION

Diagnosis and treatment of paradoxic vocal fold motion (PVFM) are challenging for the otolaryngologist and especially for the pediatric otolaryngologist. Commonly referred to as vocal cord dysfunction (VCD), PFVM is now the preferred term for the affliction. PVFM involves episodic, inappropriate adduction of the vocal folds during the inspiratory phase of the respiratory cycle resulting in intermittent (usually partial) glottic obstruction. It is important to distinguish between those patients with a true laryngeal disorder and those with other conditions that may appear to cause similar symptoms. In order to determine the etiology of this complex disorder, comprehensive neuro-laryngologic evaluation, usually including dynamic laryngeal assessment, strobovideo-laryngoscopy, and laryngeal electromyography (EMG), is essential. Consultation with a neurologist, pulmonologist, and gastroenterologist often is required. Psychological and voice therapy evaluations have proven useful, as well.

OVERVIEW

PVFM is a diagnosis that has been used widely, but the patients receiving this diagnosis actually may be suffering from one or more of a variety of disorders that may appear to impair upper respiratory tract function. Moreover, many patients who have paradoxic vocal fold adduction have been diagnosed incorrectly as having asthma. Originally described by Patterson et al[1] in 1974 as Munchausen's stridor, the etiology was first thought to be psychogenic. Other causes and exacerbating factors have been identified since that time, as well as other disorders that may present with similar symptoms. Maschka et al[2] described a classification scheme for paradoxic vocal fold motion based on 7 categories (Table 17–1), providing useful descriptions of the presenting symptoms associated with each of these diagnoses.

In addition to psychogenic causes and those listed in Table 17–1, other common diagnoses in patients referred to laryngologists for suspected PVFM include respiratory

Table 17–1. Maschka et al[2] Classification Scheme for Paradoxic Vocal Fold Motion

Feature	History	Associated Signs and Symptoms
Brainstem compression	Often otherwise unremarkable	Vagal dysfunction (velopharyngeal insufficiency, GERD)
Severe cortical injury	Static encephalopathy or cerebrovascular accident	Sialorrhea, upper airway obstruction, poor neuromuscular control
Nuclear or lower motor neuron injury	Medullary infarction, amyotrophic lateral sclerosis, myasthenia gravis	Other neurologic signs related to underlying etiology
Movement disorders	Exacerbated by stress or exertion	Other focal dystonias, tremors, rigidity, bradykinesia, decreased reflexes
Gastroesophageal reflux*	Otherwise unremarkable	May occur during calm, crying, or feeding
Factitious symptoms or malingering	Conscious effort to deceive	Underlying secondary gain
Somatiziation/conversion disorder	Unconscious manifestation of stress	Well motivated, high achievers

*Reflux is associated more commonly with laryngospasm than with true paradoxic adduction, in our experience (VD, MJH, RTS), and usually is accompanied by symptoms and signs of laryngopharyngeal reflux (LPR).

dystonia, laryngospasm, increased laryngeal irritability (usually due to reflux), and supraglottic collapse. All of these conditions are seen fairly commonly in children and adults; but in our experience, treatable organic etiologies are much more prevalent than psychogenic or serious neurologic causes.

Neurologic

Respiratory dystonia is a particularly important cause of PVFM. The condition is related to spasmodic dysphonia, but it affects respiration rather than voice. Dystonias that affect the respiratory function of the larynx may be accompanied primarily by other dystonic movements such as blepharospasm, mandibular dystonia, torticollis, spasmodic dysphonia, or upper-extremity tremors. This type of PFVM typically is better with sleep and worsens with stress and exertion. However, usually dystonic PVFM occurs alone and is called respiratory dystonia.[3,4] Patients with rhythmic adduction and abduction of the vocal folds may be found to have an associated palatal myoclonus. Kelman and Leopold[5] reported a patient with a brainstem lesion abnormality causing PVFM and suggested that the proximity of adductor and abductor neurons to each other in the nucleus ambiguus may permit inappropriate stimulation from the respiratory centers. The series reported by Maschka et al[2] also documented two patients with known central neurologic etiologies for their laryngeal movement disorders that were characterized by stridor and paradoxic vocal fold adduction during inspiration, but the patients had normal phonation.

Respiratory dystonia should be differentiated from psychogenic stridor and reflux-induced laryngeal spasm. Patients with true respiratory dystonia tend to demonstrate fairly consistent patterns of paradoxic vocal fold movement (adduction during inspiration) during respiratory and speech tasks, although the severity may vary. Many patients have worsening of their symptoms during stress and exertion. They differ from patients with reflux-induced laryngospasm who usually have acute episodes of sudden airway obstruction due to forceful vocal fold adduction, rather than chronic adduction associated with inspiration. They also differ from patients with psychogenic causes in their consistency even when they are not being observed. Respiratory dystonia is common and responds well to injection with botulinum toxin.

In children and adults, intracranial etiologies also must be investigated. Several intracranial abnormalities have been reported to give rise to PVFM, including Arnold-Chiari malformation, cerebral aqueductal stenosis, and compression of the nucleus ambiguus.[2] We have seen it associated with multiple sclerosis, as well. Static encephalopathy also may be associated with PVFM and may be accompanied by global developmental delay, hypertonia, spastic diplegia, and sialorrhea. These patients typically present as older children or adolescents, whereas those suffering from brainstem compression present typically during infancy or early childhood. The diagnosis in patients with cerebral compromise may be complicated by a narrowed airway at the level of the nasopharynx or oropharynx which causes increased inspiratory pressures and therefore may mimic PFVM, or actually cause

paradoxic adduction through Bernoulli effect. Correction of the upper airway obstruction may result in improvement and the level of the glottis in some cases.

Psychiatric

Patients may suffer episodes of airway obstruction in response to emotional stress or anxiety; and any past psychiatric history should be noted. "Munchausen's stridor," Patterson et al's original description[1] of unclassified stridor, has been supported by multiple other reports,[2,6-7] although it is likely that some of those reports inadvertently included patients with organic disorders such as respiratory dystonia that have been recognized much more recently. Vocal fold dysfunction of psychiatric origin has been called by many other names in the past including psychogenic stridor, functional stridor, and functional upper airway obstruction. It is imperative that the clinician rule out organic causes of airway obstruction and vocal fold dysfunction before attributing the respiratory symptoms to a nonorganic cause. Psychogenic PVFD is most common in young women and in members of the health care profession.[7] Over half of patients meet the diagnostic criteria for a psychological disorder, and up to 18% have a history of prior factitious disorder.[6,7] Other disorders such as anxiety, depression, personality disorders, stress disorders, or a history of sexual abuse may be present. Many of these patients have a characteristic worsening of symptoms upon observation and abatement of symptoms when they believe that they are not being observed. The main difference between a factitious/malingering disorder and a conversion disorder is that factitious/malingering disorders are expressed for secondary gain. According to the DSM-IV-TR,[8] a factitious disorder requires the presence of (1) intentional production or feigning of physical or psychological signs or symptoms, (2) motivation for the behavior is to assume the sick role, and (3) absence of external incentives for the behavior (eg, economic gain, avoiding legal responsibility, improving physical well-being, as in malingering). Malingering is not considered a medical condition and is described as the intentional production of false or exaggerated symptoms motivated by external incentives, such as obtaining compensation or drugs. Patients with conversion disorder typically have a preceding psychological or emotional incident that may have triggered an episode, although expert psychotherapy may be needed to identify the incident. Unlike malingering patients, those suffering from a conversion disorder are not aware that any underlying psychological insult is associated with their complaints. They are typically well motivated and compliant with therapy. Extensive testing in patients with conversion disorder typically yields no organic origin. Altman et al[9] documented a psychiatric illness in 70% of their patients presenting with PVFM, and other case reports have supported this observation.[6,7] This lends support to the original supposition that psychogenic or "conversion" disorder is present in some patients. However, it is not clear immediately in many cases whether there is a causal relationship between psychiatric abnormalities and PVFM, and thorough evaluation for psychiatric and organic causes is required in all cases.

Increased Laryngeal Irritability

Recent upper respiratory tract infection (URI) may have preceded the onset of symptoms and been associated with increased airway irritability that may lead to PVFM, especially if laryngopharyngeal reflux (LPR), also is present. Laryngeal hyperreactivity may be induced by LPR even without an URI, and the clinician should inquire about symptoms of laryngopharyngeal reflux including cough, throat clearing, hoarseness, globus sensation, "postnasal drip," and excess mucus production. LPR is a known cause of laryngeal irritability and has been reported in some studies to be present in up to 80% of patients with PVFM.[7,10]

The increased laryngeal irritability caused by LPR contributes to the laryngeal hypersensitivity seen in some patients with PVFM or laryngospasm mistaken for PVFM. Treatment of LPR must be accompanied by treatment of any other concomitant disorders.

Several inhaled antigens have been shown to increase laryngeal irritability and may trigger PVFM. Previously described triggers include air pollutants (dust, smoke), perfumed products (perfume, soap, detergents, and deodorants), chemical agents (paint), animal fur, and pollen.[10] Any relation between symptoms, environment and potential exposure should be investigated. An associated history of irritant exposure may be present as may a history of food or environmental allergies. A full allergy workup is warranted in patients in whom inhaled irritants are a suspected trigger. Caution must be exercised in associating PVFM with multiple chemical sensitivity disorder because of the controversies and complexities surrounding this diagnosis.

Supraglottic Collapse and Vocal Fold Hypomobility

Cystic fibrosis, partial airway obstruction, and other conditions that require high inspiratory pressures may draw the vocal folds or the supraglottic tissues toward the midline into the airway, through Bernoulli effect.[11] Careful observation should be made to see if supraglottic collapse is resulting in obstruction of airflow. This may be caused by conditions in which the laryngeal skeleton or tracheobroncheal tree is weakened, such as tracheomalacia or laryngomalacia. However, supraglottic (aryepiglottic fold and false vocal fold) collapse also may occur in children with tissue redundancy or laxity in the absence of any other abnormality. In addition, bilateral vocal fold paralysis commonly results in vocal fold adduction on inspiration. The narrow glottis causes high airflow, which in turn draws the vocal folds to the midline during inspiration (Bernoulli effect). Conditions such as cricoarytenoid joint dysfunction causing vocal fold hypomobility may present with stridor that can be confused with PFVM, as well; but the symptoms usually are less dramatic in these patients because they have innervated vocal folds with muscle tone that helps resist the Bernoulli effect. So, passive paradoxic adduction of the vocal folds usually is not seen in patients with normally innervated vocal folds.

EVALUATION

History and Physical Examination

Specific areas of questioning are necessary when working up at patient with suspected PVFM. Patients commonly are seen for otolaryngologic evaluation after they have been treated for refractory asthma unresponsive to bronchodilator or steroid therapy, or after an episode of acute respiratory distress. The patients have a history of emergency room visits for dyspnea treated with intubation

and occasionally even tracheotomy. In children, the episodes of respiratory distress often are associated with strenuous exercise, prompting an evaluation for asthma. However, unless asthma is present concurrently, methacholine challenge test may have been negative, but occasionally may be falsely positive for asthma (as discussed below). PVFM presents commonly in children during high levels of exertion, particularly in high performance athletes. This may have very severe ramifications. For example, patients may be striving to achieve an athletic scholarship and require evaluation for safety of continued participation in sports. Failure to achieve an accurate diagnosis and effective treatment may be life altering. Initially, symptoms typically are present during exertion or stress. However, as the condition progresses, symptoms may be present even at rest. PVFM episodes may be associated with stridor interpreted as wheezing, suprasternal retractions, dysphonia, or aphonia. The dysphonia or aphonia may precede the acute episode and linger after its resolution. Exercise-induced reflux may cause intermittent laryngospasm that can be mistaken for PVFM during the eliciting athletic activity, as well. If this condition is suspected, athletic activity should be performed with a multichannel pH-impedance monitor in place to confirm the diagnosis. Due to the demand of their schedules, many school athletes are prone to eating habits that may promote LPR, including eating late at night or immediately prior to an athletic event.[12,13]

A full allergic history should be taken including any respiratory inhalant allergens that have an association with the patient's dyspnea. The physician should inquire about recent respiratory infections as they may cause increased laryngeal irritability. A focused psychiatric history should be obtained with any positive answers pursued with a potential referral to a psychiatrist. Specific questions should be asked regarding stress levels and any correlation of social stress or other psychological factors with onset of respiratory symptoms. A history of throat clearing, globus sensation, excessive mucus, and hoarseness may indicate LPR as a potential etiology. Additional historical aspects of each topic were discussed with various specific etiologies.

Physical examination is the gold standard for diagnosing PVFM. A full head and neck examination should be performed including testing of the functions of all cranial nerves. Dynamic endoscopic laryngeal examination should note signs of reflux including posterior pachydermia, arytenoid erythema and edema, subglottic fullness, and vocal fold edema. Vocal fold motion should be documented and signs of upper aerodigestive tract collapse noted. Strobovideolaryngoscopy should be included even in patients who are not hoarse because the traumatic vocal fold contact that occurs during PVFM, laryngospasm, and other respiratory obstructive events results in vocal fold injury in many patients.

The presence of PVFM is confirmed through observation of vocal fold adduction during the inspiratory phase of respiration. Typically, the anterior two-thirds of the vocal folds medialize leaving a diamond-shaped posterior glottic chink, although near-complete glottic closure occurs in some patients. Observation of supraglottic or other structural collapse associated with symptoms also establishes a diagnosis. Although observation of active vocal fold adduction on inspiration confirms the diagnosis, the office examination may be normal if the patient is not placed in a situation that elicits the respiratory distress. Therefore, for patients who complain of airway distress during exercise, facilities should be present to allow the patient to perform physical activity with intensity equal to the eliciting activity. Cardiac and respiratory monitoring may be beneficial, although not necessary in all patients. This will allow for evaluation of any concomitant cardiac arrhythmias that may be present. There are case reports of patients who develop ventricular tachycardia during exertion which presents as airway obstruction (personal communication, Michael Johns, MD, 2007). In this situation, inspiration against glottic adduction allows a decrease in intrathoracic pressure which increases venous return in order to maintain cardiac output. Other maneuvers, such as repetitive rapid deep inspirations, alternating phonating the /i/ vowel, and sniffing, and other speaking tasks may elicit the abnormal laryngeal movement in some patients.[5]

Laryngeal EMG provides information regarding neuromuscular function which can be used to determine whether adductor muscles are active during the inspiratory phase of the respiratory cycle. EMG gives information regarding the amount of muscle contraction and synchrony of paired firing. In patients with a spasmodic dysphonia, a condition related to respiratory dystonia, EMG demonstrates an increase in discharge from the vocalis muscle at rest and during phonation, as well. Warnes and Allen[14] utilized EMG to determine the effectiveness of biofeedback and voice therapy. They showed that during a course of treatment, electrical discharge from the laryngeal musculature at rest decreased until a normative level was reached. This was achieved with surface electrodes which significantly increase feasibility over needle electrodes when treating children. To the best of our knowledge, similar therapy has not been tried for respiratory dystonia, but the concept seems worthy of investigation.

Airway fluoroscopy also may be used in diagnostic evaluation to determine the presence of diaphragmatic dys-synergism with the vocal folds. This results in an uncoordinated depression of the diaphragm while the vocal folds are still in the midline.

Flow-volume spirometry is very useful in supporting the diagnosis of PVFM, too. During an acute episode, "flattening" of the inspiratory limb is seen, demonstrating an extrathoracic upper airway obstruction (Fig 17–1). When the patients are asymptomatic, the flow-volume loop will return to normal. The expiratory/inspiratory flow ratio is typically greater than 2.[15] Unlike asthma and other forms of intrathoracic small airway obstruction in which FEV_1 is reduced, the FEV_1 is preserved in PVFM. Pulmonary function testing also may be used in association with methacholine challenge or bronchodilator medication to rule out concomitant asthma. Guss and Mirza[15] published a report of 7 patients sent to an otolaryngology clinic for choking and dyspnea. Only 3 patients in the study were found to have a 20% reduction in their FEV_1 consistent with the presence of asthma. Three of the other patients developed documented PVFM with methacholine challenge typically utilized for diagnosis of asthma. This is most likely due to excessive laryngeal hypersensitivity, although the mechanism has not been proven. These patients may be misdiagnosed with asthma and found to be nonresponsive to treatment. Although these patients were not the same ones diagnosed with PVFM, Newman et al[7] found that 53 of 95 patients with confirmed PVFM suffered from asthma, as well. Table 17–2 compares the various features of PVFM versus asthma.[12]

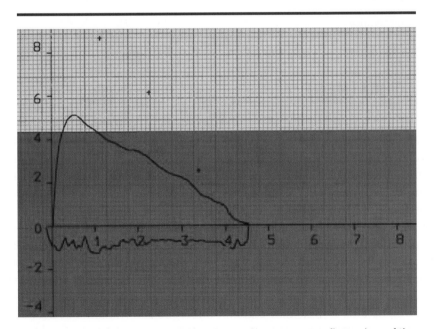

Fig 17–1. The flow-volume loop above demonstrates flattening of the inspiratory limb, demonstrating an extrathoracic airway obstruction as seen in PVFM.

Table 17–2. Distinguishing Diagnostic Features of PVFM and Asthma[12]

Diagnostic Feature	PVFM	Asthma
Chest tightness	Yes/No	Yes
Throat tightness	Yes	No
Stridor with inhalation	Yes	No
Wheezing with expiration	No	Yes
Types of triggers	Exercise, extreme temperature (hot or cold), airway irritants (GERD), emotional stressors	Exercise, extreme temperature (hot or cold), airway irritants, allergens, emotional stressors
Number of triggers	Usually one	Usually multiple
Usual onset of symptoms after beginning exercise	<5 min; however, can be variable	>5–10 min
Recovery period	5–10 min	15–60 min
Response to bronchodilators and/or systemic corticosteroids	No response	Good response
Nocturnal awakening with symptoms	Rarely	Almost always
Female preponderance	Yes	No

TREATMENT

Patients who present to the emergency room with an acute episode of respiratory distress typically are treated as a patient suffering from an asthma attack or an acute airway obstruction. Many patients receive beta-2 agonists and corticosteroids. If the symptoms do not abate, intubation, and at times emergency tracheotomy, is used to control the airway. Heliox, a combination of helium and oxygen, which has a lower molecular weight and is less dense than oxygen, can ease the dyspnea of patients with respiratory distress.[16] The lighter molecular weight gas results in less turbulence across the narrowed glottis. Christo-

pher et al[17] found that the wheezing and dyspnea resolved in all patients suffering from laryngospasm when a 20% helium/oxygen mixture was administered. However, these emergency treatments usually are used in patients in whom the diagnosis of PVFM has not been made or even suspected.

There are many different treatment approaches for the treatment of PVFM, and the most appropriate modalities depend on the cause. Biofeedback is an effective method for retraining some patients to manage an acute episode. Laryngeal image biofeedback, initially described by Bastian and Nagorsky[18] has been shown to be an effective learning tool for patients to mimic target tasks. This study demonstrated that patients can reliably alter laryngeal movements and postures using laryngeal image feedback in the absence of auditory-perceptual cues. Visual laryngoscopic biofeedback in association with speech therapy has been effective as definitive treatment in some patients, although it is only partially effective in most. A variety of other noninvasive therapeutic approaches have been used with varying success including respiratory retraining, psychological educational approaches, and other techniques to restore sensory and motor function and control. Behavioral management may be partially effective in some cases. For example, many patients have less prominent paradoxic adduction during

nasal breathing than during oral breathing, especially patients who do not have respiratory dystonia. Focusing on nasal breathing is very helpful for such patients in managing a crisis situation. Martin et al[19] described a speech therapy program which divided treatment of the acute episode into 7 steps. These steps were designed around the concepts of pitch change, diaphragmatic breathing, and extrinsic muscle tension reduction. A summary of the seven steps is included in Table 17–3.

When patients have a psychiatric component to their respiratory distress, it is often helpful not to imply initially that they

Table 17–3. 7-Step Behavioral Treatment for PVFM[19]

1. Providing the patient's slow direction and acknowledging the patient's fear and helplessness and that the stridor is real.
2. Utilizing a behavioral approach to exercises so that with self-awareness and good breathing patterns, the patients will be prepared to voluntarily control an attack when it occurs.
3. Advising use of diaphragmatic breathing, such as is used by professional singers, directs attention away from the larynx. This gives the patients a place to focus body awareness, so respiratory effort can be utilized without producing laryngeal, clavicular, or thoracic tension. The patient concentrates on pushing the lower abdomen out with inspiratory descent of the diaphragm. On expiration, the patient concentrates on utilizes support from the lower abdominal muscles.
4. Advising use of "wide-open throat" breath, concentrating on having the lips closed, the tongue lying flat on the floor of the mouth behind the lower front teeth, with the buccal areas of the mouth relaxed, releasing the jaw gently, and using diaphragmatic inhalation and exhalation techniques.
5. Advising the patient to focus on exhalation interrupts the patients' tendency to feel that they are unable to get any more breath and to hold onto their breath. They are taught to exhale, release their breath, and then allow inhalation to follow effortlessly. They are allowed to develop an exhalation count, so they know they can maintain exhalation up to that number of counts, and avoid gasping for air.
6. Increasing self-awareness of the breathing sequence of inhalation and exhalation decreases the feeling of helplessness via increased self-awareness of the correct sequence of the breathing process.
7. Interrupting effortful breathing is fostered by developing the attitude that their breathing does not have to be actively performed but is part of a natural body process that can be gradually trusted and practiced.

have a psychiatric illness that is causing their problem. First, the psychological symptoms may be secondary. Second, even if they are not, many patients and families are more willing to accept psychological consultation if it develops as an outgrowth of good rapport with a laryngologist and voice pathologist. If patients are told abruptly that their illness is psychiatric in origin, they may be resistant to voice therapy and psychotherapy; and, in addition, the diagnosis may prove to be wrong.

Although both speech-language pathologists and psychologists have a role in behavioral treatment of PVFM, a speech-language pathologist is more appropriately suited for initial treatment. In addition to addressing the emotional issues associated with this illness, speech-language pathologists are instrumental in teaching the patient how to avoid and/or deal with an acute episode of dyspnea. Initial referral to a psychologist may imply to the patient and family members that the physician believes the problem to be "in the patient's head." The anxiety associated with PVFM and related disorders is a significant component of the disorder. The need for psychologic evaluation and treatment for both the patient and the family is a concept that should be introduced gradually to ensure that the patient is openly receptive to the treatment.

Botulinum toxin has been used with success to treat respiratory dystonia. This concept was introduced in 1992 by Brin et al[3] In their series of seven patients with PVFM, four were offered vocalis muscle Botox injections with outstanding relief of laryngeal symptoms. Five of the 10 patients reported by Altman et al[9] responded at least partially to botulinum toxin injected into the thyroarytenoid muscle, and two of them had other dystonias. In our experience, EMG-confirmed adductor muscle activity during respiration, in combination with other findings that suggest respiratory dystonia, indicates that Botox has a higher likelihood of being an effective treatment. Interestingly, respiratory dystonia which is not accompanied by dysphonia responds extremely well to low doses of botulinum toxin injected into the thyroarytenoid muscle, although associated respiratory dysrhythmia may persist.

More aggressive airway management strategies have been described. Lloyd and Jones[20] have described a patient in whom an arytenoidectomy and partial cordectomy were performed. PVFM persisted 2 weeks after the procedure, and the patient then underwent a stitch lateralization of the vocal fold. The percutaneous stitch was removed after 6 weeks and the patient was symptom-free for 1 year. Eventually, she did require tracheotomy and completion arytenoidectomy. This treatment, although seemingly aggressive, may be necessary to decannulate patients who have refractory PVFM, but such intervention should be needed in exceedingly rare cases (none, in our experience).

Soft tissue surgery has proven very helpful in patients with supraglottic collapse. Excision of redundant supraglottic tissue (usually using a CO_2 laser) eliminates the collapsing tissue and alters aerodynamics resulting in cure of the symptoms in most cases, if the diagnosis is correct and if the supraglottic collapse is not being caused by stenosis or other pathology elsewhere in the respiratory tract.

CONCLUSION

PVFM is uncommon but not rare. Dystonic and psychogenic causes are encountered frequently and can be treated effectively. Supraglottic tissue collapse, reflux and other causes of laryngeal hyperirritability, and other conditions may produce PVFM or symptoms similar to those of PVFM that must be differentiated from true paradoxic adduction. Organic etiologies should be sought in all patients. Botulinum toxin provides effective control for patients with respiratory dystonia, and voice therapy and psychological intervention are valuable in many cases. Surgery is necessary only rarely for PVFM but is curative in most patients with isolated supraglottic collapse. Otolaryngologists should be able to diagnose and treat effectively virtually all patients who present with symptoms consistent with PVFM, in collaboration with an expert team of therapists and consulting physicians in other specialties.

REFERENCES

1. Patterson R, Schatz M, Horton M. Munchausen's stridor: non-organic laryngeal obstruction. *Clin Allergy*. 1974;4:307-310.
2. Maschka D, Bauman N, McGray P, Hoffman H, Karnell M, Smith R. A classification scheme for paradoxic vocal cord motion. *Laryngoscope*. 1997;107:1429-1435.
3. Brin MF, Blitzer A, Stewart C, Fahn S. Treatment of spasmodic dysphonia (laryngeal dystonia) with local injections of botulinum toxin: review and technical aspects. In: Blitzer A, Brin M, Sasaki C, et al, eds. *Neurologic Disorders of the Larynx*. New York, NY: Thieme; 1993:225.
4. Morrison M, Rammage L, Emami AJ. The irritable larynx syndrome. *J Voice*. 1999;13:447-455.
5. Kellman RM, Leopold DA. Paradoxical vocal cord motion: an important cause of stridor. *Laryngoscope*. 1982;92:58-60.
6. O'Connell M, Sklarew P, Goodman D. Spectrum of presentation of paradoxical vocal cord motion in ambulatory patients. *Ann Allergy Asthma Immunol*. 1995;14:341-344.
7. Newman KB, Mason UG, Schmaling KB. Clinical features of vocal cord dysfunction. *Am J Resp Crit Care Med*. 1995;152:1382-1386.
8. American Psychiatric Association. *Diagnostic and Statistical Manual of Mental Disorders,* 4th ed. Washington DC: Author; 1994:683.
9. Altman K, Mirza N, Ruiz C, Sataloff R. Paradoxical vocal fold motion: presentation and treatment options. *J Voice*. 2000;14:99-103.
10. Andrianopoulos M, Gallivan G, Gallivan H. PVCM, PVCD, EPL, and irritable larynx syndrome: what are we talking about and how do we treat it? *J Voice*. 2000;14:607-618.
11. Sataloff RT, Deems D. In: *Professional Voice: The Science and Art of Clinical Care*. 3rd ed. San Diego, Calif: Plural Publishing; 2005:887-902.
12. Sandage MJ, Zelany SK. Paradoxical vocal fold motion in children and adolescents. *Lang Speech Hear Serv Schools*. 2004;35(4):353-362.
13. McFadden ER, Zawadski DK. Vocal cord dysfunction masquerading as exercise-induced asthma. *Am J Respir Criti Care Med*. 1996;153:942-947.
14. Warnes E, Allen K. Biofeedback treatment of paradoxical vocal fold motion and respiratory distress in an adolescent girl. *J App Behavr Anal*. 2005;38:529-532.
15. Guss J, Mirza N. Methacholine challenge testing in the diagnosis of paradoxical vocal fold motion. *Laryngoscope*. 2006;116:1558-1561.
16. Gallivan G, Hoffman L, Gallivan H. Episodic parxysmal laryngospasm: voice and pulmonary function assessment and management. *J Voice*. 1996;10:93-105.
17. Christopher KL, Wood RP, Eckert RC, Blager FB, Raney RA, Soudhrada JF. Vocal cord dysfunction presenting as asthma. *N Eng J Med*. 1983;308:1566-1570.

18. Bastian R, Nagorsky M. Laryngeal image bio-feedback. *Laryngoscope*. 1987;97:1346–1349.

19. Martin RJ, Blager FB, Gay ML, Wood RP II. Paradoxic vocal cord motion in presumed asthmatics. *Semin Resp Med*. 1987;8:332–337.

20. Lloyd RV, Jones NS. Paradoxical vocal fold movement: a case report. *J Laryngol Otol*. 1995;109:1105–1106.

Psychiatric and Psychological Interventions for Pediatric Voice Disorders

Abigail L. Donovan
Bruce J. Masek

INTRODUCTION

In medicine, there is great temptation to classify disease as "organic" or "psychiatric."[1] However, there are many illnesses that straddle these boundaries and require a dual approach, that is, an approach informed by both medical and psychological factors. These illnesses, including pediatric voice disorders such as habit cough and paradoxical vocal fold movement (PVFM), reside somewhere in between the mind and the body. In some cases, organic disease may trigger the voice symptom, which is then maintained by psychological factors; in other cases, psychological stresses or primary psychiatric illnesses may be predominantly manifested in voice symptoms. Thus, these pediatric voice disorders are diseases in which psychological factors may play a significant role in the onset, exacerbation, or maintenance of the illness. Moreover, these disorders have been found to be responsive to psychological and psychiatric interventions when medical interventions have been unsuccessful.

BACKGROUND

Habit cough is also sometimes referred to as psychogenic cough, as the disorder frequently co-occurs with the advent of an emotional stressor in the patient's life. Habit cough typically develops after a respiratory infection, although the cough persists after the resolution of the infection for weeks, months, and, in some cases, years.[2] One hypothesis is that the physical illness triggers an irritation in the throat that leads to cough; the ongoing cough then leads to further throat irritation, which in turn produces more cough, creating a positive feedback loop. Habit cough is characterized by a repetitive, nonproductive cough which is "seal-like" or "honking." The cough can occur up to several hundred times an hour while the patient is awake, it frequently improves when the patient is distracted, and it is usually absent when the patient is asleep.[3] Adolescents account for 90% of reported cases.[4] Approximately 3 to 10% of children with a cough of unknown origin for greater than 1 month will receive a diagnosis of habit cough.[5] Chest radiographs and pulmonary function testing are usually normal and the cough is unresponsive to bronchodilators, anti-inflammatory medications, and cough suppressants. The intensity and frequency of the cough can vary greatly from patient to patient. Some patients are able to continue functioning normally, whereas others may be unable to attend school or participate in social activities.

Paradoxical vocal fold movement (PVFM), also known as vocal fold dysfunction (VFD), is characterized by the paradoxical adduction of the anterior two-thirds of the vocal cords during the inspiratory phase of the respiration cycle. PVFM presents clinically as episodic inspirational stridor and the episodes may start and resolve abruptly.[6] The episodes occur more frequently during the daytime and improve while the patient is asleep or distracted.[6] PVFM is commonly initially misdiagnosed as asthma, although it should be noted that the two disorders are not mutually exclusive. In one study of patients hospitalized for PVFM, greater than 50% also had asthma.[7] However, the symptoms of PVFM do not improve with inhaled bronchodilators or anti-inflammatory medications. The clinical presentation can be quite dramatic and may also mimic the stridor characteristic of a foreign body aspiration. The diagnosis of PVFM can be made definitively by utilizing laryngoscopy to visualize the adducted folds in the inspiration phase, during an acute

episode. The adduction is not visible when the patient is asymptomatic; thus, a normal laryngoscopy does not exclude PVFM.

In pediatrics, PVFM is most commonly seen in adolescents and it is thought to occur more frequently in females.[7,8] It has also been reported to occur in elite athletes with acute onset during sporting events.[9] One study estimates a 5% prevalence of PVFM in elite athletes.[10] PVFM may be associated with anxiety, as pediatric patients with PVFM have been found to have higher levels of anxiety and a higher number of anxiety related diagnoses by structured interview.[11]

CASE STUDIES

The most complex cases of voice disordered pediatric patients are treated at tertiary academic medical centers. The availability of pediatric otolaryngologists, pulmonologists, psychologists, and child psychiatrists allows for the multidisciplinary approach to treatment, as is illustrated in the following two cases.

Case 1: Philip

Philip is a 12-year-old Korean boy, adopted by white parents as an infant, who developed an incessant, nonproductive cough which caused him to miss 2 months of school. The medical evaluation, including larygnoscopy and endoscopy, revealed no abnormalities. Immediately prior to the onset of his cough, Philip had been asking his adoptive parents specific questions about his adoption and birth parents. Philip was diagnosed with habit cough and underwent laryngeal botulinum toxin injection, which led to a complete resolution of his cough for 10 weeks. Although he had been referred for psychiatric evaluation, he was not evaluated until his cough returned. This reoccurrence transpired shortly after his mother received information regarding abnormal lab values related to her kidney transplant, although she had been healthy for the previous 12 years.

At the time of reoccurrence, Philip was evaluated by a psychologist specializing in behavioral medicine who agreed with the diagnosis of habit cough. Philip then underwent 6 sessions of biofeedback training, with complete resolution of his symptoms. He was also referred for psychotherapy to address psychological issues related to his adoption. He remains free of symptoms 12 months after treatment.

Case 2: Mary

Mary is a 13-year-old girl with a learning disorder who was medically healthy until she developed stridor suddenly while on a school field trip. During the field trip, Mary complained of inhaling some dust. She developed inspiratory stridor that occurred with every inhalation and was absent only during sleep. Thorough medical evaluation, including neck and chest X-ray, revealed no abnormality. Laryngoscopy revealed paradoxical vocal fold movement. Mary subsequently underwent botulinum toxin injection to the thyroarytenoid muscle on two separate occasions, without relief from her symptoms. After the first injection, she was referred for biofeedback training, although treatment was discontinued after 3 sessions as her symptoms were slightly worse.

Mary then underwent four sessions of hypnosis and practiced self-hypnosis in between sessions. Each session produced a measurable decrease in both the frequency and the intensity of her stridor that lasted progressively longer (hours to days) between sessions. Concurrently, she participated both in individual psychotherapy and in family therapy. Her individual therapy was partially focused on increasing her coping skills for anxiety and stress, particularly school-based symptoms. In addition, Mary was prescribed risperidone and citalopram, to address issues of anxiety and depression. After the fourth session of hypnosis, with psychotherapy and medication, Mary's symptoms resolved completely, and have not returned at 6-month follow-up.

ASSESSMENT

Prior to referral to a mental health specialist, a thorough medical evaluation must be completed, in order to accurately make the diagnosis of habit cough or PFVM, as well as to rule out any medical illnesses. Medical evaluation should assess for asthma, infection, foreign body aspiration, chronic sinusitis, laryngopharyngeal reflux, subglottic stenosis, tracheomalacia, and adenotonsilitis. Both habit cough and PVFM may be triggered or exacerbated by medical conditions, which should be appropriately treated prior to psychological treatment. Specifically, PVFM may be triggered or exacerbated by postnasal drip, GERD, and asthma,[12,13] whereas habit cough may be triggered by a variety of infections.

Once a definitive diagnosis is made, not every patient with habit cough or PVFM will require evaluation and treatment by a mental health professional. Speech therapy can teach the patient relaxed throat breathing and diaphragmatic breathing and has been shown to be effective treatment for PVFM.[14] Reassurance by medical professionals that the symptom does not represent serious physical illness may also be therapeutic.

For patients that do require treatment by a mental health professional, appropriate referral is critical and delay can be potentially detrimental. The pediatric voice specialist should consider referral to a mental health professional under the following circumstances: when no organic etiology is found after thorough medical evaluation, when the symptoms have not responded to conventional treatment, when speech therapy has failed to produce adequate results, when the symptoms are clearly triggered by stress, when the patient appears to derive secondary gain from the symptoms, such as when school refusal is present, or when the symptoms are disproportionate to the physical signs of illness. Although there may be new and innovative procedures for the treatment of these disorders, for the patient who has failed standard treatment, it is wise to consider psychological evaluation, if available in a timely manner, prior to initiation of experimental procedures.

Research has indicated that some patients with PVFM have high levels of anxiety[11]; however, the prevalence of other psychiatric disorders in this population is not currently known. As a result, it is difficult to determine specific criteria for referral to a mental health provider in this population. Thus, the pediatric voice specialist must determine the need for psychological assessment on a case by case basis. The specialist should observe for obvious signs of anxiety or depression, as well as for the presence of clear social stressors or family discord, all of which should prompt referral to a mental health professional. However, in the absence of obvious psychopathology or psychological distress, it is wise to proceed with medical treatment and speech therapy, until these modalities of treatment have been proven unsuccessful. In addi-

tion, mental health services for children are scarce, especially outside of large medical centers. For the otolaryngologist who practices within a large medical center, it is reasonable to secure the services of a mental health practitioner for more rapid psychological assessment and ancillary treatment.

A psychological assessment of the voice disordered patient will contain standard elements. The first is a detailed Functional Behavioral Assessment (FBA) of the symptom in the context of the patient's environment. This type of assessment examines the role that the symptom plays in the patient's life and the impact that it has on the patient's environment. For example, an adolescent with habit cough may be excused from music lessons, gym class, or the entire day of school due to the cough. If the adolescent is motivated to miss these activities, then the "medical excuse" of habit cough represents a powerful negative reinforcer, as it allows escape from an undesirable aspect of the patient's environment. Or, the young child whose habit cough occurs in a specific situation in response to the attention it draws from her parents.[15] In this case, it was determined through behavioral observation and reinforcement that the frequency of the cough could be manipulated by parents using social attention or tangible rewards. By shifting their attention to cough-free intervals, they quickly extinguished the symptom permanently. Understanding the role that the symptom plays in the world of the patient may in turn lead to possible therapeutic interventions. The function of the symptom is frequently not consciously known by the patient and an explanation of the clinician's hypothesis, in nonjudgmental language, is often helpful. Then, alternative means for meeting the patient's needs must be explored. For the patient with school refusal, the reason for the school refusal needs to be examined.

This issue is often complex and a detailed assessment will need to examine the possibility of an undiagnosed learning disorder, as was the case with Mary, or social stress at school, such as bullying. This type of patient may then benefit from increased academic or social support at school. For the patient who consciously or unconsciously needs more time with a parent, setting up a schedule of daily, dedicated one-on-one time may be a successful intervention.

The second element of the psychological assessment will be a thorough evaluation of stressors in the environment that coincide with the onset of symptoms. Careful analysis is important, as adolescents may have become so desensitized to the circumstances that sometimes they do not even recognize them as stressful. In addition, thoughts and feelings about potentially stressful events may be suppressed by adolescents and denied as a cause of distress. Nonjudgmental and open-ended questions are important tools for eliciting information without putting the adolescent in a defensive position. Pertinent examples of environmental stressors from clinical practice include divorce or separation of the parents, significant medical or psychiatric illness in a parent or sibling, as was the case with Philip, moving or changing schools, and the loss of a relative or friend. Some children and adolescents are unable to express their distress in words and, therefore, unconsciously express distress through physical symptoms, such as habit cough or other voice disorders. This process is entirely unconscious and should not be confused with malingering or a factitious disorder. These patients may benefit from time-limited therapy to have an opportunity to express their distress in words, thus obviating the need for the symptom.

The third element of the psychological assessment will be a thorough evaluation for the presence of psychopathology. It should be noted that not all patients with voice disorders will have major psychopathology, but rather this group is a distinct minority. Psychiatric disorders that have been associated with voice disorders include major depressive disorder, generalized anxiety disorder, and conversion disorder. In fact, patients with PVFM may be more likely to have generalized anxiety disorder and anxiety-related diagnoses, such as Separation anxiety, when compared to asthmatic controls.[11] In addition, the symptoms of Tourette's disorder, transient tic disorder, and chronic tic disorder may mimic the symptoms of both PVFM and habit cough and should be thoughtfully evaluated by the mental health clinician.

MANAGEMENT

The psychological management of pediatric voice disorders can be divided into several categories: biofeedback, self-hypnosis, psychotherapy, and medication. Currently, there have been no clinical studies assessing the efficacies of the various treatment modalities compared to each other. However, they have individually been found to be successful with a wide variety of cases. Thus, the choice of which modality to use for a given patient is at the discretion of the clinician. Moreover, if one modality fails to produce remission of the symptoms, a second or third modality can be tried.

In addition to primary psychological management of the symptoms, patients will also benefit from regular follow-up visits with the voice specialist. These follow-up visits allow for ongoing objective assessments of symptom severity and serve to reassure the patient that no major medical illness is present. Reassuring the patient and the family on an ongoing basis is critical to the success of any psychological symptom management.

Some patients and families may be reluctant to accept the absence of organic causes or "physical" findings, or may be reluctant to accept referral to a mental health clinician for a "medical" condition. For these patients and families, it may be helpful to frame the role of psychological treatment as important for coping with illness, or with the stress that ongoing symptoms cause.

Biofeedback

A scattering of case reports document the usefulness of biofeedback alone, and in combination with psychological therapies, to treat VFD,[16,17] PVFM,[18] and habit cough.[4,19] In only two studies did biofeedback training target specific muscles thought to be involved in the production of symptoms.[16,17]

The most common application of biofeedback training is to facilitate learning relaxation techniques to modulate arousal and control muscle hypertonicity. In this paradigm, measurement of physiologic activity is achieved using noninvasive sensor technology to record muscle activity, heart rate, skin temperature, and respiration. Signals are processed by a computer and "fed back" to the patient as a readily interpretable analogue representation on a computer monitor. With this information, patients learn to lower sympathetic arousal and refine control of skeletal muscle activity as they are taught and practice relaxation techniques. How biofeedback works is a matter of conjecture, but presumably learning to control physiologic responses is educational and reinforcing.

Biofeedback has been used in the treatment of a wide range of medical and psychi-

atric disorders in children and adolescents. Patients as young as 7 years of age can learn to control maladaptive physiologic responses with the aid of biofeedback. With few exceptions, sensors attach to skin that is readily accessible using adhesive disks, Velcro, or paper tape. Patients are seated in a reclining chair facing a computer monitor in a room controlled for ambient light and sound. Initially, it is important for a parent to be present to observe the procedural aspects of biofeedback and to help the child process the learning experience outside of the session.

In Philip's case, biofeedback sessions started with attaching three self-adhesive EMG electrodes to his throat over the laryngeal muscle area, which had been wiped with an alcohol prep; a photoplethysmograph was fastened with Velcro to the volar surface of his right middle finger; and a thermistor was taped to the volar surface of his right index finger. Total preparation time of approximately 3 minutes allowed for 30 minutes of biofeedback training per session.

In all but the mildest of cases, habit cough is an intrusive and distressing symptom for the individual and those in proximity. As a result, child and adolescent patients often find themselves segregated with a 1:1 tutor outside of their normal classroom and soon thereafter with home tutoring. Philip was still attending school in his regular classroom because the symptom occurred at a low rate (1 to 2 times per minute). His ability to concentrate and retain information was deemed reasonably intact, which was an important consideration before starting treatment. In addition, his resting baseline EMG activity was well above the upper normal limit, such that it was feasible to use biofeedback training as a focused learning tool to decrease EMG activity to normal limits.

In contrast, Mary's inspirational stridor occurred 20 to 30 times per minute and was quite audible above normal room conversation. The symptom proved to be too big a distraction during biofeedback training, which made her more anxious because she had high expectations for the treatment to be successful.

Self-Hypnosis

The portrayal of hypnosis in popular culture bears little resemblance to the self-hypnosis utilized in a therapeutic setting. Hypnosis does not involve mind control, or the hypnotist causing people to perform actions against their will. In a therapeutic setting, hypnosis is more accurately described as self-hypnosis, as the patient is the active agent and actually hypnotizes him- or herself. Hypnosis is best understood as a natural mental state characterized by deep relaxation. Children may be exceptionally good candidates for the therapeutic use of hypnosis given their ability to engage in imaginary play.

Self-hypnosis has been shown to be an effective treatment for habit cough. In one recent study, 78% of patients with habit cough had complete resolution of their symptoms after a single session and an additional 12% within the next month.[2] The mechanism of action of self-hypnosis, although not fully understood, likely relates to the promotion of increased relaxation and an alteration in the perception of the cough trigger.[2] Self-hypnosis also promotes patient autonomy and self-reliance and restores the locus of control to the patient.

Self-hypnosis has also been shown to be an effective treatment for vocal fold dysfunction. At a pediatric pulmonary center, 38% percent of pediatric patients with vocal fold dysfunction had a complete resolution of their symptoms, and an additional 31% had significant improvement in their symptoms, after a single hypnosis session.[20]

In the case of Mary, self-hypnosis was successful in reducing and, with the aid of psychotherapy and medication, eventually completely resolving her symptoms after 4 sessions. Mary found self-hypnosis to be a successful coping skill and she developed a sense of mastery and self-confidence based on her ability to effectively cope with the stress in her environment.

Psychotherapy

Psychotherapy may be useful for the pediatric voice disorder patient. Psychotherapy can be used to explore the stressors in a patient's life and suggest means for modifying them. For example, the talented and highly competitive teenage athlete with PVFM may be unable to initially identify the stress that athletic performance plays in his or her life. The issue may further be complicated by the confidence that athletic achievement can bring, subtle or unspoken parental pressure to perform, or even the necessity of college scholarships. As another example, the child with habit cough may be unable to cope with the stress of a divorce and the parent's new romantic relationship. This social stress may be further complicated by feelings of jealousy, and a wish to see the parents reunite. Psychotherapy can be instrumental in untangling these compelling forces and discovering alternative solutions.

Psychotherapy may also be useful in offering the patient alternative means to cope with stress. Some patients may benefit from learning concrete methods for coping with stress, such as visualization, deep breathing, progressive muscle relaxation, and distraction. Other patients may find that the act of participating in psychotherapy, having a place to discuss the difficulty in their lives, may be a successful coping skill itself. In addition, the psychotherapist may function as a useful mediator between parents and child, and can advocate on behalf of the child for reducing or eliminating environmental stress in the form of advanced classes, highly competitive sports teams, or overly high expectations.

Medication

There has been only extremely limited research on the role of psychiatric medications in the treatment of pediatric voice disorders. There is no FDA-approved medication for the treatment of habit cough or PVFM. However, this does not mean that some patients with PVFM or habit cough will not benefit from the judicious use of psychiatric medication.

It has been reported in the literature that patients with PVFM are more likely to have anxiety disorders.[11] However, research indicates that anxiolytic medication is no more effective than placebo when treating the general population of patients with PVFM.[8] Therefore, the use of anxiolytic medication should be reserved for a smaller subset of voice disorder patients who display symptoms of anxiety independent of their voice disorder. For patients who meet full diagnostic criteria for an anxiety disorder, pharmacologic management is also indicated.

There are several pharmacologic options for the treatment of anxiety in this population, including benzodiazepines and selective serotonin reuptake inhibitors (SSRIs). Short-term use of benzodiazepines, such as lorazepam (Ativan) and clonazepam (Klonopin), may provide immediate relief,

given their quick onset of action; however, the physiologic dependence associated with these medications makes them less ideal for long-term therapy. SSRIs, including fluoxetine (Prozac), paroxetine (Paxil), sertraline (Zoloft), citalopram (Celexa), or escitalopram (Lexapro), have a more favorable side-effect profile for long-term therapy for anxiety disorders, although they can take up to 6 to 8 weeks to show efficacy. Low doses of atypical antipsychotic medications, such as risperidone (Risperdal), quetiapine (Seroquel), or olanzapine (Zyprexa), although not FDA approved for the treatment of anxiety, may also be helpful. When prescribing these medications, laboratory values such as fasting glucose, cholesterol, and prolactin may need to be monitored regularly. There is a case report of pimozide (Orap), a typical antipsychotic, being curative for habit cough,[21] although the side-effect profile, including the risk for tardive dyskinesia, makes this medication an unattractive option for most pediatric patients.

Some patients with voice disorders may endorse symptoms of anxiety that fall below the threshold of diagnosis. There has been no research examining the use of anxiolytic medication in this subpopulation, although one might hypothesize that medication could be beneficial in relieving their anxiety symptoms and decreasing their level of distress.

A subset of patients may also experience symptoms of depression either preceding their voice disorder or as a result of the voice disorder. These patients may benefit from antidepressant therapy, after thorough psychiatric evaluation. In this case, first-line therapy for uncomplicated depression would be an SSRI. Given that these medications have potentially serious side effects, they should only be prescribed by a physician well trained in their use.

CONCLUSION

Pediatric voice disorders originate in both the mind and the body. Furthermore, successful treatment may include medical interventions, psychological interventions, or both. One major quandary is when to refer pediatric voice disordered patients to behavioral medicine. The otolaryngologist should consider referral to a behavioral medicine specialist if no organic etiology is determined, if traditional medical interventions and treatments have failed to produce adequate symptom relief, or if symptoms are disproportionate to the degree of physical illness. In addition, the otolaryngologist should strongly consider referral to a behavioral medicine specialist, despite the severity or course of symptoms, if the patient has clear symptoms of anxiety or depression or severe psychosocial stress. It may be beneficial for the otolaryngologist to cultivate a strong relationship with a local mental health provider for ease of referral, to ensure ongoing communication and to promote consistent, quality care for the pediatric voice disorder patient.

REFERENCES

1. Moran MG. Vocal cord dysfunction. A syndrome that mimics asthma. *J Cardiopulm Rehabil.* 1996;16:91–92.
2. Anbar RD, Hall HR. Childhood habit cough treated with self-hypnosis. *J Pediatr.* 2004; 144:213–217.
3. Weinberg EG. "Honking": psychogenic cough tic in children. *SAMJ, S Afr Med J.* 1980: 198–200.
4. Riegel B, Warmoth JE, Middaugh SJ, et al. Psychogenic cough treated with biofeedback and psychotherapy. A review and case report. *Am J Phys Med Rehabil.* 1995;74: 155–158.
5. Holinger LD, Sanders AD. Chronic cough in infants and children: an update. *Laryngoscope.* 1991;101:596–605.
6. Julia JC, Martorell A, Armengot MA, et al. Vocal cord dysfunction in a child. *Allergy.* 1999;54:748–751.
7. Newman KB, Mason UG, Schmaling KB. Clinical features of vocal cord dysfunction. *Am J Respir Crit Care Med.* 1995;152: 1382–1386.
8. Kuppersmith R, Rosen DS, Wiatrak BJ. Functional stridor in adolescents. *J Adolesc Health.* 1993;14:166–171.
9. McFadden ER, Zawadski DK. Vocal cord dysfunction masquerading as exercise-induced asthma. a physiologic cause for "choking" during athletic activities. *Am J Respir Crit Care Med.* 1996;153:942–947.
10. Rundell KW, Spiering BA. Inspiratory stridor in elite athletes. *Chest.* 2003;123:468–474.
11. Gavin LA, Wamboldt M, Brugman S, Roesler TA, Wamboldt F. Psychological and family characteristics of adolescents with vocal cord dysfunction. *J Asthma.* 1998;35: 409–417.
12. Balkissoon R. Vocal cord dysfunction, gastroesophageal reflux disease, and nonallergic rhinitis. *Clin Allergy Immunol.* 2007; 19:411–426.
13. Wood RP 2nd, Milgrom H. Vocal cord dysfunction. *J Allergy Clin Immunol.* 1996;98: 481–485.
14. Anbar RD, Hehir DA. Hypnosis as a diagnostic modality for vocal cord dysfunction. *Pediatrics.* 2000;106:E81.
15. Watson TS, Sterling HE. Brief functional analysis and treatment of a vocal tic. *J App Behav Anal.* 1998;31: 471–474.
16. Altman KW, Mirza N, Ruiz C, et al. Paradoxical vocal fold motion: presentation and treatment options. *J Voice.* 2000;14:99–103.
17. Earles J, Kerr B, Kellar M. Psychophysiologic treatment of vocal cord dysfunction. *Ann Allergy Asthma Immunol.* 2003;90: 669–671.

18. Warnes TS, Allen KD. Biofeedback treatment of paradoxical vocal fold motion and respiratory distress in an adolescent girl. *J App Behav Anal*. 2005;38:529–532.

19. Labbe EE. Biofeedback and cognitive coping in the treatment of pediatric habit cough. *Appl Psychophysiol Biofeed*. 2006;31:167–172.

20. Anbar RD. Hypnosis in pediatrics: applications at a pediatric pulmonary center. *BMC Pediatrics*. 2002;2:11.

21. Ojoo JC, Kastelik JA, Morice AH. A boy with a disabling cough. *Lancet*. 2003;361:674.

Index